STEMI Interventions

Guest Editor

SAMEER MEHTA, MD, MBA

INTERVENTIONAL CARDIOLOGY CLINICS

www.interventional.theclinics.com

Consulting Editors
SAMIN K. SHARMA, MD
IGOR F. PALACIOS, MD

October 2012 • Volume 1 • Number 4

SAUNDERS an imprint of ELSEVIER, Inc.

W.B. SAUNDERS COMPANY
A Division of Elsevier Inc.

1600 John F. Kennedy Boulevard • Suite 1800 • Philadelphia, Pennsylvania 19103-2899

http://www.theclinics.com

INTERVENTIONAL CARDIOLOGY CLINICS Volume 1, Number 4
October 2012 ISSN 2211-7458, ISBN-13: 978-1-4557-4894-5

Editor: Barbara Cohen-Kligerman
Developmental Editor: Teia Stone

Interventional Cardiology Clinics (ISSN 2211-7458) is published quarterly by Elsevier Inc., 360 Park Avenue South, New York, NY 10010-1710. Months of issue are January, April, July, and October. Subscription prices are USD 188 per year for US individuals, USD 126 per year for US students, USD 281 per year for Canadian individuals, USD 144 per year for Canadian students, USD 281 per year for international individuals, and USD 144 per year for international students. To receive student/resident rate, orders must be accompanied by name of affiliated institution, date of term, and the *signature* of program/residency coordinator on institution letterhead. Orders will be billed at individual rate until proof of status is received. Foreign air speed delivery is included in all *Clinics* subscription prices. All prices are subject to change without notice. **POSTMASTER:** Send address changes to *Interventional Cardiology Clinics*, Elsevier Health Sciences Division, Subscription Customer Service, 3251 Riverport Lane, Maryland Heights, MO 63043. **Customer Service: Telephone: 1-800-654-2452** (U.S. and Canada); **1-314-447-8871** (outside U.S. and Canada). **Fax: 1-314-447-8029. E-mail: journalscustomerservice-usa@elsevier.com** (for print support); **journalsonlinesupport-usa@elsevier.com** (for online support).

Reprints. For copies of 100 or more of articles in this publication, please contact the Commercial Reprints Department, Elsevier Inc., 360 Park Avenue South, New York, NY 10010-1710. Tel.: 212-633-3812; Fax: 212-462-1935; E-mail: reprints@elsevier.com.

Printed and bound by CPI Group (UK) Ltd, Croydon, CR0 4YY

Transferred to digital print 2012

The cover illustration depicts the following:
Left panel, Baseline: large thrombotic lesion in mid RCA in a 65-year-old male with STEMI and TIMI I flow.
Center panel, Post AngioJet: residual 90% ulcerated lesion after thrombus removal by AngioJet with TIMI III flow (*inset;* AngioJet boing in RCA)
Right panel, Final Results: Post 4/23 mm Xience V drug oluting stent (DES) at 12 atmospheres (*inset;* DES being deployed) with excellent distal TIMI III flow and TMP grade 3 and no distal embolization.

Contributors

CONSULTING EDITORS

SAMIN K. SHARMA, MD, FSCAI, FACC
Director of Clinical Cardiology; Director of Cardiac Catheterization Laboratory, Mount Sinai Medical Center, New York, New York

IGOR F. PALACIOS, MD, FSCAI
Director of Interventional Cardiology, Cardiology Division, Heart Center, Massachusetts General Hospital; Associate Professor of Medicine, Harvard Medical School, Boston, Massachusetts

GUEST EDITOR

SAMEER MEHTA, MD, FACC, MBA
Voluntary Associate Clinical Professor of Medicine, Miller School of Medicine, University of Miami; Mercy Medical Center; Director, Lumen Foundation, Miami, Florida

AUTHORS

ANISH AMIN, MD
Cardiology Fellow, Department of Medicine, Loyola University Medical Center, Maywood, Illinois

MELISSA S.K. BLONDEAU, BSc
Coordinator, STEMI Regional Program, Department of Medicine, Division of Cardiology, University of Ottawa Heart Institute, Ottawa, Ontario, Canada

ROBERTO V. BOTELHO, MD, PhD
Instituto do Coração do Triângulo, Uberlandia, Minas Gerais, Brazil

MIGUEL A. CAMPOS-ESTEVE, MD, FACC
Director, Cardiac Catheterization Laboratories, Pavia Hospital, Santurce, Puerto Rico

CHABELY CARDENAS
Lumen Foundation, Miami, Florida

ANJAN K. CHAKRABARTI, MD
Cardiovascular Disease Fellow, Cardiovascular Division, Department of Medicine, Beth Israel Deaconess Medical Center, Harvard Medical School, Boston, Massachusetts

SALOMON COHEN, MD
Surgery Resident, Departamento de Neurocirugia, Instituto Mexicano del Seguro Social, Lomas Country, Huixquilucan Edo de Mexico, Mexico

ROBERT S. DIETER, MD, RVT
Associate Professor of Vascular & Endovascular Medicine, Department of Interventional Cardiology, Loyola University Medical Center, Maywood, Illinois; Chief of Vascular Medicine and Cardiovascular Interventions; Medical Director, Cardiovascular Collaborative Hines, VA Hospital, Illinois

BRENO A.A. FALCÃO, MD
Heart Institute (InCor), University of São Paulo, School of Medicine, Pinheiros, São Paulo, Brazil

ANTONIO FERNÁNDEZ-ORTIZ, MD, PhD
Interventional Cardiology, Cardiovascular Institute, Clínico 'San Carlos' University Hospital, Madrid, Spain

FRANCISCO FERNANDEZ, BSc
MedSolutions, São Paulo, Brazil

ANA ISABEL FLORES, MD
Research Assistant, Lumen Foundation, Miami, Florida

C. MICHAEL GIBSON, MS, MD
Associate Professor of Medicine, Harvard Medical School, Boston, Massachusetts; Chairman, PERFUSE Study Group; Founder and Chairman of the Board, WikiDoc Foundation, San Francisco, California

JASRAI GILL, MD
Cardiology Fellow, Department of Medicine, Loyola University Medical Center, Maywood, Illinois

JAVIER GOICOLEA, MD
Department of Cardiology, Puerta de Hierro Hospital, Madrid, Spain

LAKSHMI GOPALAKRISHNAN, MBBS
Research Fellow, Cardiovascular Division, Department of Medicine, Harvard Medical School; PERFUSE Angiographic Core Laboratories, Data Coordinating Center; Beth Israel Deaconess Medical Center, Boston, Massachusetts

NILUSHA GUKATHASAN, MD
Research Fellow, Mount Sinai School of Medicine, New York, New York

TIMOTHY D. HENRY, MD
Director of Research, Minneapolis Heart Institute Foundation, Abbott-Northwestern Hospital; Professor of Medicine, University of Minnesota, Minneapolis, Minnesota

DAVID A. HILDEBRANDT, RN, EMT-P
Cardiovascular Emergency Program Manager, Minneapolis Heart Institute Foundation, Abbott-Northwestern Hospital, Minneapolis, Minnesota

ANNAPOORNA S. KINI, MD
Cardiac Catheterization Laboratory of the Cardiovascular Institute, Mount Sinai Hospital, New York, New York

JENNIFER C. KOSTELA, MS, MD
Internal Medicine, New York Hospital Queens, Flushing, New York; Ross University School of Medicine, North Brunswick, New Jersey

JASON C. KOVACIC, MD, PhD
Cardiac Catheterization Laboratory of the Cardiovascular Institute, Mount Sinai Hospital, New York, New York

VARUN KUMAR, MBBS
Research Fellow, Cardiovascular Division, Department of Medicine, Harvard Medical School; PERFUSE Angiographic Core Laboratories, Data Coordinating Center; Beth Israel Deaconess Medical Center, Boston, Massachusetts

ALEXANDRA J. LANSKY, MD
Associate Professor of Medicine, Director Interventional Cardiology Research, Co-Director, Valve Program, Yale University School of Medicine, Yale University Medical Center, New Haven, Connecticut

DAVID M. LARSON, MD
Chief, Department of Emergency Medicine, Ridgeview Medical Center, Waconia, Minnesota; Associate Clinical Professor, University of Minnesota Medical School, Minneapolis, Minnesota

MICHEL R. LE MAY, MD
Director, Coronary Care Unit, Director, STEMI Regional Program, Department of Medicine, Division of Cardiology, University of Ottawa Heart Institute, Ottawa, Ontario, Canada

CARLOS MACAYA, MD, PhD
Interventional Cardiology, Cardiovascular Institute, Clínico 'San Carlos' University Hospital, Madrid, Spain

AHMED MAGDY, MD, FACC, FSCAI
Department of Cardiology, National Heart Institute, Cairo, Egypt

ROXANA MEHRAN, MD, FACC
Professor of Medicine (Cardiology), Director of Interventional Cardiovascular Research and Clinical Trials, Zena and Michael A Wiener Cardiovascular Institute, Mount Sinai School of Medicine; Cardiovascular Research Foundation, New York, New York

SAMEER MEHTA, MD, FACC, MBA
Voluntary Associate Clinical Professor of Medicine, Miller School of Medicine, University of Miami; Mercy Medical Center; Director, Lumen Foundation, Miami, Florida

AJIT S. MULLASARI, MD, DM, DNB, FRCP
Director, Department of Cardiology, Institute of Cardio Vascular Diseases, Madras Medical Mission, Chennai, Tamil Nadu, India

ARAVINDA NANJUNDAPPA, MD, FACC, FSCAI, RVT
Associate Professor of Medicine and Surgery, West Virginia University, Charleston, West Virginia

VIVIAN G. NG, MD
Associate Professor of Medicine; Director, Interventional Cardiology Research; Co-Director, Valve Program, Yale University School of Medicine, Yale University Medical Center, New Haven, Connecticut

ESTEFANIA OLIVEROS, MD
Research Fellow, Lumen Foundation, Miami, Florida

BALAJI PAKSHIRAJAN, MD, DNB
Consultant, Department of Cardiology, Institute of Cardio Vascular Diseases, Madras Medical Mission, Chennai, Tamil Nadu, India

SAMIR PANCHOLY, MD, FACC, FSCAI
Associate Professor of Medicine and Program Director, Fellowship in Cardiovascular Diseases, Department of Cardiovascular Sciences, The Commonwealth Medical College, The Wright Center for Graduate Medical Education, Scranton, Pennsylvania

NIRAJ PAREKH, MD
Cardiology Fellow, Department of Medicine, Loyola University Medical Center, Maywood, Illinois

SHALIN J. PATEL, MD
Senior Internal Medicine Resident, Cardiovascular Division, Department of Medicine, Beth Israel Deaconess Medical Center, Harvard Medical School, Boston, Massachusetts

TEJAS PATEL, MD, DM, FACC, FESC, FSCAI
Chairman, Department of Cardiovascular Sciences, Apex Heart Institute; Professor and Head, Department of Cardiovascular Sciences, Sheth K.M. School of Post Graduate Medicine and Research, Smt. NHL Municipal Medical College, Sheth V.S. General Hospital, Gujarat University, Ahmedabad, Gujarat, India

CAMILO PENA, MD
Research Assistant, Lumen Foundation, Miami, Florida

UJJWAL RASTOGI, MBBS
Research Fellow, Cardiovascular Division, Department of Medicine, PERFUSE Angiographic Core Laboratories and Data Coordinating Center; Beth Israel Deaconess Medical Center, Boston, Massachusetts

ANDER REGUEIRO, MD
Department of Cardiology, Thorax Institute, Hospital Clinic, Barcelona, Spain

ORLANDO RODRÍGUEZ-VILÁ, MD, MMS, FACC
Director, Cardiac Catheterization Laboratories, Cardiology Section, VA Caribbean Healthcare System, San Juan, Puerto Rico; Director, Cardiac Catheterization Laboratories, Auxilio Mutuo Hospital, Hato Rey, Puerto Rico

REBECCA ROWEN, BS
Ross University School of Medicine, North Brunswick, New Jersey

MANEL SABATÉ, MD, PhD
Department of Cardiology, Thorax Institute, Hospital Clinic, Barcelona, Spain

ROBERT L. SALAZAR, MD
Senior Internal Medicine Resident, Cardiovascular Division, Department of Medicine, Beth Israel Deaconess Medical Center, Harvard Medical School, Boston, Massachusetts

HISHAM SELIM, MD
National Heart Institute, Cairo, Egypt

ZIAD SERGIE, MD, MBA
Cardiology Fellow, Mount Sinai School of Medicine, New York, New York

SANJAY SHAH, MD, DM
Director, Department of Cardiovascular Sciences, Apex Heart Institute; Assistant Professor, Department of Cardiovascular Sciences, Sheth K.M. School of Post Graduate Medicine and Research, Smt. NHL Municipal Medical College, Sheth V.S. General Hospital, Gujarat University, Ahmedabad, Gujarat, India

AMIT B. SHARMA, MD
Cardiac Catheterization Laboratory of the Cardiovascular Institute, Mount Sinai Hospital, New York, New York

PRIYAMVADA SINGH, MBBS
Research Fellow, Cardiovascular Division, Department of Medicine, PERFUSE Angiographic Core Laboratories and Data Coordinating Center; Beth Israel Deaconess Medical Center, Boston, Massachusetts

VIJAYAKUMAR SUBBAN, MD, DM, FNB
Consultant, Department of Cardiology, Institute of Cardio Vascular Diseases, Madras Medical Mission, Chennai, Tamil Nadu, India

KEVIN TRETO, BS
Ross University School of Medicine, Winter Springs, Florida

THAIS WAISMAN, MD, MBA, PhD
Post Doctorate, Engineering School at University of São Paulo, INTERLAB-EPUSP, São Paulo, Brazil

MONA YOUSSEF, MD
National Heart Institute, Cairo, Egypt

JENNIFER J. YU, MBBS, FRACP
Interventional Cardiology Fellow, Mount Sinai School of Medicine, New York, New York

TRACY ZHANG, BS
Lumen Global Director, Lumen Foundation, Miami, Florida

CAFER ZORKUN, MD
Department Chief, Division of Cardiology, Yedikule Education and Research Hospital, Istanbul, Turkey

Contents

Preface: STEMI Interventions xiii

Sameer Mehta

Lessons Learned from STEMI Clinical Trials 401

Jasrai Gill, Anish Amin, Niraj Parekh, Aravinda Nanjundappa, and Robert S. Dieter

Coronary artery disease is the leading cause of the death in the United States. From 2009 to 2010, however, the rate of heart disease causing death decreased by 2.5% in part due to evolving techniques used to treat and prevent heart disease. Management of acute ST-segment elevation myocardial infarction (STEMI) has evolved accordingly and the studies investigating treatment strategies that have led to an evidence-based approach are reviewed in this article.

Pharmacoinvasive Management 409

Balaji Pakshirajan, Vijayakumar Subban, and Ajit S. Mullasari

The goal of treatment of patients with ST-segment elevation myocardial infarction (STEMI) is timely restoration of myocardial blood flow. Primary percutaneous coronary intervention (PCI) remains the treatment of choice for STEMI patients, as shown in multiple clinical trials. However, because of logistic constraints, timely primary PCI may not be possible for many STEMI patients, most of whom are treated with fibrinolysis. Debate continues as to whether, and when, patients treated with fibrinolysis should undergo subsequent PCI. Current data support the strategy of early routine PCI after fibrinolysis rather than the conservative standard-care approach or rescue PCI for failed lysis.

Optimal Anticoagulant Therapy in ST Elevation Myocardial Infarction Interventions 421

Estefania Oliveros, Sameer Mehta, Ana Isabel Flores, Camilo Pena, Salomon Cohen, Jennifer C. Kostela, Rebecca Rowen, and Kevin Treto

Bivalirudin is a direct thrombin inhibitor. It is a new recommendation for the treatment of patients with ST-elevation myocardial infarction undergoing percutaneous coronary intervention. Bivalirudin combined with aspirin and $P2Y_{12}$ inhibitors has proved to be an effective and safe choice for the management of thrombus in coronary artery disease. The use of bivalirudin compared with the combination of heparin plus glycoprotein IIb/IIIa inhibitors as anticoagulant therapy is associated with reduced severe bleeding and inpatient mortality, as well as diminished costs. There is only a slight increase of late stent thrombosis, which may be controlled with the use of thienopyridines.

Newer Pharmaceutical Agents for STEMI Interventions 429

Anjan K. Chakrabarti, Shalin J. Patel, Robert L. Salazar, Lakshmi Gopalakrishnan, Varun Kumar, Ujjwal Rastogi, Priyamvada Singh, Cafer Zorkun, and C. Michael Gibson

ST-elevation myocardial infarction (STEMI) causes 12.6% of deaths worldwide. Treatment strategies involve early revascularization by percutaneous coronary intervention and/or fibrinolytics, with adjunctive pharmacologic therapy. While antiplatelet therapy remains the cornerstone of pharmacologic management, newer antithrombotic therapies are showing benefit in the reduction of long-term thrombotic events

populations. Adherence to North American and European guidelines globally remains an unrealistic goal given the unique cultural, demographic, and fiscal dynamics in poorer countries. The authors propose a four-phased population-based strategy for global acute myocardial infarction development and a pharmacoinvasive approach to STEMI care based on socioeconomic characteristics.

Compulsive Thrombus Management in STEMI Interventions **485**

Sameer Mehta, Jennifer C. Kostela, Estefania Oliveros, Ana Isabel Flores, Camilo Pena, Salomon Cohen, Rebecca Rowen, and Kevin Treto

Thrombus is a fundamental concept in the pathophysiology of ST-elevated myocardial infarction (STEMI). Distal embolization and no reflow are associated with less angiographic success, reduced myocardial blush, less ST resolution after primary percutaneous coronary intervention, larger enzymatic infarct size, lower left ventricular ejection fraction at discharge, and higher long-term mortality. We believe that with the use of thrombectomy devices, these shortcomings can be minimized. Based on our experience from the Single Individual Community Experience Registry (SINCERE) database, we formulated a selective thrombus burden management strategy (the Mehta classification) for thrombus management.

Stenting in Acute STEMI Intervention **507**

Ahmed Magdy, Hisham Selim, and Mona Youssef

Stenting in acute myocardial infarction (AMI) has the benefits of achieving acute optimal angiographic results and correcting residual dissection to decrease the incidence of restenosis and reocclusion. Studies have shown that percutaneous transluminal coronary angioplasty for primary treatment after AMI is superior to thrombolytic therapy regarding the restoration of normal coronary blood flow. Coronary stenting improves initial success rates, decreases the incidence of abrupt closure, and is associated with a reduced rate of restenosis. In the presence of thrombus-containing lesions, coronary stenting constitutes an effective therapeutic strategy, either after failure of initial angioplasty or electively as the primary procedure.

Door-to-Balloon ST-Elevation Myocardial Infarction Interventions: Illustrated Cases **521**

Sameer Mehta, Rebecca Rowen, Estefania Oliveros, Camilo Pena, Jennifer C. Kostela, Kevin Treto, Ana Isabel Flores, and Salomon Cohen

ST-elevation myocardial infarction (STEMI) intervention comprises 2 components, the STEMI procedure and the STEMI process, which have unique aspects that can be modified and improved, ultimately affecting patient outcome. The 15 illustrated cases in this article highlight suggested improvements mainly in the STEMI procedure, with some references as to how the authors practically improved the STEMI process for the described procedure. The illustrated procedures have been meticulously selected from more than 1000 short door-to-balloon STEMI interventions recorded in the Single Individual Community Experience Registry (SINCERE) database, and are aimed at educating the reader about unique STEMI skills.

STEMI Interventions: The European Perspective and Stent for Life Initiative **559**

Ander Regueiro, Javier Goicolea, Antonio Fernández-Ortiz, Carlos Macaya, and Manel Sabaté

The Stent for Life Initiative was launched by the European Association of Percutaneous Cardiovascular Interventions (a registered branch of the ESC) and EuroPCR. The purpose of the initiative is to support the implementation of European Society

of Cardiology guidelines on management of acute myocardial infarction, help identify barriers to implementation of guidelines, and define actions to ensure that the majority of ST-segment elevation myocardial infarction (STEMI) patients in Europe have access to primary percutaneous coronary intervention. The key objectives are to define the countries with an unmet medical need in the optimal treatment of STEMI and implement an action program to increase patient access to primary percutaneous coronary intervention.

Lessons Learned from the Ottawa Regional STEMI Program **567**

Michel R. Le May and Melissa S.K. Blondeau

Percutaneous coronary intervention (PCI) has become the dominant strategy for the treatment of ST-segment elevation myocardial infarction (STEMI) when rapid access to a catheterization facility is available. In communities where primary PCI is not feasible, a pharmacoinvasive strategy has become a recommended option. At the University of Ottawa Heart Institute, a care delivery model has been developed in which primary PCI and pharmacoinvasive strategies are applied for an entire region. This article reviews the lessons learned in setting up and maintaining a regional STEMI program.

Setting Up a Population-Based Program to Optimize ST-Segment Elevation Myocardial Infarction Care **583**

Orlando Rodríguez-Vilá and Miguel A. Campos-Esteve

The development of ST-segment elevation myocardial infarction (STEMI) systems of care at the city, region, or nation levels has not only improved the speed of reperfusion but also enhanced the reach of primary angioplasty to areas far from percutaneous coronary intervention (PCI) centers. Setting up a STEMI system of care is a sophisticated process that requires a solid PCI hospital and emergency medical services infrastructure, disciplined collaboration, and a focus on outcomes measurement and continuous quality improvement. This article reviews the accumulated evidence supporting the development of STEMI systems of care and offers practical insights into this process.

The Critical Imperative: Prehospital Management of the Patient with ST-Elevation Myocardial Infarction **599**

David A. Hildebrandt, David M. Larson, and Timothy D. Henry

Prehospital care is critical to achieve the goal of timely reperfusion in patients with ST-elevation myocardial infarction. Prehospital care is delivered by emergency medical services (EMS) personnel, which include emergency medical dispatchers, first responders, and ambulance response. There is considerable variation in the training and capabilities of the EMS providers in the United States depending on the location (ie, rural vs urban) and local jurisdictions. In this article, the key components of prehospital care of the patient with ST-elevation myocardial infarction and the various levels of training and capabilities of EMS providers are discussed.

Percutaneous Left Ventricular Assist Devices **609**

Amit B. Sharma, Jason C. Kovacic, and Annapoorna S. Kini

Percutaneous left ventricular assist devices (P-LVADs) can be life saving and may permit the stabilization of a patient in cardiovascular collapse who would otherwise

face imminent demise. For specific patients and clinical indications, or where a greater degree of hemodynamic support is required, numerous studies have demonstrated the feasibility and safety of the newer generation P-LVADs. The potential applications for P-LVADs have continued to expand, now including diverse uses such as support for cardiogenic shock, bridge to and following cardiac surgery, and more novel applications such as complex electrophysiologic mapping and ablation studies of unstable ventricular rhythms.

Telemedicine: The Future of Global STEMI Care **623**

Thais Waisman, Roberto V. Botelho, Francisco Fernandez, Sameer Mehta, Estefania Oliveros, Jennifer C. Kostela, Breno A.A. Falcão, and Chabely Cardenas

Telemedicine is an innovative tool in the setting of ST-elevation myocardial infarction (STEMI), because it addresses the greatest challenge—delivering optimal reperfusion therapies in a timely manner. Telemedicine targets delays related to geography, distance, and stated prehospital systems of care. Integration of telemedicine into prehospital STEMI management has been shown to yield cost-effective improvements in patient care. Despite socioeconomic constraints, a standard prehospital network based on telemedicine is globally feasible. This article proposes 2 models that enable the use of telemedicine in the STEMI management protocol.

Index **631**

Erratum

In the article titled "Wire Strategy as a First Option: Properties of the Tools" by M. Nicholas Burke, which appeared in *Interventional Cardiology Clinics*, July 2012; 1(3):309–314, information about the source of the figure was omitted from Figures 1 through 6. The credit line for these figures is "Image courtesy of Abbott Vascular. © Abbott Laboratories 2012. All rights reserved."

INTERVENTIONAL CARDIOLOGY CLINICS

FORTHCOMING ISSUES

January 2013
Congenital and Structural Heart Disease
Damien Kenny, MD, and
Ziyad M. Hijazi, MD, MPH, *Guest Editors*

April 2013
Complex Coronary Lesions: Bypass Graft Lesions and Thrombectomy
Samir Kapadia, MD, FACC, and
Amar Krishnaswamy, MD, *Guest Editors*

July 2013
Percutaneous Ventricular Support
Howard A. Cohen, MD, and
J.P.S. Henriques, MD, PhD, *Guest Editors*

RECENT ISSUES

July 2012
Chronic Total Occlusions
William L. Lombardi, MD, *Guest Editor*

April 2012
Coronary Interventions in Women
Annapoorna S. Kini, MD, and
Roxana Mehran, MD, *Guest Editors*

January 2012
Percutaneous Approaches to Valvular Heart Disease
Samin K. Sharma, MD, and
Igor F. Palacios, MD, *Guest Editors*

ISSUES OF RELATED INTEREST

Cardiology Clinics, August 2012 (Vol. 30, No. 3)
Cardiovascular Disease in Pregnancy
Gagan Sahni, MD, and Uri Elkayam, MD, *Guest Editors*
Available at: http://www.cardiology.theclinics.com/

Heart Failure Clinics, July 2012 (Vol. 8, No. 3)
Pulmonary Hypertension
Srinivas Murali, MD, and Raymond L. Benza, MD, *Guest Editors*
Available at: http://www.heartfailure.theclinics.com/

Preface
STEMI Interventions

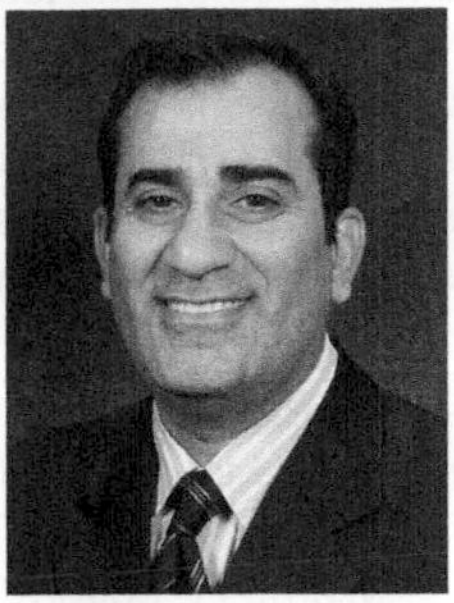

Sameer Mehta, MD, FACC, MBA
Guest Editor

It has been nearly 6 years since I published my first textbook on STEMI interventions and almost a decade since I presaged a new medical specialty of the STEMI Interventionist. Through this remarkable journey, the amazing STEMI intervention "procedure" has remained the finest indication for primary percutaneous intervention (PCI); the STEMI "process" has received global attention and spurred insightful discussions from a broad group of stakeholders involved in the care of patients with an acute myocardial infarction (AMI). Appropriately, this robust issue on STEMI interventions exhaustively transects these 2 critical components: the STEMI "process" and the "procedure," 2 central terms that I coined through the groundbreaking work with my SINCERE database, which now has data on more than 1000 short D2B procedures.

We have witnessed dramatic progress in the area of PCI, with US cardiologists having greatly contributed to this global success. Patients in our country should be pleased to learn that across the vast span of our nation, it is more than 90% likely that they will receive the finest treatment (D2B STEMI intervention) for a heart attack at any hospital 24/7/365. This is a laudable achievement for our country, a triumph that has somehow escaped its due recognition! Achieving this parameter has required the diligence and intellect of numerous cardiologists and organizations, the foremost of which are Mission Lifeline and D2B Alliance.

This issue on STEMI Interventions reflects the excellent advances made on the STEMI process and procedure. It includes a compilation of academic data by experts, a description of elegant STEMI techniques by accomplished practitioners, and insights by world authorities to deconstruct the chaotic STEMI process.

This issue features pioneering STEMI articles from a group of international experts. Dr Nanjundappa shares his thoughtful directions in approaching STEMI trials, and a triad of experts, including Drs Mehran, Gibson, and me, discusses STEMI pharmacology. Dr Mullasari has written on the important topic of pharmaco-invasive management. Dr Tejas Patel expounds on the critical aspect of radial-access STEMI intervention, making an argument for the greater adoption of transradial STEMI interventions. As stenting occupies the central theme of managing a STEMI lesion, Dr Magdy provides the essential discussions and clinical data that advocate use of either bare metal stents or drug-eluting stents.

A large component of the issue is devoted to discussing procedural enhancements. I have used my extensive STEMI work to highlight the importance of compulsive management of thrombus in STEMI lesions and have compiled a score of illustrated examples to demonstrate STEMI techniques. Dr Kini reviews the important aspects of left ventricular support, vital to managing patients with cardiogenic shock and complex STEMI procedures.

Improving the STEMI process and establishing STEMI networks are integral components of STEMI management. Shedding light on these important topics, Drs Hildebrandt, Henry, and Larson explain why improvements of the STEMI process can occur through the established prehospital triage and transfer, while Dr Waisman and I elaborate on the innovative use of telemedicine as

Intervent Cardiol Clin 1 (2012) xiii–xiv
http://dx.doi.org/10.1016/j.iccl.2012.08.001
2211-7458/12/$ – see front matter

a useful tool in optimizing the STEMI process. Furthermore, Drs Le May and Sabate enrich this issue with an international perspective on STEMI care by discussing the factors that contributed to the success of their programs. With his own global views, Dr Rodriguez-Vila lays out a rational roadmap for establishing population-based STEMI programs.

Unfortunately, wide gender disparities persist in STEMI care. Dr Lansky portrays why women are still the fragile sex in STEMI care, an appalling deficit in AMI care that must be strongly addressed in the near future. Finally, in the concluding article of this issue, I provide a comprehensive global perspective on the subject and venture "Beyond D2B Interventions" to offer a treatise on the important issues of patient education, legislation, and public advocacy for STEMI interventions.

Compiling this work has required support from several dedicated individuals. Three deserve special mention: my tireless editor, Barbara Cohen-Kligerman, and my assiduous students, Dr Estefania Oliveros and Dr Jennifer Kostela, and Tracy Zhang.

Finally, this issue is dedicated to my wife, Shoba. Without her unflinching support and deep sacrifices, all my STEMI interventions that provide the entire sustenance of this work would have never been possible!

Sameer Mehta, MD, FACC, MBA
Lumen Foundation, 55 Pinta Road
Miami, FL 33133, USA

E-mail address:
mehtas@bellsouth.net

Lessons Learned from STEMI Clinical Trials

Jasrai Gill, MD[a], Anish Amin, MD[a], Niraj Parekh, MD[a], Aravinda Nanjundappa, MD, FSCAI, RVT[b,*], Robert S. Dieter, MD, RVT[c,d]

KEYWORDS

• STEMI • Coronary artery disease • Emergency medical services
• Percutaneous coronary intervention

KEY POINTS

- Reducing door-to-balloon times in STEMI interventions results in improved mortality regardless of symptom onset or high-risk features.
- A multifaceted and multidisciplinary approach integrating the hospital administration, community and emergency medical services has been shown to reduce door-to-balloon times in STEMI interventions.
- The usefulness of Gp IIb/IIIa receptor antagonists (as part of preparatory pharmacologic strategy for patients with STEMI before their arrival in the cardiac catheterization laboratory for angiography and PCI) is uncertain.
- The current recommendations suggest rescue PCI after thrombolysis therapy for those with evidence of recurrent or ongoing ischemia, cardiogenic shock and recurrent angina without evidence of ischemia.

INTRODUCTION

Coronary artery disease is the leading cause of the death in the United States. From 2009 to 2010, however, the rate of heart disease causing death decreased by 2.5%,[1] in part due to evolving techniques used to treat and prevent heart disease. Management of acute ST-segment elevation myocardial infarction (STEMI) has evolved accordingly and the studies investigating treatment strategies that have led to an evidence-based approach are reviewed in this article.

THROMBOLYTICS

Reperfusion therapy is indicated for patients with chest pain consistent with myocardial infarction (MI) who present within 12 hours of onset of symptoms and who have ST-segment elevation greater than 0.1 mV in contiguous leads (class 1a).[2,3]

Baigent and colleagues[4] in the ISIS-2 trial investigated the use of thrombolytic therapy in 1988. They randomized more than 17,000 patients who entered an emergency department (ED) within 24 hours of an acute MI. Patients were randomized to aspirin alone, streptokinase alone, aspirin plus streptokinase, or placebo. They found that 5-week vascular mortality was lower in all 3 treatment arms versus placebo but lowest in the streptokinase plus aspirin group.

Thrombolytics do have significant limitations. Contraindications to treatment are reported as high as 27%, whereas overt treatment failure is reported at 15% and reinfarction at 90 days is 25%.[5] Cost, initially thought a benefit of thrombolytic therapy, is equal to percutaneous coronary intervention (PCI), predominately due to higher complication rates and longer duration of hospital stay in patients treated with thrombolytics.[6]

[a] Department of Medicine, Loyola University Medical Center, 2160 Maywood, IL 60153, USA; [b] West Virginia University, 3100 McCorkle Avenue Southwest, Charleston, WV 25304, USA; [c] Department of Interventional Cardiology, Loyola University Medical Center, 2160 Maywood, IL 60153, USA; [d] Cardiovascular Collaborative Hines, VA Hospital, Illinois, USA
* Corresponding author.
E-mail address: dappamd@yahoo.com

Intervent Cardiol Clin 1 (2012) 401–407
http://dx.doi.org/10.1016/j.iccl.2012.06.013
2211-7458/12/$ – see front matter

PERCUTANEOUS CORONARY INTERVENTION

PCI has been shown superior to thrombolytic therapy in regards to mortality, stroke, and heart failure and this benefit is sustained at 30-day and 6-month follow-up.[7–9] The first meta-analysis to show the mortality benefit of PCI was by Weaver and colleagues,[9] who found a 34% relative risk reduction of mortality at 30 days when treated with angioplasty. Subsequently Keeley and colleagues[8] analyzed 23 randomized controlled trials; endpoints of 30-day and 6-month mortality, reinfarction rates, and stroke were analyzed. They reinforced the survival benefit shown by Weaver and colleagues,[10] boasting 21 lives saved per 1000 patients treated. They also demonstrated that the benefit of PCI includes less recurrent ischemia, fewer revascularization procedures, and shorter hospital stay.

The benefit of PCI over thrombolytic therapy perhaps lies in the rates of Thrombolysis in Myocardial Infarction grade 3 (TIMI 3) flow in the infarct-related artery obtained. This was demonstrated by the GUSTO investigators.[5] They randomized 2400 patients to various combinations of heparin (intravenous or subcutaneous) and/or streptokinase and tissue plasminogen activator. At 90 minutes, TIMI 3 flow was achieved 54% of the time in the tissue plasminogen activator plus intravenous heparin group and approximately 40% of the time in the other groups. At 180 minutes, the patency rates were nearly equal in all groups. They also demonstrated that ventricular function mirrored the degree of revascularization, in that those with TIMI 3 flow had higher left ventricular (LV) ejection fractions.

The benefit of PCI is further enhanced by the addition of thienopyridines. The COMMIT trial randomized more than 45,000 patients within 24 hours of symptom onset to aspirin plus clopidogrel or aspirin plus placebo.[11] The treatment arm demonstrated a reduction in death, reinfarction, and stroke compared with placebo. There was a wide patient population, including those who had received thrombolytic therapy, and there were similar rates of bleeding between the groups. Clopidogrel loading (300 mg) is also shown beneficial. Patients in the treatment arm demonstrated a reduction in composite endpoint of death, recurrent MI, or recurrent ischemia without increased bleeding.[12] The pivotal trial involving prasugrel is the TRITON-TIMI 38 trial, a randomized controlled trial involving more than 13,000 patients, 3534 with STEMI.[13] The investigators compared aspirin plus clopidogrel to aspirin plus prasugrel. Prasugrel was associated with a significant 2.2% absolute reduction and a 19% relative reduction in the composite endpoint (cardiovascular mortality, nonfatal MI, and nonfatal stroke).[13]

The benefit of PCI over thrombolytic therapy is well established; however, the degree of benefit is highly dependent on timing and some investigators suggest that if the delay to PCI is long enough, mortality rates between thrombolytic therapy and PCI may become equivalent with a door-to-balloon time of 62 minutes and a composite endpoint of death, reinfarction, and stroke becomes equivalent at 93 minutes.[14] The 2 major studies aimed at investigating the optimal management strategies for those patients who present with acute ST elevation MI at community hospitals and the inherent delay in treatment were the DANAMI-2 and PRAGUE-2 trials.[15,16] In the DANAMI-2 trial, patients were randomized to intravenous alteplase or transfer to invasive hospital for PCI. The primary endpoint was a composite of death, reinfarction, and stroke at 30 days. They found that the primary endpoint was reached 8.5% versus 14.2% in the angioplasty group and the fibrinolysis group, respectively, but the benefit was only in the reinfarction rates. Death and stroke were similar among each group[15]; 96% of the patients were transferred within 2 hours of presentation; however, further resolution of the door-to-balloon time is not given.

PRAGUE-2 used the same composite endpoint, showing a lower percent of patients in the angioplasty group reaching that endpoint at 30 days; however, only those patients randomized 3 hours after symptoms started received a benefit.[16] Randomization-to-balloon time was 97 $\pm$ 27 minutes and randomization-to-needle time was approximately 12 minutes. Data from DANAMI-2 and PRAGUE-2 are difficult to apply in the United States because of quicker hospital transfer times in the geographic locations these studies were done in, lack of resolution regarding door-to-balloon time, and follow-up period of only 30 days.[10]

The hallmark study and a major driving force for aiming for shorter door-to-balloon times was done by McNamara and colleagues[17] using data from the National Registry of Myocardial Infarction. They analyzed approximately 30,000 patients treated with PCI within 6 hours of presentation. The primary endpoint was in-hospital mortality. When patients were treated within 90 minutes after arrival, mortality was 3%. Mortality increased to 4.2%, 5.7%, and 7.4% when treatment was delayed to within 120 minutes, 150 minutes, and greater than 150 minutes, respectively. Each 15-minute reduction in door-to-balloon time meant 6.3 fewer deaths per 1000 patients treated.[17]

RESCUE PCI

Despite the evidence demonstrating the benefit of PCI over thrombolytic therapy, even when treatment is delayed, thrombolytics continue to be the most used therapy for ST elevation MI, both worldwide and in the United States.[10] This is due to the inherent delays in treatment and limited access to cardiac catheterization. As discussed previously, thrombolytic failure rates are approximately 60% and associated with increased mortality and decreased LV function.[5] Rescue PCI seems a logical option given the evidence regarding the benefit of PCI in this clinical context.

Up until the early 2000s, most data regarding rescue PCI were limited to observational studies. Besides the limited data, there is ambiguity regarding the definition of "failed reperfusion." The first significant randomized controlled trials were the RESCUE and MERLIN trials.[18,19] In the RESCUE trial, patients were randomized to conservative therapy (heparin, aspirin, and intracoronary nitrates) or angioplasty; however, randomization was done after infarct-related artery was identified and TIMI grade was not improved angiographically. Therefore, RESCUE trial investigators definition was based on angiographic evidence only. Despite this limitation, patients in the angioplasty group had a lower 30-day combined endpoint of LV function, ventricular tachycardia, class III/IV heart failure, and death.[18] Some investigators also believe that this benefit is underestimated due to exclusion of patients with previous MI and inclusion of only high-risk anterior MI patients.[10]

The MERLIN trial was designed similarly and concluded that watchful waiting is the best approach[19]; however, there were several limitations to this trial, including unplanned revascularizations in the conservative treatment arm, high rate on inferior MI, excessive rate of death in both treatment arms, and underuse of proved contemporary interventions (stents and glycoprotein [Gp] IIb/IIIa inhibitors). Although the results of this trial are thought not applicable, they did define thrombolytic failure by ECG (rather than angiographically) as failure of ST-segment elevations to resolve by 50% at 60 minutes after initial ECG.

Evidence on which current guidelines are based originate from the REACT trial and a meta-analysis from Wijeysundera and colleagues.[20,21] The REACT trial defined failed thrombolysis as less than 50% resolution of ST-segment elevation after 90 minutes. The investigators demonstrated a lower combined endpoint of death, reinfarction, stroke, or severe heart failure within 6 months in the PCI treatment arm.[20] A meta-analysis of 8 trials, including more than 1100 patients, provided support for the conclusions made in the REACT trial; however, it was found that rescue PCI was associated with increased risk of stroke and minor bleeding.

The current recommendations suggest rescue PCI after thrombolysis therapy for those with evidence of recurrent or ongoing ischemia (class I), cardiogenic shock (class IIa), and recurrent angina without evidence of ischemia (class IIb).[2]

FACILITATED PCI

Facilitated PCI is another treatment concept used when immediate PCI is not available and also used in an attempt to decrease overall clot burden and distal embolization and theoretically achieve smaller infarct sizes, better recovery of LV function, and possibly lower mortality.[22] Glycoprotein IIb/IIIa receptor blockers in addition to thrombolytics are used as an adjunctive therapy with the goal of reestablishing perfusion early, before planned PCI. Although the idea seems logical and beneficial, the data are not supportive. The ASSENT-4 PCI study, the largest randomized controlled trial, was stopped early due to higher mortality rates in the facilitated PCI group; however, patients did not receive dual antiplatelet agents.[23] The FINESS trial was a double-blind, placebo-controlled trial that provided definitive evidence that not only was there no difference in all-cause mortality but also there was a trend toward increased intracranial bleeding.[24] Finally, a meta-analysis of 17 randomized controlled trials showed that although there is an improvement of TIMI 3 flow in the facilitated PCI group, there is an associated increase incidence of death, reinfarction, urgent target vessel revascularization (TVR), bleeding, and stroke in facilitated PCI group.[25] Given the current evidence, facilitated PCI is not recommended as a treatment strategy.

GLYCOPROTEIN IIB/IIIA INHIBITORS

Distal embolization rates after PCI for STEMI are reported to be 16%.[26] Theoretically, the potent antithrombotic effect of glycoprotein IIb/IIIa inhibitors, which block the final pathway of platelet aggregation, ought to decrease infarct size by preventing distal embolization and thus improve myocardial perfusion. The data are conflicting. There are 3 randomized controlled trials that question the benefit of IIb/IIIa inhibitors. The BRAVE-3 trial specifically included infarct size as a primary endpoint and found no difference in infarct size and major bleeding as well as death, MI, stroke between abciximab, and placebo.[27] ON-TIME 2 found improved ST-segment resolution with the use of tirofiban; however, it did not find any difference in TIMI flow, blush grade, death, recurrent MI, or TVR between tirofiban and placebo.[28] Similarly, the HORIZON-AMI trial was not able to show a benefit of IIb/IIIa inhibitors and found higher rates of adverse events and major bleeding.[29] The most recent meta-analyses also conclude that there was no benefit of IIb/IIIa inhibitors. There was no statistically significant difference in 30-day mortality or reinfarction and no difference in death or reinfarction at 8 months.[30,31]

Supportive data include a meta-analysis of 7 trials, and definitive data regarding abciximab is evident in 5 randomized controlled trials. A pooled analysis of more than 3000 patients demonstrates a reduction in composite endpoint of death, reinfarction, and urgent TVR; however, there was increased risk of major bleeding at 30 days.[32] This was powered by 4 randomized controlled trials displaying the benefit of abciximab specifically.[33–36] The greatest benefit was seen in the ADMIRAL trial, in which abciximab improved early and late TIMI 3 flow and was associated with higher ejection fraction and with lower composite endpoint of death, reinfarction, and urgent TVR at 30 days (6% vs 14.6% with placebo).[35]

Because of the conflicting evidence, American College of Cardiology/American Heart Association recommendations for the use of abciximab during PCI is a class IIa recommendation with level B evidence.

Current guidelines regarding use of IIb/IIIa state that it is reasonable to treat with abciximab as early as possible before primary PCI (class IIa); at the time of primary PCI (class IIa), treat with tirofiban or eptifibatide before primary PCI (class IIb). The usefulness of glycoprotein IIb/IIIa receptor antagonists (as part of preparatory pharmacologic strategy for patients with STEMI before their arrival in the cardiac catheterization laboratory for angiography and PCI) is uncertain.[2,23]

ASPIRATION THROMBECTOMY

The Thrombus Aspiration during Percutaneous Coronary Intervention in Acute Myocardial Infarction Study (TAPAS) randomized 1071 STEMI patients to manual aspiration thrombectomy (n = 535) before stenting using the Export device (Medtronic, Santa Rosa, California) or to PCI, usually with stenting but without thrombus aspiration (n = 536). The primary endpoint was the myocardial blush grade after intervention. Secondary endpoints included the degree of ST-segment elevation resolution, degree of persistent ST-segment elevation after PCI, and presence of pathologic Q waves. Patients treated with thrombus aspiration showed a higher myocardial blush grade, less-persistent ST-segment elevation, more resolution of the ST-segment elevation, and fewer pathologic Q waves. Patients with all of these characteristics of improved perfusion after thrombus aspiration showed a trend toward decreased death rates at 30 days, decreased reinfarction, and decreased combined major adverse cardiac events. At 1-year follow-up, there was a decrease in clinical events in the thrombus aspiration group versus the non–thrombus aspiration group: all-cause mortality, cardiac death, and rates of reinfarction.[37]

The results of previous studies of mechanical/rheolytic thrombectomy with the AngioJet (Possis Medical, Minneapolis, Minnesota) demonstrate that there is no significant long-term clinical benefit in the setting of STEMI. The catheter can be limited by the need for a temporary pacer wire. The gold standard, therefore, for thrombus removal is aspiration/manual thrombectomy.

REDUCING DOOR-TO-BALLOON TIMES

Immediate therapy improves survival for patients who present with STEMI. Hospitals during the past several years have looked at ways of developing and implementing systems and processes to help reduce the time between arrival at the hospital and the administration of reperfusion therapy. Over time, it has become clear that PCI is the preferred method of revascularization in this patient population. Given this, hospital systems are constantly evaluating methods to reduce door-to-balloon time, which by definition is the time interval between arrival at the hospital and the first balloon inflation during PCI. The importance of door-to-balloon time is accentuated by its inclusion as a core quality measure by both the Centers for Medicaid and Medicare Services and the Joint Commission on Accreditation of Healthcare Organizations.

Evidence from the National Registry of Myocardial Infarction shows that fewer than half of patients presenting with STEMI are treated with guideline recommended door-to-balloon times, which in the present era is 90 minutes. Door-to-balloon time reflects a complex clinical process requiring coordination across departments and disciplines to effect timely triage, diagnosis, and treatment of critically ill patients.

Research looking at hospital-based systems and methods that influence door-to-balloon times has identified several strategies that significantly affect and lower door-to-balloon times. Also, data support using a multifaceted approach, in that the more methods or protocols used resulted in incremental further reduction in times.[38]

One important variable in the practice of any individual hospital and ED is activating the cardiac catheterization laboratory. There is evidence that interval time can be reduced by an ED physician activating the cardiac catheterization laboratory without first consulting a cardiologist. Another strategy is limiting the number of pages and phone calls needed to activate the laboratory; having an ED physician activate with one single page and an operator who then simultaneously pages the interventional cardiologist as well as the laboratory staff has beem shown to significantly reduce times. Paging the interventional cardiologist and cath lab personal should be done with the expectation that arrival is in less than 20 minutes. Another key factor that played a significant role in reducing door-to-balloon times was having an attending cardiologist in the hospital on site at time of presentation or activation.[38]

A more recent community approach has been empowering emergency medical service (ie, paramedics and soon fire departments) with the ability to perform 12-lead ECGs en route to the hospital, thereby alerting the ED sooner and activating the catheterization laboratory before patients reach the hospital door. This strategy, with the addition of transmitting the infield 12-lead ECGs to a cardiologist while en route, has led to lower door-to-balloon times and helped reduce false-positive rates.[38]

In every protocol or complex hospital-based implemented strategy, feedback is important. It has been shown that hospitals that measure and record real-time data and provide constructive feedback on door-to-balloon times to staff members in the ED as well as the cardiac catheterization laboratory had faster interval times than those that did not.[38]

When interviewing specific hospital personnel and/or administrators in hospital systems that have been able to routinely achieve door-to-balloon times of less than 90 minutes, specific comments are worth noting. They note that an innovative protocol development in itself is not enough but can be effective when integrated into an environment that includes explicit goals. It is important to have engaged and visible senior management as well as clinical leaders. In addition, having collaborative, interdisciplinary teams, detailed data feedback, and a nonblaming patient-focused organization culture prove vital to success in reducing interval door-to-balloon times, resulting both in hospital and long-term mortality.[39]

The question to ask next is, Why is there such an emphasis on reducing these times and what impact does this have on patient survival and quality of life? Recent studies have shown that any delay in door-to-balloon times, even within the 90-minute allotted time frame, results in increased cardiovascular mortality both in hospital and after discharge.[40] So there seems to be a linear correlation with lower time and reduced mortality in this clinical setting.

Another study by McNamara and colleagues[17] has shown that in-hospital mortality has significantly increased with increasing door-to-balloon time. This relationship was seen in patients regardless of symptom onset–to-door time. This association between shorter door-to-balloon times and lower mortality was seen both for patients with and without American College of Cardiology/American Heart Association high-risk factors.

SUMMARY

In summary, there is substantial evidence that reducing door-to-balloon times results in improved mortality regardless of symptom onset or high-risk features. This provides even more support of the importance of reducing door-to-balloon times in patients presenting with STEMI. This approach should be multifaceted and multidisciplinary and should involve not only the hospital administration but also the community with emergency medical services all integrated in one team.

REFERENCES

1. Sherry L, Murphy BS, Jiaquan Xu MD, et al. Division of vital statistic. Deaths: preliminary data for 2010. Natl Vital Stat Rep 2012;60(4).
2. Kushner FG, Hand M, Smith SC Jr, et al. 2009 focused updates: ACC/AHA guidelines for the management of patients with ST-elevation myocardial infarction (updating the 2004 guideline and 2007 focused update) and ACC/AHA/SCAI guidelines on percutaneous coronary intervention (updating the 2005 guideline and 2007 focused update) a report of the American college of cardiology Foundation/American heart association task force on practice guidelines. J Am Coll Cardiol 2009;54(23):2205–41.
3. Guyatt GH, Norris SL, Schulman S, et al. Methodology for the development of antithrombotic therapy and prevention of thrombosis guidelines: antithrombotic therapy and prevention of thrombosis, 9th ed: American college of chest physicians evidence-based clinical practice guidelines. Chest 2012; 141(Suppl 2):53S–70S.
4. Baigent C, Collins R, Appleby P, et al. ISIS-2: 10 year survival among patients with suspected acute myocardial infarction in randomised comparison of intravenous streptokinase, oral aspirin, both, or neither. The ISIS-2 (second international study of infarct survival) collaborative group. BMJ 1988; 316(7141):1337–43.
5. The effects of tissue plasminogen activator, streptokinase, or both on coronary-artery patency, ventricular function, and survival after acute myocardial infarction. The GUSTO Angiographic Investigators. N Engl J Med 1993;329(22):1615–22.
6. Stone GW, Grines CL, Rothbaum D, et al. Analysis of the relative costs and effectiveness of primary

angioplasty versus tissue-type plasminogen activator: the primary angioplasty in myocardial infarction (PAMI) trial. The PAMI trial investigators. J Am Coll Cardiol 1997;29(5):901–7.
7. Grines C, Patel A, Zijlstra F, et al. Primary coronary angioplasty compared with intravenous thrombolytic therapy for acute myocardial infarction: six-month follow up and analysis of individual patient data from randomized trials. Am Heart J 2003;145(1):47–57.
8. Keeley EC, Boura JA, Grines CL. Primary angioplasty versus intravenous thrombolytic therapy for acute myocardial infarction: a quantitative review of 23 randomised trials. Lancet 2003;361(9351):13–20.
9. Weaver WD, Simes RJ, Betriu A, et al. Comparison of primary coronary angioplasty and intravenous thrombolytic therapy for acute myocardial infarction: a quantitative review. JAMA 1997;278(23):2093–8.
10. Mehta S, Patlola R, Cohen S, et al. STEMI interventions—a review of relevant clinical trials. Indian Heart J 2009;61(2):191–206.
11. Chen ZM, Jiang LX, Chen YP, et al. Addition of clopidogrel to aspirin in 45,852 patients with acute myocardial infarction: randomised placebo-controlled trial. Lancet 2005;366(9497):1607–21.
12. Sabatine MS, Cannon CP, Gibson CM, et al. Addition of clopidogrel to aspirin and fibrinolytic therapy for myocardial infarction with ST-segment elevation. N Engl J Med 2005;352(12):1179–89.
13. Wiviott SD, Braunwald E, McCabe CH, et al. Prasugrel versus clopidogrel in patients with acute coronary syndromes. N Engl J Med 2007;357(20):2001–15.
14. Nallamothu BK, Bates ER. Percutaneous coronary intervention versus fibrinolytic therapy in acute myocardial infarction: is timing (almost) everything? Am J Cardiol 2003;92(7):824–6.
15. Maeng M, Nielsen PH, Busk M, et al. Time to treatment and three-year mortality after primary percutaneous coronary intervention for ST-segment elevation myocardial infarction-a DANish trial in acute myocardial infarction-2 (DANAMI-2) substudy. Am J Cardiol 2010;105(11):1528–34.
16. Widimsky P, Bilkova D, Penicka M, et al. Long-term outcomes of patients with acute myocardial infarction presenting to hospitals without catheterization laboratory and randomized to immediate thrombolysis or interhospital transport for primary percutaneous coronary intervention. Five years' follow-up of the PRAGUE-2 trial. Eur Heart J 2007;28(6):679–84.
17. McNamara RL, Wang Y, Herrin J, et al. Effect of door-to-balloon time on mortality in patients with ST-segment elevation myocardial infarction. J Am Coll Cardiol 2006;47(11):2180–6.
18. Ellis SG, da Silva ER, Heyndrickx G, et al. Randomized comparison of rescue angioplasty with conservative management of patients with early failure of thrombolysis for acute anterior myocardial infarction. Circulation 1994;90(5):2280–4.
19. Sutton AG, Campbell PG, Graham R, et al. A randomized trial of rescue angioplasty versus a conservative approach for failed fibrinolysis in ST-segment elevation myocardial infarction: the middlesbrough early revascularization to limit INfarction (MERLIN) trial. J Am Coll Cardiol 2004;44(2):287–96.
20. Gershlick AH, Stephens-Lloyd A, Hughes S, et al. Rescue angioplasty after failed thrombolytic therapy for acute myocardial infarction. N Engl J Med 2005; 353(26):2758–68.
21. Wijeysundera HC, Vijayaraghavan R, Nallamothu BK, et al. Rescue angioplasty or repeat fibrinolysis after failed fibrinolytic therapy for ST-segment myocardial infarction: a meta-analysis of randomized trials. J Am Coll Cardiol 2007;49(4):422–30.
22. Stone GW, Cox D, Garcia E, et al. Normal flow (TIMI-3) before mechanical reperfusion therapy is an independent determinant of survival in acute myocardial infarction: analysis from the primary angioplasty in myocardial infarction trials. Circulation 2001;104(6): 636–41.
23. Assessment of the Safety, Efficacy of a New Treatment Strategy with Percutaneous Coronary Intervention (ASSENT-4 PCI) investigators. Primary versus tenecteplase-facilitated percutaneous coronary intervention in patients with ST-segment elevation acute myocardial infarction (ASSENT-4 PCI): randomised trial. Lancet 2006;367(9510):569–78.
24. Ellis SG, Tendera M, de Belder MA, et al. Facilitated PCI in patients with ST-elevation myocardial infarction. N Engl J Med 2008;358(21):2205–17.
25. Keeley EC, Boura JA, Grines CL. Comparison of primary and facilitated percutaneous coronary interventions for ST-elevation myocardial infarction: quantitative review of randomised trials. Lancet 2006;367(9510):579–88.
26. Henriques JP, Zijlstra F, Ottervanger JP, et al. Incidence and clinical significance of distal embolization during primary angioplasty for acute myocardial infarction. Eur Heart J 2002;23(14):1112–7.
27. Mehilli J, Kastrati A, Schulz S, et al. Abciximab in patients with acute ST-segment-elevation myocardial infarction undergoing primary percutaneous coronary intervention after clopidogrel loading: a randomized double-blind trial. Circulation 2009; 119(14):1933–40.
28. Van't Hof AW, Ten Berg J, Heestermans T, et al. Prehospital initiation of tirofiban in patients with ST-elevation myocardial infarction undergoing primary angioplasty (on-TIME 2): a multicentre, double-blind, randomised controlled trial. Lancet 2008; 372(9638):537–46.
29. Stone GW, Witzenbichler B, Guagliumi G, et al. Bivalirudin during primary PCI in acute myocardial infarction. N Engl J Med 2008;358(21):2218–30.
30. Gurm HS, Tamhane U, Meier P, et al. A comparison of abciximab and small-molecule glycoprotein IIb/IIIa

inhibitors in patients undergoing primary percutaneous coronary intervention: a meta-analysis of contemporary randomized controlled trials. Circ Cardiovasc Interv 2009;2(3):230–6.

31. De Luca G, Ucci G, Cassetti E, et al. Benefits from small molecule administration as compared with abciximab among patients with ST-segment elevation myocardial infarction treated with primary angioplasty: a meta-analysis. J Am Coll Cardiol 2009; 53(18):1668–73.
32. Kandzari DE, Hasselblad V, Tcheng JE, et al. Improved clinical outcomes with abciximab therapy in acute myocardial infarction: a systematic overview of randomized clinical trials. Am Heart J 2004;147(3):457–62.
33. Brener SJ, Barr LA, Burchenal JE, et al. Randomized, placebo-controlled trial of platelet glycoprotein IIb/IIIa blockade with primary angioplasty for acute myocardial infarction. ReoPro and primary PTCA organization and randomized trial (RAPPORT) investigators. Circulation 1998;98(8):734–41.
34. Neumann FJ, Kastrati A, Schmitt C, et al. Effect of glycoprotein IIb/IIIa receptor blockade with abciximab on clinical and angiographic restenosis rate after the placement of coronary stents following acute myocardial infarction. J Am Coll Cardiol 2000;35(4):915–21.
35. Montalescot G, Barragan P, Wittenberg O, et al. Platelet glycoprotein IIb/IIIa inhibition with coronary stenting for acute myocardial infarction. N Engl J Med 2001;344(25):1895–903.
36. Stone GW, Grines CL, Cox DA, et al. Comparison of angioplasty with stenting, with or without abciximab, in acute myocardial infarction. N Engl J Med 2002; 346(13):957–66.
37. Svilaas T, Vlaar PJ, Van der Horst IC, et al. Thrombus aspiration during primary percutaneous intervention. N Engl J Med 2008;358:557–67.
38. Bradley EH, Herrin J, Wang Y, et al. Strategies for reducing the door-to-balloon time in acute myocardial infarction. N Engl J Med 2006;355(22):2308–20.
39. Bradley EH, Curry LA, Webster TR, et al. Achieving rapid door-to-balloon times: how top hospitals improve complex clinical systems. Circulation 2006; 113(8):1079–85.
40. Rathore SS, Curtis JP, Chen J, et al. Association of door-to-balloon time and mortality in patients admitted to hospital with ST elevation myocardial infarction: national cohort study. BMJ 2009;338: b1807.

Pharmacoinvasive Management

Balaji Pakshirajan, MD, DNB,
Vijayakumar Subban, MD, DM, FNB,
Ajit S. Mullasari, MD, DM, DNB, FRCP*

KEYWORDS

• ST-segment elevation myocardial infarction • Primary percutaneous coronary intervention
• Thrombolysis • Total ischemic time

KEY POINTS

- Pharmacoinvasive management is a strategy of routine or adjunctive percutaneous coronary intervention (PCI) between 3 and 24 hours after fibrinolysis in patients with ST-segment elevation myocardial infarction (STEMI).
- Pharmacoinvasive management appears to be a more effective and practical way of treating STEMI patients for whom the option of primary PCI is not available because of logistic constraints.
- Randomized trials and meta-analyses suggest that the early invasive strategy is more beneficial than the current conservative/ischemia-guided approach or rescue PCI.
- The optimal time to perform PCI after fibrinolysis is still a question of debate; PCI may be harmful when performed within 2 hours of lytic therapy, as shown in trials of facilitated PCI.
- Given the consistent benefit observed in the randomized trials of pharmacoinvasive therapy, fibrinolysis should be followed by an early invasive approach on a nonemergency basis except in failed thrombolysis.

INTRODUCTION

Rapid restoration of adequate blood flow in the occluded infarct–related artery by either pharmacologic or mechanical therapy is central to optimal treatment of patients with ST-elevation myocardial infarction (STEMI). Timely reperfusion minimizes myocardial damage by reducing infarct size, preserving left ventricular function and thereby reducing the morbidity and mortality.[1]

Despite the decline in mortality in patients with STEMI in the last 2 decades, 30% of patients still do not get reperfusion therapy acutely.[2] Primary percutaneous coronary intervention (PCI) is the preferred reperfusion strategy for patients with STEMI if it can be performed in a timely manner and by experienced operators.[3,4] Fibrinolytic therapy is an alternative to primary PCI, but as many as 40% of patients are ultimately resistant to infarct artery reperfusion.[5] The various strategies that combine these 2 reperfusion therapies are:

- Rescue PCI for failed reperfusion
- Facilitated PCI (transfer for immediate angiography and PCI)
- Pharmacoinvasive approach (immediate transfer and or routine angiography within 24 hours of successful reperfusion)
- Ischemia-/symptom-guided PCI

Thus, the definitive goal in STEMI management is early, complete, and sustained reperfusion, which in turn results in better short-term and long-term outcomes.[6] Because of the challenges

Disclosures: None.
Department of Cardiology, Institute of Cardio Vascular Diseases, Madras Medical Mission, 4A Dr. JJ Nagar, Mogappair, Chennai 600037, India
* Corresponding author.
E-mail address: icvddoctors@mmm.org.in

Intervent Cardiol Clin 1 (2012) 409–419
http://dx.doi.org/10.1016/j.iccl.2012.06.010
2211-7458/12/$ – see front matter

related to delivering primary PCI worldwide, it is better to combine the best of both reperfusion therapies with early upstream administration of fibrinolytic therapy, anticoagulants, and antiplatelet agents to establish initial reperfusion, followed by final stabilization of the infarct artery with PCI. Trials testing the hypothesis of routine but nonemergent PCI versus the standard-care approach after successful fibrinolytic therapy, which comprise the focus of this review, have shown benefit when delays between fibrinolysis and PCI were 3 to 24 hours.[7]

TOTAL ISCHEMIC TIME: WHY IS IT IMPORTANT?

Infarct size increases proportionately with the increase in ischemic time because of microvascular obstruction. The extent of myocardial salvage decreased significantly when the ischemic times were longer than 90 minutes. Similarly, in patients with ischemic times of less than 90 minutes, the ejection fraction improved over time, whereas they worsened in patients with ischemic times greater than 360 minutes.[8]

The amount of myocardial salvage per unit time from the moment of coronary artery occlusion is curvilinear, with the maximum amount of salvage occurring in the first few hours after the onset of infarction and sharp reductions in the amount of salvage thereafter.[9] Thus, total ischemic time is of paramount importance regardless of whether reperfusion is attempted with a fibrinolytic or by PCI.[10,11] After symptom onset, for every 30-minute delay before reperfusion the relative mortality risk increases by 7.5%.[11]

The European Myocardial Infarction Project Group found that there were 15 more lives saved at 30 days per 1000 patients treated because of treatment 1 hour earlier.[12] Boersma and colleagues[10] showed that in patients presenting within 60 minutes of symptom onset, there were 65 fewer deaths per 1000 patients treated when compared with patients with longer duration of symptoms; moreover, the greatest impact of fibrinolysis was seen when it was administered within the first 2 hours of symptom onset.

In the study by De Luca and colleagues[13] in patients with STEMI treated by primary PCI, the main finding was that symptom onset to balloon time, but not door to balloon time, affects 1-year mortality, particularly in high-risk patients and in the absence of preprocedural flow of Thrombolysis In Myocardial Infarction (TIMI) grade 2 to 3. A symptom onset to balloon time longer than 4 hours has been shown to be an independent predictor of 1-year mortality.

The impact of total ischemic time on the short-term and long-term outcomes underscores the need for effective and timely reperfusion.

REPERFUSION STRATEGIES: AN OVERVIEW

Thrombolysis Versus Primary PCI

Multiple randomized clinical trials demonstrated the superiority of rapid primary PCI over thrombolysis in STEMI.[14,15] Primary PCI was shown to have lower rates of nonfatal reinfarction, stroke, and short-term mortality than thrombolysis in a meta-analysis of data from 23 randomized trials enrolling thrombolytic-eligible patients with STEMI.[4] Primary PCI would be the universal "dominant default strategy" for prompt early reperfusion if not limited by resource and logistical constraints. The American College of Cardiology/American Heart Association (ACC/AHA) and European Society of Cardiology (ESC) STEMI guidelines recommend PCI as the initial approach to management of STEMI, at centers with a skilled PCI laboratory and rapid initiation.[14,15]

The Danish Acute Myocardial Infarction 2 Trial (DANAMI-2) showed that primary PCI when compared with thrombolysis reduced the risk of reinfarction (13% vs 18.5%; hazard ratio [HR], 0.66; 95% confidence interval [CI], 0.49–0.89) and mortality (26.7% vs 33.3%; HR, 0.78; 95% CI, 0.63–0.97) among patients randomised at invasive centers within 120 minutes.[16]

CAPTIM (Comparison of Angioplasty and Prehospital Thrombolysis in Acute Myocardial Infarction)[17] and PRAGUE-2 (Primary Angioplasty in Patients Transported From General Community Hospitals to Specialized PTCA Units With or Without Emergency Thrombolysis 2)[18] trials have shown that there is no strong preference between PCI and thrombolysis in STEMI patients who present within 3 hours after symptom onset, as the mortality is similar or lower in both groups.[17,18] An analysis of 21 trials showed that as PCI-related time delay increased, absolute mortality reduction at 4 to 6 weeks favoring primary PCI versus thrombolysis decreased (0.94% decrease per additional 10-minute delay; $P = .006$).[19] STEMI guidelines indicate that thrombolysis is generally preferred over primary PCI when the door-to-balloon time minus door-to-needle time exceeds 1 hour.[14]

Prehospital Thrombolysis

Early reperfusion results in optimum myocardial salvage. Prehospital fibrinolysis, an important method to initiate early reperfusion strategy, reduces total ischemic time and might enhance the therapeutic benefits of thrombolysis[20] when compared with the delay in implementing primary PCI.[17,21]

Randomized clinical trials and meta-analysis provide clear evidence that earlier treatment with prehospital fibrinolysis is safe and improves survival compared with in-hospital administration.[22–24]

The Comparison of Angioplasty and Prehospital Thrombolysis In acute Myocardial infarction (CAPTIM) trial, which compared prehospital thrombolysis and primary PCI in patients with STEMI, showed no difference in the combined end point of death, reinfarction, and disabling stroke at 30 days between the 2 groups. Cardiogenic shock was less frequent and survival better with lytic therapy than with primary PCI (1.3% vs 5.3%, $P = .032$) when treatment was established within 2 hours of symptom onset, whereas the rates were similar in patients randomized later. Patients randomized less than 2 hours after symptom onset had a strong trend toward lower 30-day mortality with prehospital thrombolysis in comparison with those randomized to primary PCI (2.2% vs 5.7%, $P = .058$), whereas mortality was similar in patients randomized later than 2 hours after symptom onset (5.9% vs 3.7%, $P = .47$).[10,21]

Rescue PCI

The options of management for failed thrombolysis as suggested by ongoing chest pain and/or persistent ST-segment elevation at 60 to 90 minutes include repeat fibrinolysis and rescue angioplasty. Two recent studies on rescue PCI showed potential benefits of rescue PCI regarding mortality.[25,26]

In the Middlesbrough Early Vascularization to Limit Infarction (MERLIN) trial, 307 patients who failed thrombolytic therapy were randomized to either rescue PCI or conservative treatment. There was no difference in the all-cause mortality at 30 days, but the composite secondary end point of death/reinfarction/stroke/subsequent revascularization/heart failure occurred less frequently in the rescue group (37.3% vs 50%, $P = .02$), driven mainly by reduction in subsequent revascularization rates (6.5% vs 20.1%, $P<.01$), and was also observed during 1-year follow-up.[25,27]

In the Rescue Angioplasty versus Conservative Treatment or Repeat Thrombolysis (REACT) trial, 427 patients who had failed fibrinolysis were randomized to conservative management, repeat fibrinolysis, or emergency PCI. The primary end point (death, reinfarction, stroke, hospitalization for heart failure) at 6 months was observed in 29.8% of the conservative arm, 31.0% of the repeat-thrombolysis arm, and 15.3% of the rescue PCI arm ($P<.01$). At 6 months, there was a significant decrease in repeat revascularization in the rescue PCI group compared with conservative-therapy and repeat-thrombolysis groups (86.2%,77.6%, and 74.4%, respectively; overall $P = .05$).[26]

In the meta-analysis of Wijeysundera and colleagues,[28] when compared with conservative treatment rescue PCI was associated with significant risk reductions in heart failure and reinfarction, but showed no significant reduction in all-cause mortality.

Facilitated PCI

Facilitated PCI is a strategy of planned immediate catheterization after administration of an initial pharmacologic regimen including high-dose heparin, platelet glycoprotein (GP) IIb/IIIa inhibitors, full-dose or reduced-dose thrombolytic therapy, and the combination of a GP IIb/IIIa inhibitor with a reduced-dose thrombolytic agent before PCI.

The largest study comparing facilitated PCI and primary PCI is the Assessment of the Safety and Efficacy of a New Treatment Strategy with Percutaneous Coronary Intervention (ASSENT-4 PCI), which randomized patients with STEMI of 6 hours' duration to primary PCI (n = 838) or full-dose tenecteplase-facilitated PCI (n = 829). This study was terminated early because of increased in-hospital mortality in the facilitated PCI arm compared with the primary PCI group (6% vs 3%, $P = .0105$), largely attributable to higher rates of total stroke ($P = .0001$) and hemorrhagic stroke ($P = .0037$). The primary end point of death, congestive heart failure, or shock within 90 days was 19% in the facilitated PCI group versus 13% in the primary PCI group ($P = .0045$).[29]

The Facilitated Intervention with Enhanced Reperfusion Speed to Stop Events (FINESSE) study compared STEMI patients treated with conventional primary PCI, abciximab-facilitated PCI, or half-dose reteplase/abciximab-facilitated PCI, and showed no difference in all-cause mortality at 90 days (5.2%, 5.5%, and 4.5%, respectively, $P = .49$). Early ST-segment resolution occurred with combination-facilitated PCI (43.9%) in comparison with abciximab-facilitated PCI (33.1%) or primary PCI (31.0%; $P = .01$ and $P = .003$, respectively), with no significant difference in the primary end point (9.8%, 10.5%, and 10.7%, respectively, $P = .55$) and significantly higher rates of bleeding for the abciximab/lytic-facilitated PCI strategy compared with primary PCI.[30]

Meta-analysis and systematic reviews of several randomized trials demonstrated no advantage of facilitated PCI over primary PCI, and even possible harm.[31–33] Two important factors that were considered for the excess reinfarction rates observed in the facilitated PCI arm include insufficient antithrombotic therapy (low dose of heparin and minimal use of GP IIb/IIIa inhibitors) and performance of PCI at a time (median time 104 minutes after fibrinolysis) when platelet reactivity was still higher.[31–33]

PCI guidelines do not recommend full-dose thrombolytic therapy followed by immediate catheterization.[34]

PHARMACOINVASIVE THERAPY: A NEW PARADIGM

Pharmacoinvasive therapy is a strategy of initial pharmacologic reperfusion followed by timely planned PCI between 3 and 24 hours. In addition to reducing the total ischemic time by early reperfusion therapy, an important rationale for this strategy is that it results in higher TIMI flow grades (2 or 3) before PCI, thereby achieving better clinical outcomes.[35–38]

Pharmacoinvasive strategy yields early and 1-year survival rates that are comparable with those of primary PCI. Appropriate time delay between fibrinolysis and PCI neutralizes the hemorrhagic effect of thrombolysis and also allows the antiplatelet agents to act maximally, yielding better outcomes. This approach appears to be a more effective and practical way of treating STEMI patients for whom immediate PCI is not available.[39]

Several new studies conducted to assess safety and benefits of routine early angiography/PCI versus a conservative approach in STEMI patients treated with thrombolysis have shown benefit with this early invasive therapy when compared with fibrinolytic therapy.[39–46]

OVERVIEW OF PHARMACOINVASIVE TRIALS

PRAGUE-1 Study

In this trial, patients with STEMI were randomized in non-PCI hospitals to streptokinase alone (group A, n = 99), streptokinase followed by systematic transfer for immediate PCI (group B, n = 100), and immediate transportation for primary PCI without pretreatment with thrombolysis (group C, n = 101). (An overview of the trials discussed here is given in **Table 1**.) Revascularization was performed within 30 days in 14% (including rescue PCI in 7%) of the streptokinase alone group. The occurrences of death, reinfarction, and stroke at 30 days were 14%, 10%, and 1%, respectively, in the streptokinase-alone group versus 12%, 7%, and 3%, respectively, in the streptokinase plus immediate PCI group and 7%, 1%, and 0%, respectively, in the primary PCI group. The composite primary end point of death/reinfarction/stroke at 30 days were respectively 23%, 15%, and 8% in groups A, B, and C (P = .02). The end point of death and reinfarction was reported as 30% in the streptokinase-alone group versus 18% in the pharmacoinvasive group (relative risk 0.59; 95% CI, 0.36–0.99; P = .04). Limitations of this study are the use of a fibrinolytic strategy generally considered to be inferior, and the relatively small number of patients.[40,41]

SIAM III Trial

In the Southwest German Interventional Study in Acute Myocardial Infarction (SIAM III) trial, 197 STEMI patients were treated with full-dose reteplase (<12 hours) and randomized to either immediate stenting (median time, 3.5 hours) or elective stenting after 2 weeks. Immediate stenting resulted in a reduction in the primary composite end point of death, reinfarction, target lesion revascularization, and recurrent ischemic events after 30 days (8.5% vs 30.9%, P = .001) and at 6 months (25.6% vs 50.6%; relative risk 0.51; 95% CI, 0.33–0.78; P = .001) without significant difference in bleeding risk. The difference between the 2 groups was driven by ischemic events (4.9% vs 28.4%; relative risk 0.17; 95% CI, 0.06–0.47; P = .001), more than by death or reinfarction (7.3% vs 13.6%; relative risk 0.54; 95% CI, 0.21–1.39; P = .146).[7]

GRACIA-1 Trial

In Grupo de Analisis de la Cardiopatia Isquemica Aguda (GRACIA-1) study, patients were randomized to angiography and intervention if indicated within 24 hours (median time 17 hours) of thrombolysis with accelerated-dose alteplase (n = 248), or to an ischemia-guided conservative approach (n = 252). In the interventional arm, 80% underwent stenting of the infarct-related artery, 2% underwent coronary artery bypass grafting and 16% were treated medically. Amongst patients treated conservatively 20% underwent angiography, and 19% underwent PCI. The primary end point at 1 year was lower in the interventional arm (9% vs 21%; risk ratio [RR] 0.44, P = .0008), with much of the reduction driven by a lower revascularization rate in the intervention arm (4% vs 12%, RR 0.30, P = .001), they tended to have a reduced rate of death or reinfarction (7% vs 12%, RR 0·59 [95% CI 0·33–1·05], P = 0·07), and there was no increase in bleeding rates. The limitations include unbalanced use of clopidogrel in the 2 groups, as

Table 1
Summary of pharmacoinvasive trials

Serial No.	Trial	No. of Patients	Pharmacologic Strategy	Time Interval Between TT and PCI (h)	Primary Outcomes (Pharmacoinvasive vs Conservative Strategy)
1	SIAM III Trial[7]	197	Reteplase	3.5 ± 2.3 (mean ± SD)	Composite of death, reinfarction, ischemic events, and TLR at 6 mo: 25.6% vs 50.6% (P = .001)
2	GRACIA-1[42]	500	tPA	16.7 ± 5.6 (mean ± SD)	Composite of death, reinfarction, and revascularization at 1 y: 9% vs 21% (P = .0008)
3	CAPITAL AMI Trial[43]	170	TNK	1.6 (median)	Composite of death, reinfarction, recurrent ischemia, and stroke at 6 mo: 11.6% vs 24.4% (P = .04)
4	WEST study[44]	204	TNK	4.9 (median)	Composite of death, reinfarction, refractory ischemia, congestive cardiac failure, cardiogenic shock, and ventricular arrhythmias at 30 d: 25% vs 24% (P = NS)
5	CARESS in AMI Trial[45]	600	Half-dose reteplase + abciximab	2.2 (median)	Composite of death, reinfarction, refractory ischemia: 4.4% vs 10.7% (P = .004)
6	TRANSFER AMI trial[39]	1059	TNK	3.9 (median)	Composite of death, reinfarction, recurrent ischemia, and cardiogenic shock at 30 d: 11% vs 17% (P = .004)
7	NORDI-STEMI Trial[46]	266	TNK	2.7 (median)	Composite of death, reinfarction, stroke, or new ischemia at 1 y: 21% vs 27% (P = .19)

Abbreviations: CAPITAL AMI, Combined Angioplasty and Pharmacologic Intervention versus Thrombolysis Alone in Acute Myocardial Infarction; CARESS in AMI, Combined Abciximab Reteplase Stent Study in Acute Myocardial Infarction; GRACIA-1, Grupo de Analisis de la Cardiopatia Isquemica Aguda; NORDI-STEMI, Norwegian Study on District Treatment of ST-Elevation Myocardial Infarction trial; NS, not significant; SIAM III, Southwest German Interventional Study in Acute Myocardial Infarction; STK, streptokinase; TLR, target lesion revascularization; TNK, tenecteplase; tPA, tissue plasminogen activator; TRANSFER AMI, Trial of Routine Angioplasty and Stenting After Fibrinolysis to Enhance Reperfusion in Acute Myocardial Infarction; TT, thrombolytic therapy; WEST, Which Early ST-elevation myocardial infarction Therapy.

well as a lower enzyme threshold (3 times the normal value of creatine kinase MB isoenzyme) for defining reinfarction within 48 hours of fibrinolysis compared with that of invasive intervention (5 times the normal value).[42]

CAPITAL AMI Trial

In the Combined Angioplasty and Pharmacologic Intervention versus Thrombolysis Alone in Acute Myocardial Infarction (CAPITAL AMI) study, 170 patients with high-risk STEMI treated with thrombolysis (full-dose tenecteplase) were randomized to either immediate angiography/PCI (n = 86) or a conservative approach (n = 84). The primary composite end point of death, reinfarction, recurrent unstable ischemia, or stroke at 6 months was 24.4% in the tenecteplase-alone group versus 11.6% in the tenecteplase-facilitated angioplasty group (P = .04). This difference was driven by a reduction in the rate of recurrent unstable ischemia (20.7% vs 8.1%, P = .03). There was a trend toward a lower reinfarction rate with tenecteplase-facilitated angioplasty (14.6% vs 5.8%, P = .07), with no difference in frequency of major bleedings. The relatively small numbers in the study and the unbalanced use of clopidogrel (91% in the pharmacoinvasive arm compared with 57% in the fibrinolysis-alone arm) are limitations.[43]

WEST Study

Which Early ST-elevation myocardial infarction Therapy (WEST) was a 4-city Canadian, open-label, randomized feasibility study of 304 STEMI patients, randomized to fibrinolysis with tenecteplase and usual care, tenecteplase and mandatory invasive study within 24 hours, including rescue PCI for reperfusion failure, and primary PCI with a 300-mg loading dose of clopidogrel. The primary composite end point of death, reinfarction, refractory ischemia, congestive heart failure, cardiogenic shock, and major ventricular arrhythmia, at 30 days was 25% in the fibrinolysis-alone group, 24% in the pharmacoinvasive group, and 23% in the primary PCI group (relative risk 0.96; 95% CI, 0.59–1.56; *P* = .87). A reduced composite end point of death and reinfarction was not significant between the 2 groups (6.7% in the pharmacoinvasive versus 13.0% in the fibrinolysis-alone group). These data suggest that fibrinolysis, when delivered rapidly and coupled with a strategy of rescue/pharmacoinvasive therapy, may not be different from timely expert PCI.[44]

CARESS in AMI Trial

The Combined Abciximab Reteplase Stent Study in Acute Myocardial Infarction (CARESS in AMI) trial randomized 600 patients with STEMI, aged 75 years or younger, after receiving half-dose reteplase and abciximab, to a pharmacoinvasive approach (median time from thrombolysis initiation to angiography in immediate PCI group = 135 minutes) or standard ischemia-guided management (including rescue PCI). Ninety-seven percent of patients assigned to immediate PCI underwent angiography and 85% received PCI, and 30% of patients in the standard care/rescue PCI group underwent PCI. This randomized trial showed that transfer of high-risk STEMI patients with at least one high-risk feature (sum of ST-segment elevation or depression more than 15 mm in 12-lead electrocardiogram or new-onset complete left bundle branch block, prior myocardial infarction, Killip class 2 or 3, and left ventricular ejection fraction <35%) for early routine PCI soon after the administration of abciximab and half-dose reteplase reduces the risk of recurrent ischemia and all ischemic complications (death, repeat myocardial infarction, recurrent ischemia) (immediate PCI group versus standard care/rescue PCI group: 4.4% vs 10.7%, *P* = .004) at 30 days (relative risk 0.41; 95% CI, 0.22–0.77; *P* = .005). This reduction is driven mainly by reduced refractory ischemia (0.3% in the pharmacoinvasive group versus 4.3% in the standard care/rescue group; *P* = .003) without a significant increase in major bleeding complications (pharmacoinvasive PCI group versus standard care/rescue PCI group: 3.4% vs 2.3%; *P* = .47), as well as stroke (0.7% vs 1.3%, *P* = .50).[45]

TRANSFER AMI Trial

In the Trial of Routine Angioplasty and Stenting After Fibrinolysis to Enhance Reperfusion in Acute Myocardial Infarction (TRANSFER AMI), 1059 high-risk patients who had STEMI and who were receiving fibrinolytic therapy at centers that did not have the capability of performing PCI were assigned to either standard treatment (including rescue PCI, if required, or delayed angiography; n = 522) or a strategy of immediate transfer to another hospital and PCI within 6 hours after fibrinolysis (n = 537) and a recommendation that cardiac catheterization be performed in all patients within 2 weeks. All patients received standard-dose tenecteplase, heparin, and aspirin 160 to 325 mg. Either unfractionated heparin or enoxaparin was used based on institutions' standard practice, using weight-adjusted dosing consistent with published STEMI guidelines. Clopidogrel loading (300 mg for patients ≤75 years of age, and 75 mg if >75 years) was strongly encouraged in all study patients. GP IIb/IIIa inhibitors were used at the interventional centers, at the discretion of the operator. PCI of the culprit lesion was performed if at least 70% stenosis or high-risk features were present (ie, thrombus, ulceration, dissection). Stents were used whenever technically feasible (bare metal: 79.3%). Cardiac catheterization was performed in 98.5% of patients in the pharmacoinvasive arm and in 88.7% of patients in the standard treatment arm. The median time to administration of tenecteplase from onset of symptoms was about 2 hours in both arms, whereas the median time from tenecteplase to catheterization was 2.8 hours in the pharmacoinvasive arm and 32.5 hours in the standard treatment arm. PCI was performed in 84.9% of the patients in the pharmacoinvasive arm and in 67.4% in the standard therapy arm. The primary composite 30-day end point of death, reinfarction, congestive heart failure, severe recurrent ischemia, and shock occurred in 11.0% of the immediate PCI arm and 17.2% of the standard arm (relative risk 0.64; 95% CI, 0.47–0.87; *P* = .004), the difference mainly being due to reduced rate of recurrent ischemia (0.2% vs 2.1%; relative risk 0.09; 95% CI, 0.01–0.68; *P* = .003) and reinfarction (3.4% vs 5.7%; relative risk 0.57; 95% CI, 0.33–1.04; *P* = .06). At 6 months, there was no significant difference in death or reinfarction between the 2 groups (8.9% in the routine early group versus 10.6% in the standard group; relative risk 0.83; 95% CI, 0.55–1.25; *P* = .36). The results of this large randomized clinical trial indicate that in patients presenting with STEMI to centers without timely access to a catheterization laboratory, a pharmacoinvasive approach consisting of full-dose thrombolytics, followed by emergent transfer for cardiac catheterization within 6 hours, is safe and efficacious in comparison with treatment with thrombolytics and transfer for rescue PCI only.[39]

NORDI-STEMI Trial

The Norwegian Study on District Treatment of ST-Elevation Myocardial Infarction (NORDI-STEMI) trial compared a strategy of immediate transfer for PCI with an ischemia-guided approach with early transfer, only if indicated for rescue or clinical deterioration after fibrinolysis with full-dose tenecteplase (prehospital in 57%) in 266 patients situated too far away for timely primary PCI (>90 minutes transfer delay). All patients were treated with aspirin, enoxaparin, and clopidogrel. At 30 days, the combined incidence of death, reinfarction, stroke, or new ischemia was significantly reduced in the early invasive group compared with the conservative group (10% vs 21%; relative risk 0.49; 95% CI, 0.27 to 0.89; $P = .03$) with no significant difference in the risk of bleeding between the 2 groups. Median infarct size, estimated as percentage of the left ventricle using single-photon emission computed tomography at 3 months, was 7% (interquartile range 0%–24%) in the early invasive group compared with 6% (interquartile range 0%–19%) in the conservative group ($P = .29$). The primary composite end point of death, reinfarction, stroke, or new ischemia at 12 months was reached in 28 patients (21%) in the early invasive group compared with 36 (27%) in the conservative group (HR 0.72; 95% CI, 0.44–1.18; $P = .19$). The composite of death, reinfarction, or stroke at 12 months was significantly reduced in the early invasive group compared with the conservative group (6% vs 16%; HR 0.36; 95% CI, 0.16 to 0.81; $P = .01$). These data suggest that an early invasive strategy may be the preferred option in patients receiving thrombolytic therapy, especially in those with long transfer delays.[46]

STREAM Study

In the Strategic Reperfusion Early After Myocardial Infarction (STREAM) study, an ongoing open-label, prospective, randomized, parallel, comparative, international multicenter trial, acute STEMI patients presenting early after symptom onset in whom PCI is not feasible within 60 minutes of first medical contact were randomized to fibrinolysis with tenecteplase combined with enoxaparin, clopidogrel, and aspirin, and cardiac catheterization within 6 to 24 hours or rescue coronary intervention for failed reperfusion within 90 minutes of fibrinolysis versus PCI performed according to local guidelines. Composite efficacy end points at 30 days include death, shock, heart failure, and reinfarction. Safety end points include ischemic stroke, intracranial hemorrhage, and major nonintracranial bleeding with 1-year follow-up of all-cause mortality. The STREAM results will provide useful additional data on therapeutic decisions in many patients who fail to achieve the desired reperfusion times of 90 to 120 minutes after first medical contact.[47]

PHARMACOINVASIVE THERAPY: META-ANALYSIS OF THE CURRENT TRIALS

The recent meta-analyses by Borgia and colleagues,[48] D'Souza and colleagues,[49] and Bogaty and colleagues[50] showed that in patients with STEMI, routine early referral for PCI after thrombolysis leads to a significant reduction in the composite end point of mortality, reinfarction, and ischemia at 1 year. This reduction appeared to be driven mainly by the decrease in reinfarction rates and recurrent ischemia, but not mortality. The benefits of early routine PCI after thrombolysis occurs without increased risk of adverse events such as stroke or major bleeding. The results of these meta-analyses suggest that the early invasive strategy is more beneficial when compared with current conservative/ischemia-guided approach or rescue PCI after thrombolysis in STEMI patients for whom PCI is not readily available.

PHARMACOINVASIVE THERAPY: WHAT IS THE OPTIMAL TIME WINDOW?

The optimal time to perform angiography/PCI after lytic administration is still open for debate. It has been shown to be harmful when performed within 2 hours of initiation of fibrinolytic therapy.[29,51] Various trials on early invasive strategy showed different median time to PCI from about 2 hours in CARESS in AMI, 3.5 hours in SIAM III, 3 hours in TRANSFER AMI, to almost 17 hours in GRACIA-1.[39–46] Because most of the reocclusion and reinfarction occurs in the initial 24 hours, the recent guidelines recommend routine postthrombolytic PCI between 3 and 24 hours. Pharmacoinvasive strategy results in timely, sustained, and more complete reperfusion, improved myocardial salvage and, consequently, a decrease in adverse cardiac events.[51,52]

PHARMACOINVASIVE THERAPY: GUIDELINES

The 2009 focused updates of the ACC/AHA guidelines for the management of patients with STEMI and the ACC/AHA/Society for Cardiovascular

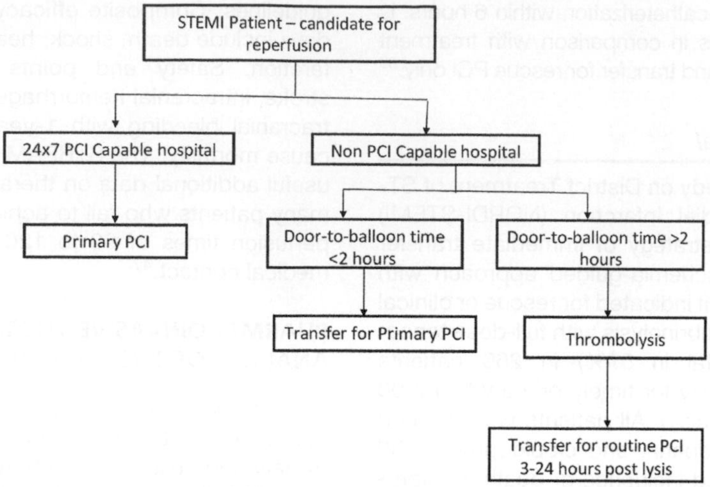

Fig. 1. Current reperfusion strategy for ST-segment elevation myocardial infarction (STEMI). PCI, percutaneous coronary intervention.

Angiography and Interventions (SCAI) guidelines on PCIs consider early routine postthrombolysis PCI a class IIb recommendation (level of evidence: C). Only high-risk patients receive a class IIa recommendation (level of evidence: B). The guidelines use the term "facilitated PCI" instead of "early routine postthrombolysis PCI."[34] The 2008 ESC guidelines recommend an early routine coronary angiogram 3 to 24 hours after successful thrombolysis with a class IIa level of recommendation (level of evidence: A).[3] With the availability of more evidence from recent trials, the latest 2011 American College of Cardiology Foundation/AHA/SCAI guidelines[51] for PCI upgraded the recommendation to class IIa (level of evidence: A) irrespective of the risk category, and the ESC/European School for Cardiothoracic Surgery/European Association for Percutaneous Cardiovascular Interventions guidelines[52] have given class I (Level of Evidence: B) recommendation for pharmacoinvasive therapy.

The current reperfusion strategy for STEMI is summarized in **Fig. 1**.

SUMMARY

Timely primary PCI remains the choice of reperfusion therapy for STEMI patients. All efforts should be made to shorten transfer delays and to increase the number of centers with experienced operators to perform primary PCI round the clock, so that most patients can be treated with primary PCI. However, because of logistic constraints, most patients will still be treated by fibrinolysis. Prehospital thrombolysis improves the efficacy of pharmacologic therapy by shortening the total ischemic time. Published trials have showed that in STEMI treatment, pharmacoinvasive therapy when compared with the conservative standard-care approach results in significant reduction in the composite end point of death, reinfarction, or stroke, and is also safe, with an acceptable bleeding risk. Given the consistent benefit observed in the randomized trials of an early invasive approach optimally timed between 3 and 24 hours, fibrinolysis should not be the end of reperfusion therapy in STEMI, and should be followed by an early invasive approach on a nonemergency basis except in the event of failed thrombolysis.

REFERENCES

1. Boden WE, Eagle K, Granger CB. Reperfusion strategies in acute ST-segment elevation myocardial infarction: a comprehensive review of contemporary management options. J Am Coll Cardiol 2007;50:917–29.
2. Eagle KA, Goodman SG, Avezum A, et al. Practice variation and missed opportunities for reperfusion in ST-segment-elevation myocardial infarction: findings from the Global Registry of Acute Coronary Events (GRACE). Lancet 2002;359:373–7.
3. Van de Werf F, Bax J, Betriu A, et al. Management of acute myocardial infarction in patients presenting with persistent ST segment elevation: the Task Force on the Management of ST Segment Elevation Acute Myocardial Infarction of the European Society of Cardiology. Eur Heart J 2008;29:2909–45.
4. Keeley EC, Boura JA, Grines CL. Primary angioplasty versus intravenous thrombolytic therapy for acute myocardial infarction: a quantitative review of 23 randomized trials. Lancet 2003;361:13–20.

5. The GUSTO Investigators. The effects of tissue plasminogen activator, streptokinase, or both on coronary-artery patency, ventricular function, and survival after acute myocardial function. N Engl J Med 1993;329:1615–22.
6. Ndrepepa G, Mehilli J, Schulz S, et al. Prognostic significance of epicardial blood flow before and after percutaneous coronary intervention in patients with acute coronary syndromes. J Am Coll Cardiol 2008;52:512–7.
7. Scheller B, Hennen B, Hammer B, et al. Beneficial effects of immediate stenting after thrombolysis in acute myocardial infarction. J Am Coll Cardiol 2003; 42:634–41.
8. Francone M, Bucciarelli-Ducci C, Carbone I, et al. Impact of primary coronary angioplasty delay on myocardial salvage, infarct size, and microvascular damage in patients with ST-segment elevation myocardial infarction: insight from cardiovascular magnetic resonance. J Am Coll Cardiol 2009;54: 2145–53.
9. Gersh BJ, Stone GW, White HD, et al. Pharmacological facilitation of primary percutaneous coronary intervention for acute myocardial infarction: is the slope of the curve the shape of the future? JAMA 2005;293:979–86.
10. Boersma E, Maas AC, Deckers JW, et al. Early thrombolytic treatment in acute myocardial infarction: reappraisal of the golden hour. Lancet 1996; 348:771–5.
11. De Luca G, Suryapranata H, Ottervanger JP, et al. Time delay to treatment and mortality in primary angioplasty for acute myocardial infarction: every minute of delay counts. Circulation 2004;109:1223–5.
12. The European Myocardial Infarction Project Group. Prehospital thrombolytic therapy in patients with suspected acute myocardial infarction. N Engl J Med 1993;329:383–9.
13. De Luca G, Suryapranata H, Zijlstra F, et al. Symptom-onset-to-balloon time and mortality in patients with acute myocardial infarction treated by primary angioplasty. J Am Coll Cardiol 2003;42:991–7.
14. Antman EM, Hand M, Armstrong PW, et al. 2007 Focused Update of the ACC/AHA 2004 Guidelines for the Management of Patients With ST-Elevation Myocardial Infarction: a report of the American College of Cardiology/American Heart Association Task Force on Practice Guidelines: 2007 Writing Group to Review New Evidence and Update the ACC/AHA 2004 Guidelines for the Management of Patients With ST-Elevation Myocardial Infarction. J Am Coll Cardiol 2008;51:210–47.
15. Silber S, Albertsson P, Fernandez-Aviles F, et al. Guidelines for percutaneous coronary interventions. The Task Force for Percutaneous Coronary Interventions of the European Society of Cardiology. Eur Heart J 2005;26:804–47.
16. Nielsen PH, Maeng M, Busk M, et al. Primary angioplasty versus fibrinolysis in acute myocardial infarction, long-term follow-up in the Danish Acute Myocardial Infarction 2 trial. Circulation 2010;121: 1484–91.
17. Steg PG, Bonnefoy E, Chabaud S, et al. Impact of time to treatment on mortality after prehospital fibrinolysis or primary angioplasty: data from the CAPTIM randomized clinical trial. Circulation 2003;108: 2851–6.
18. Widimský P, Budesínský T, Vorác D, et al, 'PRAGUE' Study Group Investigators. Long distance transport for primary angioplasty vs immediate thrombolysis in acute myocardial infarction: final results of the randomized national multicenter trial 'PRAGUE-2'. Eur Heart J 2003;23:94–104.
19. Nallamothu BK, Bates ER. Percutaneous coronary intervention versus fibrinolytic therapy in acute myocardial infarction: is timing (almost) everything? Am J Cardiol 2003;92:824–6.
20. Fibrinolytic Therapy Trialist (FTT) Collaborative Group. Indications for fibrinolytic therapy in suspected acute myocardial infarction: collaborative overview of early mortality and major morbidity results from all randomised trials of more than 1000 patients. Lancet 1994;343:311–22.
21. Bonnefoy E, Lapostolle F, Leizorovicz A, et al. Primary angioplasty versus prehospital fibrinolysis in acute myocardial infarction: a randomised study. Lancet 2002;360:825–9.
22. Morrison L, Verbeek P, McDonald A, et al. Mortality and pre-hospital thrombolysis for acute myocardial infarction. A meta-analysis. JAMA 2000;283:2686–92.
23. Danchin N, Durand E, Blanchard D. Pre-hospital thrombolysis in perspective. Eur Heart J 2008;29: 2835–42.
24. Bonnefoy E, Steg PG, Bouititie F, et al, for the CAPTIM Investigators. Comparison of primary angioplasty and pre-hospital fibrinolysis in acute myocardial infarction (CAPTIM) trial: a 5-year follow-up. Eur Heart J 2009;30:1598–606.
25. Sutton AG, Campbell PG, Graham R, et al. A randomized trial of rescue angioplasty versus conservative approach for failed fibrinolysis in ST-segment elevation myocardial infarction: the Middlesbrough Early Revascularization to Limit Infarction (MERLIN) trial. J Am Coll Cardiol 2004; 44:287–96.
26. Gershlick AH, Stephens-Lloyd A, Hughes S, et al. Rescue angioplasty after failed thrombolytic therapy for acute myocardial infarction. N Engl J Med 2005; 353:2758–68.
27. Sutton AG, Campbell PG, Graham R, et al. One year results of the Middlesbrough Early Revascularisation to Limit Infarction (MERLIN) trial. Heart 2005;91: 1330–7.

28. Wijeysundera HC, Vijayaraghavan R, Nallamothu BK, et al. Rescue angioplasty or repeat fibrinolysis after failed fibrinolytic therapy for ST-segment myocardial infarction: a meta-analysis of randomized trials. J Am Coll Cardiol 2007;49:422–30.
29. Keeley EC, Boura JA, Grines CL. Comparison of primary and facilitated percutaneous coronary interventions for ST-elevation myocardial infarction: quantitative review of randomised trials. Lancet 2006;367:579–88.
30. Collet JP, Montalescot G, Le May M, et al. Percutaneous coronary intervention after fibrinolysis: a multiple metaanalyses approach according to the type of strategy. J Am Coll Cardiol 2006;48: 1326–35.
31. Kiernan TJ, Ting HH, Gersh BJ. Facilitated percutaneous coronary intervention: current concepts, promises, and pitfalls. Eur Heart J 2007;28:1545–53.
32. Assessment of the Safety, and Efficacy of a New Treatment Strategy with Percutaneous Coronary Intervention (ASSENT-4 PCI) Investigators. Primary versus tenecteplase-facilitated percutaneous coronary intervention in patients with ST-segment elevation acute myocardial infarction (ASSENT-4 PCI): randomised trial. Lancet 2006;367:569–78.
33. Ellis SG, Tendera M, de Belder MA, et al. Facilitated PCI in patients with ST-segment elevation myocardial infarction. N Engl J Med 2008;358:2205–17.
34. Kushner FG, Hand M, Smith SC Jr, et al. 2009 focused updates: ACC/AHA Guidelines for the Management of Patients With ST-Elevation Myocardial Infarction (updating the 2004 Guideline and 2007 Focused Update) and ACC/AHA/SCAI Guidelines on Percutaneous Coronary Intervention (updating the 2005 Guideline and 2007 Focused Update): a report of the American College of Cardiology Foundation/American Heart Association Task Force on Practice Guidelines. Circulation 2009;120:2271–306.
35. Ross AM, Coyne KS, Reiner JS, et al. A randomized trial comparing primary angioplasty with a strategy of short-acting thrombolysis and immediate planned rescue angioplasty in acute myocardial infarction: the PACT trial. PACT Investigators. Plasminogen-Activator Angioplasty Compatibility Trial. J Am Coll Cardiol 1999;34:1954–62.
36. Brodie BR, Stuckey TD, Hansen C, et al. Benefit of coronary reperfusion before intervention on outcomes after primary angioplasty for acute myocardial infarction. Am J Cardiol 2000;85:13–8.
37. Stone GW, Cox D, Garcia E, et al. Normal flow (TIMI-3) before mechanical reperfusion therapy is an independent determinant of survival in acute myocardial infarction: analysis from the Primary Angioplasty in Myocardial Infarction trials. Circulation 2001;104: 636–41.
38. De Luca G, Ernst N, Zijlstra F, et al. Preprocedural TIMI flow and mortality in patients with acute myocardial infarction treated by primary angioplasty. J Am Coll Cardiol 2004;43:1363–7.
39. Cantor WJ, Fitchett D, Borgundvaag B, et al. Routine early angioplasty after fibrinolysis for acute myocardial infarction. N Engl J Med 2009;360:2705–18.
40. Widimsky P, Groch L, Zelizko M, et al. Multicentre randomized trial comparing transport to primary angioplasty vs immediate thrombolysis vs combined strategy for patients with acute myocardial infarction presenting to a community hospital without a catheterization laboratory. The PRAGUE study. Eur Heart J 2000;21:823–31.
41. Bednar F, Widimsky P, Krupicka J, et al. Interhospital transport for primary angioplasty improves the long-term outcome of acute myocardial infarction compared with immediate thrombolysis in the nearest hospital (one-year follow-up of the PRAGUE- 1 study). Can J Cardiol 2003;19:1133–7.
42. Fernandez-Avilés F, Alonso JJ, Castro-Beiras A, et al. Routine invasive strategy within 24 hours of thrombolysis versus an ischaemia guided conservative approach for acute myocardial infarction with ST-segment elevation (GRACIA-1): a randomized controlled trial. Lancet 2004;364:1045–53.
43. So DY, Ha AC, Davies RF, et al. ST segment resolution in patients with tenecteplase-facilitated percutaneous coronary intervention versus tenecteplase alone: insights from the Combined Angioplasty and Pharmacological Intervention versus Thrombolysis ALone in Acute Myocardial Infarction (CAPITAL AMI) trial. Can J Cardiol 2010;26:e7–12.
44. Armstrong PW, WEST Steering Committee. A comparison of pharmacologic therapy with/without timely coronary intervention vs. primary percutaneous intervention early after ST-elevation myocardial infarction: the WEST (Which Early ST-elevation myocardial infarction Therapy) study. Eur Heart J 2006;27:1530–8.
45. Di Mario C, Dudek D, Piscione F, et al. Immediate angioplasty versus standard therapy with rescue angioplasty after thrombolysis in the Combined Abciximab REteplase Stent Study in Acute Myocardial Infarction (CARESS-in-AMI): an open, prospective, randomised, multicentre trial. Lancet 2008;371:559–68.
46. Bohmer E, Hoffmann P, Abdelnoor M, et al. Efficacy and safety of immediate angioplasty versus ischemia-guided management after thrombolysis in acute myocardial infarction in areas with very long transfer distances results of the NORDISTEMI (NORwegian study on DIstrict treatment of ST-Elevation Myocardial Infarction). J Am Coll Cardiol 2010;55:102–10.
47. Armstrong PW, Gershlick A, Goldstein P, et al, STREAM Steering Committee. The Strategic Reperfusion Early After Myocardial Infarction (STREAM) study. Am Heart J 2010;160:30–5.
48. Borgia F, Goodman SG, Halvorsen S, et al. Early routine percutaneous coronary intervention after

fibrinolysis vs. standard therapy in ST-segment elevation myocardial infarction: a meta-analysis. Eur Heart J 2010;31:2156–69.
49. D'Souza SP, Mamas MA, Fraser DG, et al. Routine early coronary angioplasty versus ischaemia-guided angioplasty after thrombolysis in acute ST-elevation myocardial infarction: a meta-analysis. Eur Heart J 2011;32:972–82.
50. Bogaty P, Filion KB, Brophy JM. Routine invasive management after fibrinolysis in patients with ST-elevation myocardial infarction: a systematic review of randomized clinical trials. BMC Cardiovasc Disord 2011;11:34. Available at: http://www. biomedcentral. com/1471-2261/11/34. Accessed February 12, 2012.
51. Levine GN, Bates ER, Blankenship JC, et al. 2011 ACCF/AHA/SCAI Guideline for Percutaneous Coronary Intervention: a report of the American College of Cardiology Foundation/American Heart Association Task Force on Practice Guidelines and the Society for Cardiovascular Angiography and Interventions. J Am Coll Cardiol 2011;58:e44–122.
52. Wijns W, Kolh P, Danchin N, et al, Task Force on Myocardial Revascularization of the European Society of Cardiology (ESC) and the European Association for Cardio-Thoracic Surgery (EACTS), European Association for Percutaneous Cardiovascular Interventions (EAPCI). Guidelines on myocardial revascularization. Eur Heart J 2010;31:2501–55.

Optimal Anticoagulant Therapy in ST Elevation Myocardial Infarction Interventions

Estefania Oliveros, MD[a], Sameer Mehta, MD, MBA[a,b,c,*],
Ana Isabel Flores, MD[a], Camilo Pena, MD[a],
Salomon Cohen, MD[d], Jennifer C. Kostela, MS, MD[e,f],
Rebecca Rowen, BS[f], Kevin Treto, BS[g]

KEYWORDS

• STEMI • Anticoagulant • Bivalirudin • PCI

KEY POINTS

- Optimal anticoagulant therapy combined with an adequate reperfusion therapy in patients with ST elevation myocardial infarction (STEMI) is associated with lower mortality, reduced bleeding episodes, and lower hospitalization costs.
- Bivalirudin is a direct thrombin inhibitor that has proved to be useful in the management of STEMI in patients undergoing percutaneous coronary intervention.
- Bivalirudin is an anticoagulant with favorable pharmacokinetic and numerous pharmacodynamic benefits compared with unfractionated heparin.

INTRODUCTION

According to the World Health Report, 17.3 million deaths per year were caused by cardiovascular diseases (CVDs) in 2008, representing 30% of global deaths. CVDs represent the largest cause of death and disability in the world. Of these, an estimated 7.3 million (42%) were caused by coronary artery disease and 6.2 million (35.8%) were caused by stroke. By 2030, 23.6 million people are predicted to die from CVDs, leaving coronary artery disease as the leading cause of death.[1]

The pathophysiology of acute coronary syndromes is characterized by disruption of atherosclerotic plaques, activation and aggregation of platelets, and formation of an arterial thrombus (**Fig. 1**A–C).[2] Thrombus formation can produce transient or persistent occlusion. Inhibition of the different pathways of platelet activation might offer the best management conduct. Antithrombotic therapy and mechanical reperfusion have changed the management of acute coronary syndromes by improving the outcome and survival rates of the patients. Anticoagulants prevent thrombus formation at the site of arterial lesion, the guidewire, and in the catheters used for percutaneous coronary intervention (PCI).[3] Anticoagulation combined with antiplatelet therapy is considered the gold

Disclosure: Sameer Mehta is Chief Medical Officer, Asia Pacific, for the Medicines Company. The rest of the authors report no conflict of interest regarding the content herein.
[a] Lumen Foundation, 55 Pinta Road, Miami, FL 33133, USA; [b] Miller School of Medicine, University of Miami, 1400 Northwest 12th Avenue, Miami, FL 33136, USA; [c] Mercy Medical Center, 3663 South Miami Avenue, Miami, FL 33133, USA; [d] Departamento de Neurocirugia, Instituto Mexicano del Seguro Social, Avenida Club de Golf#3 Torre A Dep. 1501, Lomas Country, Huixquilucan Edo de Mexico, 52779, Mexico; [e] Internal Medicine, New York Hospital Queens, 56-45 Main Street, Flushing, NY 11355, USA; [f] Ross University School of Medicine, 630 US Highway 1, North Brunswick, NJ 08902, USA; [g] Ross University School of Medicine, 786 Seneca Meadows Road, Winter Springs, FL 32708, USA
* Corresponding author. 185 Shore Drive South, Miami, FL 33133.
E-mail address: mehtas@bellsouth.net

Intervent Cardiol Clin 1 (2012) 421–428
http://dx.doi.org/10.1016/j.iccl.2012.06.002
2211-7458/12/$ – see front matter

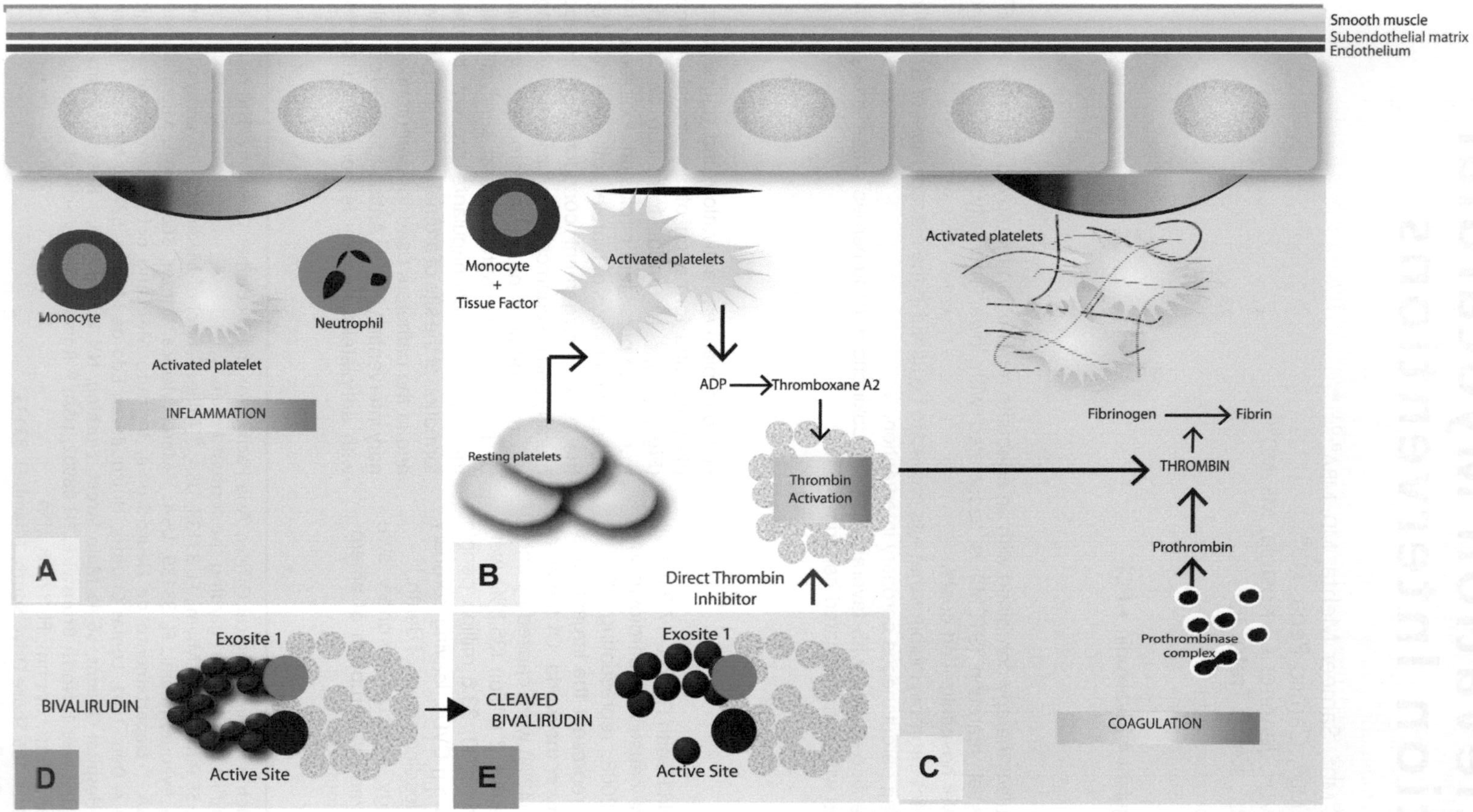

Fig. 1. Role of thrombin and bivalirudin. (*A*) Thrombin is involved in inflammation. It activates neutrophils and platelets, releasing cytokines, chemotactic factors, and growth factors. (*B*) Monocytes express tissue factor, triggering the extrinsic pathway of the coagulation cascade, thereby activating platelets. It leads to the activation of thrombin. (*C*) Thrombin is a trypsinlike serine protease produced by the enzymatic cleavage of 2 sites on prothrombin by factor Xa, which is enhanced by binding of the prothrombinase complex (factor Va). Prothrombin is proteolytically cleaved to form thrombin. Thrombin converts soluble fibrinogen into insoluble strands of fibrin (cross-linked framework). (*D*) Bivalirudin directly inhibits thrombin by binding to the active catalytic site and to the anion-binding exosite 1 of circulating and clot-bound thrombin. (*E*) The binding is reversible because thrombin cleaves the bivalirudin-thrombin bond, resulting in the recovery of the thrombin active binding site. ADP, adenosine diphosphate.

standard for adequate management according to recent guidelines.[4,5] At present, the antiplatelet therapy consists of aspirin, a $P2Y_{12}$ receptor inhibitor, and a platelet glycoprotein (GP) IIb/IIIa inhibitor. When selecting the most appropriate therapy, the physician must consider which reperfusion option can be delivered most promptly, with the least recurrence of adverse ischemic events, as well as assessing the bleeding risk of an aggressive pharmacologic agent that may lead to mortality.

New drugs have been introduced considering the previous factors. Bivalirudin (Angiomax, the Medicines Company, Parsippany, NJ) is a reversible direct thrombin inhibitor. The active substance is a synthetic peptide with 20 amino acids. Bivalirudin has been investigated as an adjunct antithrombotic therapy in patients undergoing PCI, because it allows on-off administration during the procedure (see **Fig. 1**D, E). **Box 1** shows the benefits of bivalirudin compared with unfractionated heparin (UFH) for ST elevation myocardial infarction (STEMI). The following clinical studies evaluated the role of bivalirudin in patients with STEMI (**Table 1**).

CLINICAL TRIALS: BIVALIRUDIN AND STEMI

Hirulog Early Reperfusion/Occlusion Trials

Hirulog Early Reperfusion/Occlusion (HERO)-1 was a landmark trial that included 412 patients with STEMI who underwent reperfusion therapy with streptokinase. The subjects received aspirin and streptokinase, and were randomized in a double-blind manner to receive up to 60 hours of heparin, low-dose bivalirudin, or high-dose bivalirudin. The higher dosage of bivalirudin, a 0.25-mg/kg bolus followed by 0.5 mg/kg/h for 12 hours followed by 0.25 mg/kg/h for up to 60 hours, was associated with an increased in the Thrombolysis in Myocardial Infarction (TIMI) grade 3 flow at 90 to 120 minutes compared with UFH (48% vs 35%, $P = .03$). Major bleeding was significantly lower with bivalirudin than with UFH (27% vs 19%, $P<.01$).[6] These TIMI grade 3 flow rates were not as high as those of more fibrin-specific thrombolytics in combination with UFH, reported in the Global Use of Strategies to Open Occluded Coronary Arteries in Acute Coronary Syndromes (GUSTO)-1 trial with alteplase (48%–60%) and the Reteplase (r-PA) versus Alteplase Patency Investigation during Myocardial Infarction (RAPID)-2 with rerelease (59.9%).[7,8]

HERO-2 was a large randomized trial that involved 17,000 patients. The patients randomly received UFH or bivalirudin, given 3 minutes before streptokinase administration.[9] All patients received aspirin. The primary end point was 30-day mortality, and its major secondary end points were investigator-adjudicated reinfarction and bleeding. The patient population came from Russia, Asia, eastern Europe, and South America. The decrease in reinfarction rates was an important result of the HERO-2 trial; early reinfarction after fibrinolysis was associated with an increased risk of further reinfarction, heart failure, and death.

In HERO-2, the overall 30-day mortality of 10.8% was higher than that seen in other similar trials (Assessment of the Safety and Efficacy of a New Thrombolytic [ASSENT]-3 and GUSTO V),[10,11] which might be because the patients in HERO-2 were older, and greater proportions were female and had anterior myocardial infarction or Killip class III or IV heart failure. Furthermore, the mortality in the Western countries in HERO-2 was 6.7%, which is similar to the rates seen in the other studies. The differences in the severe bleeding and intracranial hemorrhage rates were not statistically significant in the bivalirudin and UFH groups (1.32, $P = .05$). This trial showed that bivalirudin is at least as effective as UFH and not inferior when combined with streptokinase for the treatment of STEMI.[6,7]

Harmonizing Outcomes with Revascularization and Stents in Acute Myocardial Infarction

Harmonizing Outcomes with Revascularization and Stents in Acute Myocardial Infarction (HORIZONS-AMI) is the largest study to focus on the appropriate use of anticoagulation medications

Box 1
Advantages of bivalirudin compared with unfractionated heparin

1. Bivalirudin has more predictable pharmacokinetics and pharmacodynamics
2. Not activated by PF4
3. No cofactor required for activity
4. Not inhibited by plasma proteins
5. Does not activate platelets
6. Not associated with thrombocytopenia
7. Can be used in cases of heparin-induced thrombocytopenia
8. No anticoagulation tests are required for monitoring
9. Reduced bleeding compared with UFH plus GP IIb/IIIa inhibitors

Table 1
Clinical trials of bivalirudin used in patients with STEMI

Study, Year	Aim	Type	N	Primary End Points	Results
HERO-1, 1997	Comparison of bivalirudin vs heparin in patients receiving streptokinase and ASA for AMI	Randomized, double blind	412	Patency at 90–120 min as measured by TIMI 3 flow. Patency at 2–3 d, left ventricular function, ejection fraction, end systolic volume, regional wall motion, incidence of death, stroke, reinfarction, and cardiogenic shock (35 after treatment)	48% of patients who received bivalirudin with streptokinase had TIMI grade 3 flow in the infarct-related artery, compared with 35% of patients who received heparin with streptokinase (P<.05)
HERO-2, 1998	Bivalirudin plus ASA before streptokinase decreases mortality vs heparin plus ASA for AMI	Randomized, double blind	17,000	30-d mortality, reinfarction, and bleeding	Bivalirudin vs heparin: death, 10.0% vs 10.9%, P = .46; death/nonfatal disabling stroke, 10.6% vs 11.1%, P = .36; death/reinfarction (investigator reported), 12.9% vs 14.2%, P = .023; death/reinfarction (adjudicated), 12.6% vs 13.6%, P = .07; reinfarction within 96 h, 1.6% vs 2.3%, P = .001; death/reinfarction/nonfatal disabling stroke, 12.7% vs 13.8%, P = .049
HORIZONS-AMI, 2011	Comparing bivalirudin monotherapy with heparin plus a GPI and paclitaxel-eluting stents with bare-metal stents in STEMI plus primary PCI strategy	Prospective, open-label, randomized, multicenter trial	3602	Major bleeding and net adverse clinical events, such as death, reinfarction, stroke, or ischemic target vessel revascularization and major bleeding at 30 d	At 30 d, major bleeding occurred in 5.1% of patients in the bivalirudin group and 8.8% of patients in the heparin plus GP IIb/IIIa inhibitor group. At 1 y, 5.8% bivalirudin group vs 9.2% in the other group

Abbreviations: AMI, acute myocardial infarction; ASA, aspirin; GPI, GP inhibitor; HERO, Hirulog Early Reperfusion/Occlusion; HORIZONS-AMI, Harmonizing Outcomes with Revascularization and Stents in AMI; TIMI, Thrombolysis in Myocardial Infarction.

and stents in patients experiencing STEMI and undergoing primary PCI.[12] This landmark study was conducted in 11 countries recruiting 3602 patients with STEMI intended for a primary PCI. The trial is ongoing and has at least 3 years of follow-up data available at this time.[13] HORIZONS-AMI was a prospective, open-label, factorial, randomized, multicenter trial comparing bivalirudin monotherapy with heparin plus a GP IIb/IIIa and paclitaxel-eluting stents with bare-metal stents in patients with STEMI undergoing a primary PCI management strategy. Both treatment arms received aspirin. Patients were stratified by administration of prerandomization heparin, administration of clopidogrel 300 mg or 600 mg or ticlopidine 500 mg before catheterization, planned administration of abciximab versus eptifibatide if randomized to the control group, and US study site versus non-US study site. Consecutive patients aged 18 years or older with a symptom duration of 20 to 720 minutes and ST-segment elevation of 1 mm or more in 2 or more contiguous leads, new left bundle branch block, or true posterior myocardial infarction were eligible for enrollment.

The 2 primary end points of the trial were major bleeding and net adverse clinical events, a composite of major adverse cardiovascular events (death, reinfarction, stroke, or ischemic target vessel revascularization) and major bleeding at 30 days. The major secondary end point was major adverse cardiovascular events at 30 days. For the primary outcome of major adverse cardiovascular events, bivalirudin was not inferior to heparin plus GP IIb/IIIa inhibitor at 30 days and 1 year. In both treatment groups, around 5.5% of patients had a major adverse cardiovascular event after 30 days and about 12% after 1 year. For the primary outcome of major bleeding, there was a statistically significant difference ($P<.0001$) between the treatment groups at 30 days and at 1 year. At 30 days, major bleeding occurred in 5.1% of patients in the bivalirudin group and 8.8% of patients in the heparin plus GP IIb/IIIa inhibitor group ($P<.0001$). At 1 year, major bleeding occurred in 5.8% of patients in the bivalirudin group and 9.2% of patients in the other group ($P<.0001$).[14]

For the secondary outcomes of all-cause mortality and cardiac mortality, there were statistically significant differences between treatment with bivalirudin and treatment with heparin plus GP IIb/IIIa inhibitor. After 1 year of follow-up, all-cause mortality was 3.5% in the bivalirudin group and 4.8% in the comparator group ($P = .037$). The 1-year results for cardiac mortality were 2.1% for bivalirudin and 3.8% for comparator ($P = .005$).[14]

A slightly higher percentage of patients in the bivalirudin group had a target vessel revascularization than in the heparin plus GP IIb/IIIa inhibitor group (7.2% compared with 5.9% at 1 year), but this difference was not statistically significant. The overall rate of any stent thrombosis at 30 days and at 1 year was identical in the bivalirudin and the heparin plus GP IIb/IIIa inhibitor groups. However, more stent thrombosis events occurred in the bivalirudin group within the first 24 hours of PCI. Investigators reported comparable rates of adverse events between the treatment groups, with a trend toward fewer events in the bivalirudin group and significantly reduced rates of drug-related adverse events ($P<.0001$). Significantly fewer thrombocytopenia events occurred in the bivalirudin group (1.4%) than in the heparin plus GP IIb/IIIa inhibitor group (3.9%; $P<.0001$).[14]

At the 3-year follow-up, 1802 patients received heparin plus a GP IIb/IIIa inhibitors, and 1800 patients received bivalirudin monotherapy showing lower rates of all-cause mortality (5.9% vs 7.7%, $P = .03$), cardiac mortality (2.9% vs 5.1%, $P = .001$), reinfarction (6.2% vs 8.2%, $P = .04$), and major bleeding not related to bypass graft surgery (6.9% vs 10.5%, $P = .0001$), with no significant differences in ischemia-driven target vessel revascularization, stent thrombosis, or composite adverse events (**Table 2**).[13] Bivalirudin monotherapy and paclitaxel-eluting stenting were effective and safe at 3 years for patients with STEMI undergoing primary PCI.[13]

The HORIZONS-AMI cardiac magnetic resonance imaging (CMRI) substudy included 51 randomized patients with STEMI from a single center. They received bivalirudin or UFH plus GP IIb/IIIa. CMRI was performed within 7 days and 6 months after primary PCI. The results did not show significant differences in infarct size, microvascular obstruction, left ventricular ejection fraction, or left ventricular volume indices in patients

Table 2
HORIZONS-AMI 3-year outcomes

	Bivalirudin (%) (n = 1800)	Heparin + GPI (%) (n = 1802)	*P* Value
Major bleeding	6.9	10.5	.0001
Reinfarction	6.2	8.2	.04
Cardiac mortality	2.9	5.1	.001
All-cause mortality	5.9	7.7	.03

treated with bivalirudin compared with patients treated with UFH plus abciximab.[15]

Guidelines Supporting the Use of Bivalirudin

In 2009, the American College of Cardiology (ACC)/American Heart Association (AHA) guidelines added a new recommendation for patients with STEMI undergoing PCI who were at high risk of bleeding: drugs such as bivalirudin may be used (class I, level of evidence B).[4] In 2010, the European Guidelines on Myocardial Revascularization recommended bivalirudin as an anticoagulant during PCI in patients with acute coronary syndrome (non-ST and ST elevation) at high risk of bleeding (class I, level of evidence B).[16] In 2011, the American College of Cardiology Foundation (ACCF)/AHA/Society for Cardiovascular Angiography and Interventions (SCAI) guidelines[5] still suggested the use of bivalirudin for patients with STEMI undergoing PCI, as a recommendation class I, level of evidence B. The recommendation for dosing of parental bivalirudin during PCI depends whether the patient receives prior anticoagulant therapy or not. For those patients who receive UFH, a waiting time of 30 minutes is recommended, followed by 0.75 mg/kg intravenous (IV) bolus, then 1.75 mg/kg/h IV infusion. If the patient did not received prior anticoagulant treatment, then bivalirudin should be given in a 0.75 mg/kg bolus, followed by 1.75 mg/kg/h IV infusion. Both ways have been shown to be beneficial for patients undergoing PCI. Lower bleeding rates were associated with bivalirudin used concomitantly with a GP IIb/IIIa inhibitor.

Single Individual Community Experience Registry for Primary PCI Database

Based on the medical evidence, the Single Individual Community Experience Registry for Primary PCI (SINCERE) group adopted bivalirudin as part of the pharmacotherapy used.[17] A total of 1034 patients at 5 community hospitals underwent primary PCI for STEMI. Bivalirudin was used in 98.5% of them in a bolus followed by a drip, with no massive bleeding complications. The benefits of using bivalirudin instead of combined therapy with heparin and GP IIb/IIIa inhibitors are well established in terms of less bleeding risk and lower long-mortality, as shown in the studies discussed, and corroborated with SINCERE. Bivalirudin shows linear pharmacokinetics following IV administration, with a more consistent and more rapid achievement of therapeutic antithrombin effects compared with UFH.[18] It is predictable and simple to monitor, which makes it beneficial, reducing the need for multiple anticoagulation tests. It can also be used in cases of heparin-induced thrombocytopenia, in which bivalirudin or argatroban are recommended to replace UFH (level of evidence B).[5] The standard of use in SINCERE is to use both a bolus and a drip to target anticoagulation tests between 300 and 350 seconds. The angiographic drip is stopped when an acceptable angiographic result is obtained, facilitating earlier sheath removal.[17]

Choosing an adequate anticoagulant regimen may also affect the overall cost of treatment of patients with STEMI, so a cost-benefit comparison using bivalirudin versus UFH and a GP IIb/IIIa inhibitor was made. The use of bivalirudin reduces the overall costs of treating patients with STEMI with the following end points: reduction in bleeding (P<.001), length of hospital stay (P<.03), and hospital costs (P<.04).[19] Pinto and colleagues[20] compared bivalirudin versus heparin plus a GP IIb/IIIa inhibitor; the primary outcome was in-hospital death, which was reduced in the bivalirudin arm (3.2% vs 4%). Secondary outcomes were clinically apparent bleeding, 6.9% versus 10.5%; transfusion, 5.9% versus 7.6%; mean cost ($), 18,640 $\pm$ 15,174 versus 19,967 $\pm$ 15,772. European cost-effectiveness studies also concur in suggesting bivalirudin as more beneficial than heparin plus a GP IIb/IIIa inhibitor, by showing increased survival years and reduced patient lifetime costs with the use of bivalirudin.[21] These studies support a lower mortality, lower bleeding risk, and a lower cost for patients with STEMI undergoing primary PCI.

The concern is the slight increase in the risk of stent thrombosis with the use of bivalirudin, which might be counteracted by the use of the new thienopyridine agents, like prasugrel. The combination of prasugrel and bivalirudin needs to be further evaluated in randomized controlled trials, but may offer a solution. In the Therapeutic Outcomes by Optimizing Platelet Inhibition with Prasugrel–Thrombolysis in Myocardial Infarction (TRITON-TIMI) 38 study, both drugs were used in 3% of the patients, achieving good results. The ongoing Randomized Trial of Prasugrel Plus Bivalirudin versus Clopidogrel Plus Heparin in Acute STEMI (BRAVE) 4 may also retrieve some answers to the use of this combination. Anderson and colleagues[22] addressed this concern by proposing a 2-hour infusion of bivalirudin following STEMI PCI. They did a multicenter prospective study at a single PCI center. The registry included 128 patients receiving a preload of dual antiplatelet therapy and 75% a UFH bolus before PCI. They used bivalirudin in a bolus followed by a 2-hour infusion in 92% of the patients. Nine percent of the patients stopped using GP IIb/IIIa inhibitors, and 1 of these patients presented with probable or definite acute stent thrombosis. Major bleeding occurred in 1.7%. The investigators suggested that prolonged bivalirudin infusion might lessen the acute stent thrombosis after STEMI PCI. The Swedish Coronary Angiography and Angioplasty Registry (SCAAR) enrolled 2996 patients undergoing PCI caused by STEMI who received a bivalirudin strategy. Patients were divided into 2 groups, 1928 (64%) received only bivalirudin and 1068 (36%) received bivalirudin plus a bolus dose of UFH. The primary combined end point of death or target lesion thrombosis at 30 days happened more frequently in the bivalirudin arm (11.3% vs 6.5%, $P<.001$). Death at 30 days and definite target lesion thrombosis at 30 days did not differ between the 2 groups (9.2% vs 5.1%, $P = .07$). The researchers concluded that adding a bolus dose of UFH is associated with a lower rate of death or definite target lesion thrombosis at 30 days in patients undergoing primary PCI with bivalirudin.[23]

Long-term follow-up of the bivalirudin studies suggests that small or nominal increases in ischemic events have not turned into long-standing consequences and that treatment at or before the time of PCI with clopidogrel may diminish any increment in early ischemic risk.[3,14,24]

SUMMARY

Current guidelines encourage the use of bivalirudin in patients with STEMI who undergo PCI. Establishing a prompt and effective anticoagulation strategy improves the procedure outcome. Bivalirudin is an anticoagulant with a pharmacokinetic and pharmacodynamic advantage compared with UFH. The net adverse clinical events (combined major adverse cardiac event and bleeding) are lower with the use of the bivalirudin strategy. The higher cost of this drug may require evaluation; however, it is key to consider that there are lower bleeding risks and hospitalization complications, which reduce costs.

REFERENCES

1. Mendis S, Puska P, Norvrving B, editors. Global atlas on cardiovascular disease prevention and control. Geneva (Switzerland): World Health Organization; 2011.
2. Falk E, Shah PK, Fuster V. Coronary plaque disruption. Circulation 1995;92(3):657–71.
3. Smith SC Jr, Feldman TE, Hirshfeld JW Jr, et al. ACC/AHA/SCAI 2005 guideline update for percutaneous coronary intervention: a report of the American College of Cardiology/American Heart Association Task Force on Practice Guidelines (ACC/AHA/SCAI Writing Committee to Update 2001 Guidelines for Percutaneous Coronary Intervention. Circulation 2006;113(7):e166–286.
4. Kushner FG, Hand M, Smith SC Jr, et al. 2009 Focused Updates: ACC/AHA guidelines for the management of patients with ST-elevation myocardial infarction (updating the 2004 Guideline and 2007 Focused Update) and ACC/AHA/SCAI Guidelines on Percutaneous Coronary Intervention (updating the 2005 Guideline and 2007 Focused Update): a report of the American College of Cardiology Foundation/American Heart Association Task Force on Practice Guidelines. Circulation 2009;120(22): 2271–306.
5. Levine GN, Bates ER, Blankenship JC, et al. 2011 ACCF/AHA/SCAI Guideline for Percutaneous Coronary Intervention: a report of the American College of Cardiology Foundation/American Heart Association Task Force on Practice Guidelines and the Society for Cardiovascular Angiography and Interventions. Circulation 2011;124(23):e574–651.
6. White HD, Aylward PE, Frey MJ, et al. Randomized, double-blind comparison of hirulog versus heparin in patients receiving streptokinase and aspirin for acute myocardial infarction (HERO). Hirulog Early Reperfusion/Occlusion (HERO) Trial Investigators. Circulation 1997;96(7):2155–61.
7. An international randomized trial comparing four thrombolytic strategies for acute myocardial infarction. The GUSTO investigators. N Engl J Med 1993;329(10):673–82.
8. Bode C, Smalling RW, Berg G, et al. Randomized comparison of coronary thrombolysis achieved with double-bolus reteplase (recombinant plasminogen activator) and front-loaded, accelerated alteplase (recombinant tissue plasminogen activator) in patients with acute myocardial infarction. The RAPID II Investigators. Circulation 1996;94(5):891–8.
9. White H. Thrombin-specific anticoagulation with bivalirudin versus heparin in patients receiving fibrinolytic therapy for acute myocardial infarction: the HERO-2 randomised trial. Lancet 2001;358(9296): 1855–63.
10. Topol EJ. Reperfusion therapy for acute myocardial infarction with fibrinolytic therapy or combination reduced fibrinolytic therapy and platelet glycoprotein IIb/IIIa inhibition: the GUSTO V randomised trial. Lancet 2001;357(9272):1905–14.
11. Efficacy and safety of tenecteplase in combination with enoxaparin, abciximab, or unfractionated heparin: the ASSENT-3 randomised trial in acute myocardial infarction. Lancet 2001;358(9282): 605–13.
12. Mehran R, Brodie B, Cox DA, et al. The Harmonizing Outcomes with RevasculariZatiON and Stents in Acute Myocardial Infarction (HORIZONS-AMI)

Trial: study design and rationale. Am Heart J 2008;156(1):44–56.
13. Stone GW, Witzenbichler B, Guagliumi G, et al. Heparin plus a glycoprotein IIb/IIIa inhibitor versus bivalirudin monotherapy and paclitaxel-eluting stents versus bare-metal stents in acute myocardial infarction (HORIZONS-AMI): final 3-year results from a multicentre, randomised controlled trial. Lancet 2011;377(9784):2193–204.
14. Mehran R, Lansky AJ, Witzenbichler B, et al. Bivalirudin in patients undergoing primary angioplasty for acute myocardial infarction (HORIZONS-AMI): 1-year results of a randomised controlled trial. Lancet 2009;374(9696):1149–59.
15. Wohrle J, Merkle N, Kunze M, et al. Effect of bivalirudin compared with unfractionated heparin plus abciximab on infarct size and myocardial recovery after primary percutaneous coronary intervention: the horizons-AMI CMRI substudy. Catheter Cardiovasc Interv 2012;79(7):1083–9.
16. Wijns W, Kolh P, Danchin N, et al. Guidelines on myocardial revascularization: the Task Force on Myocardial Revascularization of the European Society of Cardiology (ESC) and the European Association for Cardio-Thoracic Surgery (EACTS). Eur Heart J 2010;31(20):2501–55.
17. Mehta S. Textbook of STEMI Interventions. 2nd edition. Malvern (PA): HMP Communications; 2010.
18. Angiomax (bivalirudin) prescribing information. Parsippany (NJ): The Medicine Company; 2005.
19. Kessler DP, Kroch E, Hlatky MA. The effect of bivalirudin on costs and outcomes of treatment of ST-segment elevation myocardial infarction. Am Heart J 2011;162(3):494–500.e492.
20. Pinto DS, Ogbonnaya A, Sherman SA, et al. Bivalirudin therapy is associated with improved clinical and economic outcomes in ST-elevation myocardial infarction patients undergoing percutaneous coronary intervention: results from an observational database. Circ Cardiovasc Qual Outcomes 2012;5(1):52–61.
21. Schwenkglenks M, Toward TJ, Plent S, et al. Cost-effectiveness of bivalirudin versus heparin plus glycoprotein IIb/IIIa inhibitor in the treatment of acute ST-segment elevation myocardial infarction. Heart 2012;98(7):544–51.
22. Anderson PR, Gogo PB, Ahmed B, et al. Two hour bivalirudin infusion after PCI for ST elevation myocardial infarction. J Thromb Thrombolysis 2011;31(4):401–6.
23. Koutouzis M, Lagerqvist B, James S, et al. Unfractionated heparin administration in patients treated with bivalirudin during primary percutaneous coronary intervention is associated lower mortality and target lesion thrombosis: a report from the Swedish Coronary Angiography and Angioplasty Registry (SCAAR). Heart 2011;97(18):1484–8.
24. Dangas G, Mehran R, Guagliumi G, et al. Role of clopidogrel loading dose in patients with ST-segment elevation myocardial infarction undergoing primary angioplasty: results from the HORIZONS-AMI (harmonizing outcomes with revascularization and stents in acute myocardial infarction) trial. J Am Coll Cardiol 2009;54(15):1438–46.

Newer Pharmaceutical Agents for STEMI Interventions

Anjan K. Chakrabarti, MD[a], Shalin J. Patel, MD[a], Robert L. Salazar, MD[a], Lakshmi Gopalakrishnan, MBBS[a,b], Varun Kumar, MBBS[a,b], Ujjwal Rastogi, MBBS[b], Priyamvada Singh, MBBS[b], Cafer Zorkun, MD[b,c], C. Michael Gibson, MS, MD[a,d,*]

KEYWORDS

• STEMI • Fibrinolytics • Thienopyridines • Thrombin inhibitors

KEY POINTS

- Pharmaceutical agents currently used in clinical practice for early management of ST elevation myocardial infraction (STEMI) act primarily on the two pathways of clot formation: platelet aggregation and the coagulation cascade.
- Although percutaneous coronary intervention is the standard therapy for revascularization, new fibrinolytic drugs are being developed to provide increased safety and efficacy through a longer plasma half-life, more fibrin specificity, and resistance to plasminogen activator inhibitor-1.
- Antiplatelet therapies useful for early and extended management of STEMI include acetylsalicylic acid, glycoprotein IIb/IIIa inhibitors (eptifibatide, tirofiban, and abciximab), the thienopyridines (clopidogrel and prasugrel), and contemporary agents (ticagrelor, cangrelor, elinogrel, and vorapaxar).
- Novel therapies for long-term inhibition of thrombin formation following STEMI include factor Xa inhibitors, such as rivaroxaban and apixaban.
- Emerging areas of STEMI treatment include pharmacotherapy that specifically targets reperfusion injury and cardiomyoplasty, which involves the use of hematopoietic stem cell therapy or growth factors to induce proliferation and differentiation of cardiac myocytes.

INTRODUCTION

Ischemic heart disease is one of the most common causes of death and is responsible for 12.6% of deaths worldwide. ST elevation myocardial infarction (STEMI) is the most severe presentation of ischemic heart disease and affects 500,000 people in the United States each year.[1] Even though the management of patients with STEMI has evolved significantly over the last several decades with the advent of fibrinolytic agents and percutaneous coronary intervention (PCI), the morbidity and mortality associated with STEMI remains a significant problem in the United States.

Historically, bed rest and morphine were cornerstones in the management of patients with STEMI before the discovery of fibrinolytics.[2] Pharmacologic therapy for STEMI has seen numerous advances since that time. The current management strategies of STEMI aim to achieve two goals: prompt restoration of blood to the ischemic heart tissue and pharmacologic therapy to improve long-term prognosis.[1] Various pharmaceutical agents currently used in clinical practice

[a] Cardiovascular Division, Department of Medicine, Beth Israel Deaconess Medical Center, Harvard Medical School, 185 Pilgrim Road, Deaconess 319, Boston, MA 02215, USA; [b] Cardiovascular Division, Department of Medicine, PERFUSE Angiographic Core Laboratories, Data Coordinating Center, Beth Israel Deaconess Medical Center, 185 Pilgrim Road, Deaconess 319, Boston, MA 02215, USA; [c] Division of Cardiology, Yedikule Education and Research Hospital, Istanbul, Turkey; [d] WikiDoc Foundation (a 509 (a)(1) Charitable Organization), San Francisco, California

* Corresponding author. Cardiovascular Division, Department of Medicine, Beth Israel Deaconess Medical Center, 185 Pilgrim Road, Deaconess 319, Boston, MA 02215.

E-mail address: mgibson@perfuse.org

Intervent Cardiol Clin 1 (2012) 429–440
http://dx.doi.org/10.1016/j.iccl.2012.06.005

for early management of STEMI act primarily on the two pathways of clot formation: platelet aggregation and the coagulation cascade (**Fig. 1**). Antiplatelet agents impair platelet function, whereas fibrinolytic agents and anticoagulants exert their effects by inhibiting the clotting factors. The use of these agents in conjunction with PCI has further enhanced the treatment of STEMI.

THROMBOLYTICS

Fibrinolytic therapy has evolved significantly since the discovery of streptokinase in 1933. Although primary PCI has since become the preferred treatment in STEMI when administered in a timely fashion, fibrinolytic therapy remains effective owing to its ease of administration, standardized dosing regimens, and widespread accessibility.[3]

Four fibrinolytics are currently available (**Table 1**): first-generation streptokinase, second-generation alteplase, and third-generation reteplase and tenecteplase. First-generation fibrinolytics lack fibrin specificity, are immunogenic, and have a short half-life, which led to the development of the second-generation drugs, which are more fibrin specific but have an increased incidence of intracranial hemorrhage and a modest mortality benefit.[4] The third-generation agents were developed to improve the efficacy, safety, and ease of administration and have been shown to have superior angiographic patency.[5] New fibrinolytic drugs are being developed to provide a longer plasma half-life, more fibrin specificity, and resistance to plasminogen activator inhibitor-1 (**Table 2**).[6–9]

ANTIPLATELET AGENTS

Prevention of platelet aggregation is an important strategy in the management of patients with STEMI. Currently used antiplatelet agents are classified into thromboxane inhibitors (acetylsalicylic acid [ASA]), P2Y12 receptor antagonists (thienopyridines), glycoprotein IIb/IIIa inhibitors, and, most recently, thrombin-receptor (protease-activated receptor-1) antagonists.

Aspirin

In 2002, the Antithrombotic Trialists' Collaboration demonstrated a 30% relative risk reduction with aspirin (ASA) use for acute coronary syndrome (ACS).[10] This benefit is primarily due to an irreversible inhibition of platelet cyclooxygenase-1 enzyme, which subsequently inhibits thromboxane-A2 in a nonlinear fashion. Additionally, ASA spares other platelet pathways, including P2Y12 and PAR1 receptors, which is the rationale behind dual or triple antiplatelet therapies.[11]

A dose-dependent increase in the bleeding risk associated with ASA has led to an ongoing debate concerning its optimal dose. Recent studies have demonstrated that increased doses of ASA do not necessarily correlate with increased efficacy but do cause an increased risk of bleeding.[12] The Clopidogrel Optimal Loading Dose Usage to Reduce Recurrent Events/Optimal Antiplatelet Strategy for Interventions (CURRENT-OASIS-7) trial demonstrated that among ACS patients undergoing an invasive strategy, there was no significant

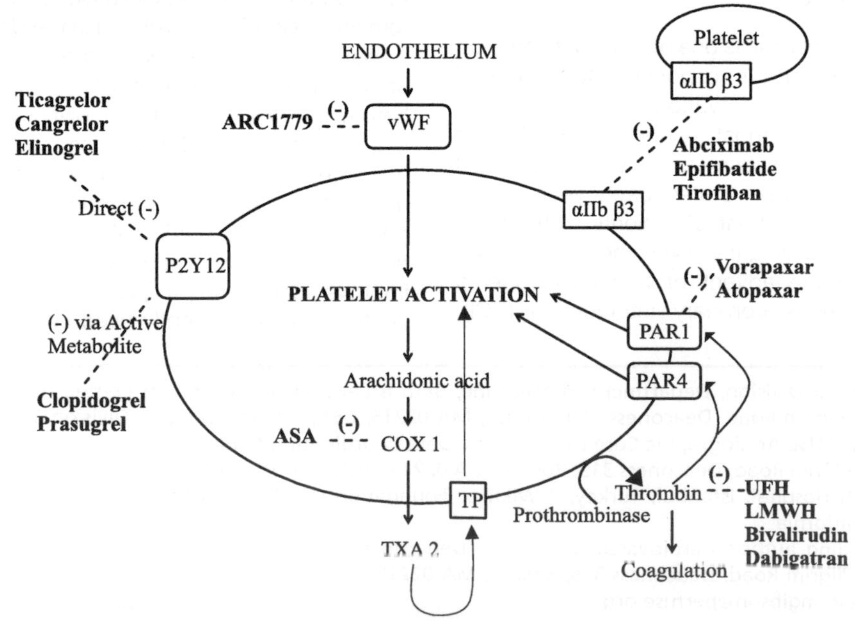

Fig. 1. STEMI therapy targets.

Table 1
Fibrinolytic agents

	First-Generation		Second-Generation			Third-Generation			
	Streptokinase	Urokinase	Alteplase	Anistreplase	Saruplase	Reteplase	Tenecteplase	Lanoteplase	Staphylokinase
Source	Group C Streptococci	Recombinant, human fetal kidney	Recombinant human	Group C Streptococci	Prodrug from protease	Recombinant human mutant type PA	Variant of tPA-rearranging gene sequence.	Chinese hamster ovary cells	PA of bacterial origin-strains of *Staphylococus aureus*
Dose	1.5 MU over 30–60 min	3 MU over 30–60 min	<100 mg in 90 min (weight-based regimen)*	30 units IV over 2–5 min	Up to 80 mg in 60 min	10 IU × 2 (30 min apart), each over 2 min	30–50 mg (weight-based regimen)¥	120 IU/Kg bolus	5 mg bolus
Bolus administration	No	No	Yes	Yes	Yes	Double, Yes	Single, Yes	Yes	Yes
Plasma half life (min)	25 €	~15	4–8	70–120	9	11–18	20	23–45	6–15
Immunogenicity	Yes	No	No	Yes	No	No	No	No	Yes
Relative fibrin specificity	–	+	++	+	±	+	+++	+	+++(+)
Fibrin affinity	–		++			+	++++	—	—
90 min patency	—	—	+++	—	+++	++++	+++(+?)	++++	+++(+?)
TIMI flow grade 3, (%)	~30	—	~50	—	—	~60	~50	—	—
TIMI flow grade 2/3, (%)	~55	—	~75	—	—	~83	~50	—	—
Metabolism	Renal	Renal	Hepatic	Hepatic	—	Renal	Hepatic	Hepatic	Hepatic
Intracranial hemorrhage (%)	—	—	0.62–0.94	—	—	0.77–1.2	0.93	—	Not well studied
Advantages	Lower cost	Nonantigenic	Good efficacy for anterior MI	—	—	Lower bleeding risk Nonantigenic	Good efficacy	Not further developed	—
Disadvantages	Immunogenic	—	Higher % of strokes	Immunogenic	—	Higher cost	—	—	Immunogenic

Abbreviations: MI, myocardial infraction; MU, million units; TIMI, thrombolysis in myocardial infarction; tPA, tissue-type plasminogen activator.

Table 2
Newer fibrinolytic agents

Drug	Direct/Indirect Inhibitor	Mechanism of Action	Stage of Development
Alfimeprase	Direct	Directly degrades fibrin and fibrinogen	Halted
BB10153	Direct	Thrombin activated plasminogen variant	Phase II
Desmoteplase	Indirect but has high fibrin specificity	A variant of tPA with enhanced fibrin specificity	Phase III
Plasmin	Direct	Directly degrades fibrin and fibrinogen	Phase III

difference in cardiovascular morbidity and mortality or major bleeding observed between the two aspirin doses (300–325 mg/day or 75–100 mg/day).[13] However, high-dose ASA was associated with a significant increase in the risk of minor bleeding and gastrointestinal bleeding, solidifying 81 mg/day as the preferred dose in the United States.

Clopidogrel

Clopidogrel is a first-generation thienopyridine derivative that irreversibly binds to P2Y12 receptors to inhibit adenosine diphosphate (ADP)-induced platelet aggregation. Its effectiveness depends on the conversion of the prodrug to an active metabolite through cytochrome P450 enzyme CYP2C19 in the liver. The clinical benefit of dual antiplatelet therapy with clopidogrel and aspirin among patients with STEMI is well established.[14,15] Proper dosing of clopidogrel in ACS has been a topic of debate; the 600 mg loading dose has been shown to provide superior platelet inhibition when compared with 300 mg daily.[16,17] However, this did not translate into clinical benefit in the CURRENT-OASIS-7[13] and Gauging Responsiveness with A VerifyNow Assay—Impact on Thrombosis and Safety (GRAVITAS) trials.[18]

Monitoring of clopidogrel by platelet function assays revealed interindividual pharmacodynamic variability that may be attributed to genetic predisposition and/or interactions with proton pump inhibitors, particularly omeprazole, a potent CYP2C19 inhibitor.[19,20] Furthermore, poor clopidogrel response has been associated with increased incidence of recurrent major cardiovascular events and stent thrombosis, particularly post-PCI.[21]

Prasugrel

Prasugrel is a third-generation thienopyridine that irreversibly inhibits P2Y12 receptors. Like clopidogrel, prasugrel is a prodrug that undergoes initial metabolism via esterases and subsequent hepatic metabolism to form an active metabolite.[22] Higher bioavailability and faster activation has resulted in more rapid and constant platelet inhibition observed with prasugrel when compared with clopidogrel.

The Trial to Assess Improvement in Therapeutic Outcomes by Optimizing Platelet Inhibition with Prasugrel–Thrombolysis in Myocardial Infarction 38 (TRITON–TIMI 38) a large phase III trial designed to assess prasugrel versus clopidogrel in patients undergoing PCI,[23] demonstrated a significant reduction in the frequency of ischemic events with prasugrel (10.0% vs 12.4%). There was no apparent excess in bleeding with prasugrel, except for an increase in thrombolysis in myocardial infarction (TIMI) major bleeding observed in the less than 4% of patients who underwent coronary artery bypass graft (CABG) (18.8% vs 2.7%). Additionally, a subanalysis of the study demonstrated significant reductions in both early and late stent thrombosis associated with prasugrel use, irrespective of the type of stent implanted.[24]

Ticagrelor

Ticagrelor is an orally active direct and reversible P2Y12 receptor blocker. As a cyclopentyl-triazolo-pyrimidine compound, ticagrelor represents a new class of drug that does not require metabolic activation and, therefore, has a more rapid onset of action and achieves higher levels of platelet inhibition with faster offset following discontinuation.[25] A subgroup analysis[26] of the Platelet Inhibition and Patient Outcomes (PLATO) study involving 7544 ACS patients with STEMI, demonstrated that ticagrelor was superior to clopidogrel in significantly reducing the primary composite endpoint of myocardial infraction (MI), stroke, and cardiovascular death (10.8% vs 9.4%) and several secondary endpoints, including total mortality and definite stent thrombosis. However, an increased risk of stroke was observed with ticagrelor, which was consistent with the overall trial results.

The pending concern with ticagrelor is its failure to demonstrate benefit among the 1814 subjects enrolled in the United States and Canada, despite demonstrating superiority over clopidogrel among the remaining patient population enrolled worldwide.[27] Possible explanations include the fact that United States and Canadian patients more commonly used high-dose ASA. Further clinical outcome studies, including the now active Prevention of Cardiovascular Events in Patients With Prior Heart Attack Using Ticagrelor Compared to Placebo on a Background of Aspirin (PEGASUS)-TIMI-54 trial, may provide answers and better evaluate the long term benefits associated with ticagrelor.[28]

Cangrelor and Elinogrel

Similar to ticagrelor, cangrelor and elinogrel are direct and reversible P2Y12 receptor blockers with very rapid onset of action, greater platelet inhibition, and rapid reversal of antiplatelet effects following drug discontinuation.[29,30] The favorable pharmacokinetic properties of cangrelor coupled with no significant increase in bleeding risk when compared with clopidogrel or abciximab led to the study of this drug in two phase III trials: Cangrelor versus Standard Therapy to Achieve Optimal Management of Platelet Inhibition (CHAMPION) PCI[31] and CHAMPION-PLATFORM,[19] both of which were stopped at interim analysis due to a lack of efficacy. Another new drug in this class is elinogrel, which can be administered both orally and intravenously. Following the successful demonstration of a single oral dose of elinogrel to reversibly overcome high-platelet reactivity observed in patients on clopidogrel who carry the CYP2C19*2 allele and the subsequent phase II a randomized, double-blind, active controlled trial to evaluate intravenous and oral PRT060128 (elinogrel), a selective and reversible P2Y12 receptor inhibitor vs clopidogrel as a novel antiplatelet therapy in patients undergoing nonurgent percutaneous coronary interventions (INNOVATE) PCI study,[20] the drug is currently in the planning stage for a phase III trial.

Glycoprotein IIb/IIIa Inhibitors: Abciximab, Eptifibatide, and Tirofiban

Among the various antiplatelet agents, inhibitors of glycoprotein IIb/IIIa receptors (GPRs) have had a significant clinical impact in STEMI care because these receptors mediate the final stage of platelet activation. Glycoprotein IIb/IIIa inhibitors (GPIs) have also been associated with disaggregation of preexisting clot.[32] Abciximab, eptifibatide, and tirofiban are key agents used in ACS. Compared with eptifibatide and tirofiban, abciximab has a separate and distinct binding site on the GPR complex with distinct pharmacokinetic and pharmacodynamic properties.[33]

Several studies have demonstrated that the administration of abciximab during PCI in STEMI patients was associated with improved myocardial perfusion, coronary blood flow, left ventricular function, and ST segment resolution.[34,35] A meta-analysis evaluating periprocedural use of abciximab demonstrated a significant mortality benefit with a significantly lower frequency of reinfarction and no change in major bleeding risk.[36]

The intracoronary (IC) route of administration of glycoprotein IIb/IIIa inhibitor (GPI) as an adjunctive therapy to PCI has demonstrated improved myocardial perfusion with a smaller infarct size in comparison to the intravenous (IV) route.[37] This may be attributed to higher local GPR occupancy as demonstrated in the ICE trial, which evaluated IC administration of eptifibatide.[34] The CICERO trial reported that there was a significant improvement in infarct size and myocardial reperfusion as assessed by myocardial blush among patients treated with IC abciximab compared with IV abciximab, though no difference was noted between the two groups in relation to myocardial reperfusion as assessed by resolution of ST segment.[38] Most recently, the Intracoronary Abciximab Infusion and Aspiration Thrombectomy in Patients Undergoing Percutaneous Coronary Intervention for Anterior ST Segment Elevation Myocardial Infarction (INFUSE-AMI) study demonstrated IC administration of abciximab delivered to the infarct lesion site resulted in a significant but mild reduction in infarct size in patients presenting with a large anterior STEMI.[39] There was not, however, any improvement in myocardial reperfusion, ST segment resolution, or 30-day clinical event rates, leaving the clinical utility of this therapy unclear.

ANTITHROMBIN AGENTS

Bivalirudin

Direct thrombin inhibitors have shown significant benefit in the acute treatment of STEMI. Bivalirudin, a direct reversible thrombin inhibitor that produces an immediate dose and concentration dependent anticoagulation effect when administered intravenously, has been extensively studied in the Randomized Evaluation in PCI Linking Angiomax to Reduced Clinical Events (REPLACE-2)[40] and the Harmonizing Outcomes with Revascularization and Stents in Acute Myocardial Infarction (HORIZONS-AMI)[41] trials. The REPLACE-2 trial found bivalirudin to be noninferior to unfractionated heparin

(UFH) plus GPI in the combined endpoint of death, MI, or urgent revascularization. In addition, the frequency of major hemorrhage was significantly lower in the bivalirudin group (2.4% vs 4.1%). Similar bleeding results were demonstrated in the HORIZONS-AMI trial, with significantly lower 30-day rates of all cause death in the bivalirudin plus provisional GPI group compared with UFH plus GPI group (1.8% vs 2.9%).

Factor Xa Inhibitors: Rivaroxaban and Apixaban

Extended anticoagulation therapy is an important consideration for STEMI patients as there is an increased risk of recurrent thrombotic events secondary to persistent thrombin-generation long after the acute event has occurred.[42] Therefore, continued suppression of the coagulation cascade following an acute event may be required among this population. Warfarin plus ASA has been shown to be beneficial in this population but with an increased risk of major bleeding.[43]

Improved results were observed with newer anticoagulant therapy using direct factor Xa (FXa) inhibitors, such as apixaban and rivaroxaban, which demonstrated promising results among ACS patients for secondary prevention in the Apixaban for Prevention of Acute Ischemic and Safety Events-I (APPRAISE-I)[44] and Anti-Xa Therapy to Lower cardiovascular events in addition to Aspirin with/without thienopyridine therapy in Subjects with Acute Coronary Syndrome (ATLAS ACS) TIMI-46[45] trials. These results mostly reflect the ability of FXa inhibitors to not only inhibit clot-bound FXa, but also to target FXa within the prothrombinase complex, which, therefore, helps in reducing thrombin production during the propagation phase of the coagulation cascade and also prevent subsequent clot formation. Additionally, these agents do not require the presence of antithrombin cofactor for exerting their anticoagulation effects, in contrast to unfractionated and low-molecular-weight heparin. Despite these advantages, a phase II study of darexaban among ACS patients demonstrated a dose-dependent twofold to fourfold increase in bleeding risk without any reduction in ischemic events.[46] Similarly, the increased incidence of major bleeding (HR 2.59, $P = .001$) lead to the premature termination of APPRAISE-II phase III trial evaluating apixaban.[47] The ATLAS ACS2 TIMI-51 study was the first to demonstrate that oral FXa inhibitor in addition to dual-antiplatelet therapy resulted in a significant 34% relative risk reduction in cardiovascular (CV) mortality and a 32% relative risk reduction in total mortality.[48] However, this trial also demonstrated a dose-dependent increase in TIMI major bleeding with no increase in fatal bleeds. Of note, the doses evaluated in this trial include much lower doses of rivaroxaban (2.5 mg BID and 5 mg BID) than those used for stroke prophylaxis, such as in atrial fibrillation (30 mg daily).

OTHER THERAPIES USED IN STEMI

Magnesium

The utility of membrane stabilizers has been studied in several clinical trials. In the Magnesium in Coronaries (MAGIC) and The Fourth International Study of Infarct Survival (ISIS-4) trials, IV magnesium showed no benefit compared with placebo in patients with STEMI.[49,50] The 2004 American College of Cardiology Foundation/American Heart Association guidelines recommended that IV magnesium should not be used routinely, except for those with documented magnesium deficiency and in patients with polymorphic ventricular tachycardia.

Calcium Channel Blockers

Currently available evidence suggests that calcium channel blockers have a limited role in the management of patients with acute myocardial infarction and there is no indication for using these agents in the acute phase.[51] However, dihydropyridines like verapamil may be used as an alternative for secondary prevention in situations in which a beta-blocker is contraindicated or not tolerated.[51]

Insulin

The importance and management of hyperglycemia among STEMI patients is an evolving concept. The prevalence of admission hyperglycemia in different epidemiologic studies ranges from 25% to greater than 50% of patients admitted with ACS.[52] Currently, there is a lack of consensus on the optimal blood glucose target in hyperglycemic patients with STEMI. Several trials have attempted to address the value of intensive insulin therapy in this subset of patients; unfortunately, none of these trials were conclusive due to inherent shortcomings in the study designs.[53,54]

FUTURE AND EMERGING THERAPIES FOR STEMI

Therapies Targeting Reperfusion Injury

An understanding of the pathophysiology of STEMI and the subsequent dysfunctional remodelling observed has identified new therapeutic targets for STEMI treatment. Myocardial injury during STEMI is a product of MI due to flow limiting stenosis in coronary epicardial vessels and reperfusion injury following restoration of blood flow. Reperfusion injury has a complex pathophysiology that involves the combination of free radical formation, endothelial dysregulation, and aggregation of inflammatory mediators with activation of a proapoptotic signaling cascade, complement activation, and platelet activation.[55] There are several novel antiinflammatory agents currently under evaluation as adjunct therapy to PCI in patients with STEMI.

Preclinical trials in animal models have demonstrated that antiinflammatory agents, when added to traditional reperfusion therapy, reduced MI size in STEMI.[56,57] The Limitation of Myocardial Infarction Following Thrombolysis in Acute Myocardial Infarction (LIMIT AMI) study looked to translate the benefit of reducing inflammatory changes during STEMI with the anti-CD 18 antibody but was not able to show any beneficial effect on coronary blood flow or infarct size.[56] Similarly, the Assessment of Pexelizumab in Acute Myocardial Infarction (APEX AMI) trial evaluated the role of pexelizumab, a monoclonal antibody to the complement C5 component of complement, as adjunctive therapy to PCI, but was not able to show a morbidity or mortality benefit at 30 or 90 days following STEMI.[57] A cardiac magnetic resonance (CMR) substudy of the APEX-AMI trial did show a reduction in myocardial infarct size and higher left ventricular ejection fractions.[58]

Adenosine, which was evaluated in the Acute Myocardial Infarction STudy of ADenosine (AMISTAD) and AMISTAD 2 trials, showed reduced infarct size when used in conjunction with thrombolysis or primary PCI; however, its benefit was not translated into morbidity or mortality benefit at 6 months.[59–61] Similarly, cyclosporine was evaluated in small pilot study of 58 patients with single intravenous bolus before primary PCI and resulted in significant reduction of cardiac biomarkers and infarct size when measured by CMR though its potential clinical outcomes remain to be determined.[62]

Erythropoietin is another example of an agent used to reduce reperfusion injury owing to its antiinflammatory, antiapoptotic, and angiogenic properties. In the Reduction of Infarct Expansion and Ventricular Remodeling With Erythropoietin After Large Myocardial Infarction (REVEAL) trial, erythropoietin given within 4 hours of successful PCI for STEMI did not show any effect on infarct size or left ventricular mass measured by CMR.[63]

Cardiomyoplasty

Another promising field in STEMI management is cellular cardiomyoplasty, which involves the use of hematopoietic stem cell therapy or growth factors to induce proliferation and differentiation of cardiac myocytes. The BOne marrOw transfer to enhance ST-elevation infarct regeneration (BOOST) trial, which involved IC infusion of bone marrow harvest, and the Reinfusion of Enriched Progenitor Cells and Infarct Remodeling in Acute Myocardial Infarction (REPAIR-AMI) trial, which involved intracoronary infusion of autologous mononuclear progenitor cells in infarct-related artery of STEMI patients undergoing PCI, demonstrated improvement in left ventricular ejection fraction (LVEF) compared with patients undergoing PCI alone. Additionally, a meta-analysis of cellular cardiomyoplasty within 9 days of STEMI showed a small (2.70%) but statistically significant improvement in LVEF in the short term with cellular cardiomyoplasty when compared with placebo.[64] Stem cell therapy is a promising emerging therapy for STEMI; however, it has faced limitations, including choice of ideal cell type, timing of delivery, and method of cell delivery with less than 3% of stem cells actually implanted with current techniques.[65]

Emerging Antiplatelet Therapies

Protease-activated receptors (PARs) are new potential targets in drug therapy for STEMI. Thrombin is a potent activator of platelets via its interactions with the platelet surface receptors PAR-1 and PAR-4—with PAR-1 exhibiting a higher thrombin affinity than PAR-4.[66] Two agents studied in this class are vorapaxar and atopaxar. Vorapaxar is a potent oral PAR-1 receptor antagonist that was recently evaluated in the Thrombin Receptor Antagonist in Secondary Prevention of Atherothrombotic Ischemic Events (TRA 2P-TIMI 50) trial, which demonstrated that vorapaxar reduced the risk of cardiovascular death or ischemic events in patients with stable atherosclerosis who were receiving standard therapy. There was, however, an increased risk of moderate or severe bleeding, including intracranial hemorrhage.[67]

Another target for platelet inhibition is von Willebrand factor (vWF) induced platelet adhesion. The anti-vWF agent ARC1779 is an aptamer that when intravenously administered has been shown to produce a dose-dependent inhibition of the A1 domain of vWF resulting in the inhibition of platelet activation. In addition, this anti-vWF agent has a rapid onset and offset of action with the restoration of normal platelet function within 12 to 24 hours following termination.[68] Although the drug has been shown to reduce thromboembolism in humans, clinically relevant studies demonstrating its efficacy in STEMI are forthcoming.

Table 3
Clinical trials of antiplatelet and anticoagulants in STEMI

Trial	Agent	Number of Patients	Primary Endpoint	Bleeding Events
CURRENT OASIS-7	Double dose (600 mg/150 mg/75 mg) vs standard dose clopidogrel (300 mg/75 mg)	25,086	Reduction in stent thrombosis associated with double dose regimen (1.6% vs 2.3%, *P* = .001)	Significant increase in major bleeding events (2.5% vs 2.0%, *P* = .01)
TRITON TIMI-38	Prasugrel (10 mg) vs clopidogrel (300 mg/75 mg)	3534	Reduction in frequency of ischemic events with prasugrel (10.0% vs 12.4%, *P* = .0221)	Significant increase in TIMI Major bleeding after CABG with prasugrel (*P* = .0033)
PLATC	Ticagrelor (180 mg) vs clopidogrel (300 mg/75 mg)	7544 patients with STEMI or LBBB	Reduction in cardiovascular events with ticagrelor (9.4% vs 10.8%, *P* = .07)	Higher risk of stroke with ticagrelor (1.7% vs 1.0%, *P* = .02)
ATLAS ACS 2 TIMI 51	Rivaroxaban (2.5 mg vs 5 mg) vs placebo	15,526	Significant reduction in CV mortality, MI, or stroke with rivaroxaban (8.9% vs 10.7%, *P* = .008)	Significant increase in non–CABG-related major bleeding (2.1% vs 0.6%, $P \leq 0.001$) and ICH (0.6% vs 0.2%, *P* = .009)
TRAP-2P TIMI 50	Vorapaxar (2.5 mg) vs placebo	26,449	CV mortality, MI, or stroke (9.3% vs 10.5%) (HR, 0.87; CI, 0.80–0.94; *P*<.001)	Moderate or severe (4.2% vs 2.5%) (HR, 1.66; CI, 1.43–1.93; *P*<.001). Increase in the rate of ICH (1.0%, vs 0.5%, *P*<.001)

Abbreviations: ICH, intracranial hemorrhage; LBBB, left bundle branch block.

SUMMARY

STEMI continues to be a source of considerable morbidity and mortality worldwide. The management and treatment of STEMI has improved considerably through an evidence-based approach to management incorporating new therapeutic agents. Current acute management of STEMI aims to restore and maintain perfusion to the occluded coronary artery and prevent ischemia, arrhythmic complications, and subsequent dysfunctional remodeling. Anticoagulants useful in early STEMI treatment include the indirect thrombin inhibitors unfractionated and low-molecular-weight heparin, as well as the direct thrombin inhibitor bivalirudin. Antiplatelet therapies useful for early and extended management of STEMI include ASA, glycoprotein IIb/IIIa inhibitors (eptifibatide, tirofiban and abciximab), the thienopyridines clopidogrel and prasugrel, and contemporary agents (ticagrelor, cangrelor and elinogrel), all of which show promising clinical data (**Table 3**). Going forward, state-of-the-art STEMI treatment will likely include FXa inhibitors, such as rivaroxaban and apixaban, for improvement in long-term outcomes following an MI and, potentially, further platelet-inhibiting therapies such as vorapaxar. With all of these pharmacologic agents at the clinician's disposal, there remains a great deal of research in emerging areas of STEMI treatment, including those targeted to reperfusion injury and cardiomyoplasty, both of which could have a significant clinical impact on STEMI treatment.

REFERENCES

1. Antman EM, Anbe DT, Armstrong PW, et al. ACC/AHA guidelines for the management of patients with ST-elevation myocardial infarction; a report of the American College of Cardiology/American Heart Association task force on practice guidelines (Committee to Revise the 1999 Guidelines for the Management of Patients with Acute Myocardial Infarction). J Am Coll Cardiol 2004;44:E1–211.
2. Mukau L. A critical appraisal of the evolution of ST elevation myocardial infarction (STEMI) therapy and the evidence behind the current treatment guidelines. Am J Clin Med 2011;8:15–36.
3. Llevadot J, Giugliano RP, Antman EM. Bolus fibrinolytic therapy in acute myocardial infarction. JAMA 2001;286:442–9.
4. ISIS-3: a randomised comparison of streptokinase vs tissue plasminogen activator vs anistreplase and of aspirin plus heparin vs aspirin alone among 41,299 cases of suspected acute myocardial infarction. ISIS-3 (Third International Study of Infarct Survival) Collaborative Group. Lancet 1992;339: 753–70.
5. Bode C, Smalling RW, Berg G, et al. Randomized comparison of coronary thrombolysis achieved with double-bolus reteplase (recombinant plasminogen activator) and front-loaded, accelerated alteplase (recombinant tissue plasminogen activator) in patients with acute myocardial infarction. The RAPID II Investigators. Circulation 1996;94:891–8.
6. Witt W, Maass B, Baldus B, et al. Coronary thrombolysis with desmodus salivary plasminogen activator in dogs. Fast and persistent recanalization by intravenous bolus administration. Circulation 1994;90:421–6.
7. Curtis LD, Brown A, Comer MB, et al. Pharmacokinetics and pharmacodynamics of bb-10153, a thrombin-activatable plasminogen, in healthy volunteers. J Thromb Haemost 2005;3:1180–6.
8. Shah AR, Scher L. Drug evaluation: alfimeprase, a plasminogen-independent thrombolytic. IDrugs 2007;10:329–35.
9. Marder VJ. Thrombolytic therapy for deep vein thrombosis: potential application of plasmin. Thromb Res 2009;123(Suppl 4):S56–61.
10. Collaborative meta-analysis of randomised trials of antiplatelet therapy for prevention of death, myocardial infarction, and stroke in high risk patients. BMJ 2002;324:71–86.
11. Kushner FG, Hand M, Smith SC Jr, et al. 2009 focused updates: ACC/AHA guidelines for the management of patients with ST-elevation myocardial infarction (updating the 2004 guideline and 2007 focused update) and ACC/AHA/SCAI guidelines on percutaneous coronary intervention (updating the 2005 guideline and 2007 focused update): a report of the American College of Cardiology Foundation/American Heart Association task force on practice guidelines. Circulation 2009;120:2271–306.
12. Topol EJ, Easton D, Harrington RA, et al. Randomized, double-blind, placebo-controlled, international trial of the oral IIB/IIIA antagonist lotrafiban in coronary and cerebrovascular disease. Circulation 2003;108:399–406.
13. Mehta SR, Bassand JP, Chrolavicius S, et al. Dose comparisons of clopidogrel and aspirin in acute coronary syndromes. N Engl J Med 2010;363: 930–42.
14. Sabatine MS, Cannon CP, Gibson CM, et al. Effect of clopidogrel pretreatment before percutaneous coronary intervention in patients with ST-elevation myocardial infarction treated with fibrinolytics: the PCI-clarity study. JAMA 2005;294: 1224–32.
15. Mehta SR, Yusuf S, Peters RJ, et al. Effects of pretreatment with clopidogrel and aspirin followed by long-term therapy in patients undergoing percutaneous coronary intervention: the PCI-cure study. Lancet 2001;358:527–33.
16. Patti G, Colonna G, Pasceri V, et al. Randomized trial of high loading dose of clopidogrel for reduction of

periprocedural myocardial infarction in patients undergoing coronary intervention: results from the armyda-2 (Antiplatelet therapy for reduction of MYocardial Damage during Angioplasty) study. Circulation 2005;111:2099–106.

17. Gurbel PA, Bliden KP, Zaman KA, et al. Clopidogrel loading with eptifibatide to arrest the reactivity of platelets: results of the clopidogrel loading with eptifibatide to arrest the reactivity of platelets (clear platelets) study. Circulation 2005; 111:1153–9.
18. Price MJ, Berger PB, Teirstein PS, et al. Standard- vs high-dose clopidogrel based on platelet function testing after percutaneous coronary intervention: the GRAVITAS randomized trial. JAMA 2011;305: 1097–105.
19. Bhatt DL, Lincoff AM, Gibson CM, et al. Intravenous platelet blockade with cangrelor during PCI. N Engl J Med 2009;361:2330–41.
20. Leonardi S, Rao SV, Harrington RA, et al. Rationale and design of the randomized, double-blind trial testing intravenous and oral administration of elinogrel, a selective and reversible p2y(12)-receptor inhibitor, versus clopidogrel to evaluate tolerability and efficacy in nonurgent percutaneous coronary interventions patients (innovate-PCI). Am Heart J 2010;160:65–72.
21. Bonello L, Tantry US, Marcucci R, et al. Consensus and future directions on the definition of high on-treatment platelet reactivity to adenosine diphosphate. J Am Coll Cardiol 2010;56:919–33.
22. Angiolillo DJ, Capranzano P. Pharmacology of emerging novel platelet inhibitors. Am Heart J 2008;156:S10–5.
23. Wiviott SD, Braunwald E, McCabe CH, et al. Prasugrel versus clopidogrel in patients with acute coronary syndromes. N Engl J Med 2007;357: 2001–15.
24. Wiviott SD, Braunwald E, McCabe CH, et al. Intensive oral antiplatelet therapy for reduction of ischaemic events including stent thrombosis in patients with acute coronary syndromes treated with percutaneous coronary intervention and stenting in the TRITON-TIMI 38 trial: a subanalysis of a randomised trial. Lancet 2008;371:1353–63.
25. Gurbel PA, Bliden KP, Butler K, et al. Randomized double-blind assessment of the onset and offset of the antiplatelet effects of ticagrelor versus clopidogrel in patients with stable coronary artery disease: the onset/offset study. Circulation 2009; 120:2577–85.
26. Steg PG, James S, Harrington RA, et al. Ticagrelor versus clopidogrel in patients with ST-elevation acute coronary syndromes intended for reperfusion with primary percutaneous coronary intervention: A Platelet Inhibition and Patient Outcomes (PLATO) trial subgroup analysis. Circulation 2010;122:2131–41.
27. Wallentin L, Becker RC, James SK, et al. The PLATO trial reveals further opportunities to improve outcomes in patients with acute coronary syndrome. Editorial on Serebruany. "Viewpoint: Paradoxical excess mortality in the PLATO trial should be independently verified"(thromb haemost 2011; 105.5). Thromb Haemost 2011;105:760–2.
28. Sabatine MS. Prevention of cardiovascular events (eg, death from heart or vascular disease, heart attack, or stroke) in patients with prior heart attack using ticagrelor compared to placebo on a background of aspirin. 2011. Available at: http://ClinicalTrials.gov/show/NCT01225562. Accessed March 27, 2012.
29. Cattaneo M. New P2Y(12) inhibitors. Circulation 2010;121:171–9.
30. Wallentin L. P2Y(12) inhibitors: differences in properties and mechanisms of action and potential consequences for clinical use. Eur Heart J 2009; 30:1964–77.
31. Harrington RA, Stone GW, McNulty S, et al. Platelet inhibition with cangrelor in patients undergoing PCI. N Engl J Med 2009;361:2318–29.
32. Gibson CM, Buros J, Ciaglo LN, et al. Impact of iodinated contrast injections on percent diameter coronary arterial stenosis and implications for trials of intracoronary pharmacotherapies in patients with ST-elevation myocardial infarction. Am J Cardiol 2007;100:13–7.
33. Phillips DR, Scarborough RM. Clinical pharmacology of eptifibatide. Am J Cardiol 1997;80: 11B–20B.
34. Deibele AJ, Jennings LK, Tcheng JE, et al. Intracoronary eptifibatide bolus administration during percutaneous coronary revascularization for acute coronary syndromes with evaluation of platelet glycoprotein IIb/IIIa receptor occupancy and platelet function: the Intracoronary Eptifibatide (ICE) Trial. Circulation 2010;121:784–91.
35. Gibson CM, Jennings LK, Murphy SA, et al. Association between platelet receptor occupancy after eptifibatide (integrilin) therapy and patency, myocardial perfusion, and ST-segment resolution among patients with ST-segment-elevation myocardial infarction: an integriti (Integrilin and Tenecteplase in Acute Myocardial Infarction) substudy. Circulation 2004;110:679–84.
36. De Luca G, Suryapranata H, Stone GW, et al. Abciximab as adjunctive therapy to reperfusion in acute ST-segment elevation myocardial infarction: a meta-analysis of randomized trials. JAMA 2005; 293:1759–65.
37. Thiele H, Schindler K, Friedenberger J, et al. Intracoronary compared with intravenous bolus abciximab application in patients with ST-elevation myocardial infarction undergoing primary percutaneous coronary intervention: the randomized Leipzig immediate percutaneous coronary intervention

abciximab IV versus IC in ST-elevation myocardial infarction trial. Circulation 2008;118:49–57.
38. Gu YL, Kampinga MA, Wieringa WG, et al. Intracoronary versus intravenous administration of abciximab in patients with ST-segment elevation myocardial infarction undergoing primary percutaneous coronary intervention with thrombus aspiration: the comparison of intracoronary versus intravenous abciximab administration during emergency reperfusion of ST-segment elevation myocardial infarction (CICERO) trial. Circulation 2010;122:2709–17.
39. Stone GW, Maehara A, Witzenbichler B, et al. Intracoronary abciximab and aspiration thrombectomy in patients with large anterior myocardial infarction: the INFUSE-AMI randomized trial. JAMA 2012;307: 1817–26.
40. Lincoff AM, Kleiman NS, Kereiakes DJ, et al. Long-term efficacy of bivalirudin and provisional glycoprotein IIB/IIIA blockade vs heparin and planned glycoprotein IIB/IIIA blockade during percutaneous coronary revascularization: replace-2 randomized trial. JAMA 2004;292:696–703.
41. Stone GW, Witzenbichler B, Guagliumi G, et al. Bivalirudin during primary PCI in acute myocardial infarction. N Engl J Med 2008;358:2218–30.
42. Merlini PA, Bauer KA, Oltrona L, et al. Persistent activation of coagulation mechanism in unstable angina and myocardial infarction. Circulation 1994; 90:61–8.
43. Rothberg MB, Celestin C, Fiore LD, et al. Warfarin plus aspirin after myocardial infarction or the acute coronary syndrome: meta-analysis with estimates of risk and benefit. Ann Intern Med 2005; 143:241–50.
44. Alexander JH, Becker RC, Bhatt DL, et al. Apixaban, an oral, direct, selective factor XA inhibitor, in combination with antiplatelet therapy after acute coronary syndrome: results of the Apixaban for Prevention of Acute Ischemic and Safety Events (APPRAISE) trial. Circulation 2009;119:2877–85.
45. Mega JL, Braunwald E, Mohanavelu S, et al. Rivaroxaban versus placebo in patients with acute coronary syndromes (ATLAS ACS-TIMI 46): a randomised, double-blind, phase II trial. Lancet 2009;374:29–38.
46. Steg PG, Mehta SR, Jukema JW, et al. RUBY-1: a randomized, double-blind, placebo-controlled trial of the safety and tolerability of the novel oral factor XA inhibitor darexaban (YM150) following acute coronary syndrome. Eur Heart J 2011;32: 2541–54.
47. Alexander JH, Lopes RD, James S, et al. Apixaban with antiplatelet therapy after acute coronary syndrome. N Engl J Med 2011;365:699–708.
48. Mega JL, Braunwald E, Wiviott SD, et al. Rivaroxaban in patients with a recent acute coronary syndrome. N Engl J Med 2012;366:9–19.
49. Flather M, Pipilis A, Collins R, et al. Randomized controlled trial of oral captopril, of oral isosorbide mononitrate and of intravenous magnesium sulphate started early in acute myocardial infarction: safety and haemodynamic effects. ISIS-4 (Fourth International Study of Infarct Survival) Pilot Study Investigators. Eur Heart J 1994;15:608–19.
50. Cooper HA, Domanski MJ, Rosenberg Y, et al. Acute ST-segment elevation myocardial infarction and prior stroke: an analysis from the Magnesium in Coronaries (MAGIC) trial. Am Heart J 2004; 148:1012–9.
51. Yusuf S, Held P, Furberg C. Update of effects of calcium antagonists in myocardial infarction or angina in light of the second Danish verapamil infarction trial (davit-II) and other recent studies. Am J Cardiol 1991;67:1295–7.
52. Kosiborod M, Rathore SS, Inzucchi SE, et al. Admission glucose and mortality in elderly patients hospitalized with acute myocardial infarction: implications for patients with and without recognized diabetes. Circulation 2005;111:3078–86.
53. Prasad A, Stone GW, Stuckey TD, et al. Impact of diabetes mellitus on myocardial perfusion after primary angioplasty in patients with acute myocardial infarction. J Am Coll Cardiol 2005;45:508–14.
54. Timmer JR, van der Horst IC, de Luca G, et al. Comparison of myocardial perfusion after successful primary percutaneous coronary intervention in patients with ST-elevation myocardial infarction with versus without diabetes mellitus. Am J Cardiol 2005;95:1375–7.
55. Chiong M, Wang ZV, Pedrozo Z, et al. Cardiomyocyte death: mechanisms and translational implications. Cell Death Dis 2011;2:e244.
56. Baran KW, Nguyen M, McKendall GR, et al. Double-blind, randomized trial of an anti-cd18 antibody in conjunction with recombinant tissue plasminogen activator for acute myocardial infarction: Limitation of Myocardial Infarction Following Thrombolysis in Acute Myocardial Infarction (LIMIT AMI) study. Circulation 2001;104:2778–83.
57. Armstrong PW, Granger CB, Adams PX, et al. Pexelizumab for acute ST-elevation myocardial infarction in patients undergoing primary percutaneous coronary intervention: a randomized controlled trial. JAMA 2007;297:43–51.
58. Patel MR, Worthley SG, Stebbins A, et al. Pexelizumab and infarct size in patients with acute myocardial infarction undergoing primary percutaneous coronary intervention: a delayed enhancement cardiac magnetic resonance substudy from the APEX-AMI trial. JACC Cardiovasc Imaging 2010;3: 52–60.
59. Mahaffey KW, Puma JA, Barbagelata NA, et al. Adenosine as an adjunct to thrombolytic therapy for acute myocardial infarction: results of a multicenter,

randomized, placebo-controlled trial: the Acute Myocardial Infarction STudy of ADenosine (AMISTAD) trial. J Am Coll Cardiol 1999;34:1711–20.
60. Ross AM, Gibbons RJ, Stone GW, et al. A randomized, double-blinded, placebo-controlled multicenter trial of adenosine as an adjunct to reperfusion in the treatment of acute myocardial infarction (AMISTAD-II). J Am Coll Cardiol 2005;45:1775–80.
61. Kloner RA, Forman MB, Gibbons RJ, et al. Impact of time to therapy and reperfusion modality on the efficacy of adenosine in acute myocardial infarction: the AMISTAD-2 trial. Eur Heart J 2006;27:2400–5.
62. Piot C, Croisille P, Staat P, et al. Effect of cyclosporine on reperfusion injury in acute myocardial infarction. N Engl J Med 2008;359:473–81.
63. Najjar SS, Rao SV, Melloni C, et al. Intravenous erythropoietin in patients with ST-segment elevation myocardial infarction: REVEAL: a randomized controlled trial. JAMA 2011;305:1863–72.
64. Zimmet H, Porapakkham P, Sata Y, et al. Short- and long-term outcomes of intracoronary and endogenously mobilized bone marrow stem cells in the treatment of ST-segment elevation myocardial infarction: a meta-analysis of randomized control trials. Eur J Heart Fail 2012;14:91–105.
65. Traverse JH. Using biomaterials to improve the efficacy of cell therapy following acute myocardial infarction. J Cardiovasc Transl Res 2012;5:67–72.
66. Coughlin SR. Protease-activated receptors in hemostasis, thrombosis and vascular biology. J Thromb Haemost 2005;3:1800–14.
67. Morrow DA, Braunwald E, Bonaca MP, et al. Vorapaxar in the secondary prevention of atherothrombotic events. N Engl J Med 2012;366:1404–13.
68. Diener JL, Daniel Lagasse HA, Duerschmied D, et al. Inhibition of von Willebrand factor-mediated platelet activation and thrombosis by the anti-von Willebrand factor A1-domain aptamer ARC1779. J Thromb Haemost 2009;7:1155–62.

The Use of Bivalirudin in ST-Segment Elevation Myocardial Infarction

Advantages and Limitations

Ziad Sergie, MD, MBA[a], Nilusha Gukathasan, MD[a], Jennifer J. Yu, MBBS, FRACP[a], Roxana Mehran, MD[a,b,*]

KEYWORDS

• Bivalirudin • Acute coronary syndrome • ST-segment elevation myocardial infarction
• Percutaneous coronary intervention • Thrombin • Antithrombin

KEY POINTS

- Although the incidence of STEMI is declining, it remains a common emergent complication of coronary artery disease, with significant risk for subsequent ischemic or bleeding events.
- The use of bivalirudin in this setting has been shown to decrease major bleeding, including in-hospital, access-site, and non–access-site bleeding, with a correlated and sustained decrease in 3-year cardiac mortality.
- Early stent thrombosis (in the first 24 hours) was seen in STEMI patients treated with bivalirudin, and was partially mitigated by a preprocedural bolus of heparin.
- Periprocedural pharmacotherapy can be most effectively optimized by an individualized approach, balancing each patient's risk for major bleeding, recurrent ischemia, and stent thrombosis.

INTRODUCTION

Coronary heart disease is common in the United States, affecting roughly 16 million individuals older than 20 years, a prevalence of 7%.[1] In 2012, approximately 1.3 million people in the United States will experience a coronary event, and close to a third of all cases will be classified as ST-segment elevation myocardial infarction (STEMI).[1] The number of STEMI cases as a percentage of all myocardial infarctions (MIs) has declined in recent years, from 47% in 1999 to 30% in 2008 according to a recent analysis of more than 46,000 patients.[2] Despite significant reductions in in-hospital and 30-day mortality rates attributable to MI over the past 2 decades,[3,4] cardiovascular disease is the still the leading cause of death in the United States and worldwide. However, improvements in patient outcomes after acute coronary syndrome (ACS) reflect an evolution of the management of ACS, including the use of early invasive strategies coupled with potent antiplatelet and anticoagulant therapies. Furthermore, in the case of STEMI dedicated care networks have been developed to optimize the timing of treatment and intervention.[5]

Disclosures: Z. Sergie, N. Gukathasan, J.J. Yu: None. R. Mehran: research funding: the Medicines Company, BMS/Sanofi; consulting: AstraZeneca, Janssen.
[a] Zena and Michael A Wiener Cardiovascular Institute, Mount Sinai School of Medicine, One Gustave L. Levy Place, Box 1030, New York, NY 10029, USA; [b] Cardiovascular Research Foundation, 111 East 59th Street, New York, NY 10022, USA
* Corresponding author. Zena and Michael A Wiener Cardiovascular Institute, Mount Sinai School of Medicine, One Gustave L. Levy Place, Box 1030, New York, NY 10029.
E-mail address: roxana.mehran@mountsinai.org

Intervent Cardiol Clin 1 (2012) 441–451
http://dx.doi.org/10.1016/j.iccl.2012.06.003
2211-7458/12/$ – see front matter Published by Elsevier Inc.

This review focuses on the impact of optimal anticoagulation on outcomes after STEMI and discusses the recent trials evaluating bivalirudin, a direct thrombin inhibitor, in this setting.

MYOCARDIAL INFARCTION: A PROTHROMBOTIC STATE

Considerable progress in elucidating the mechanisms of acute MI has been made since the early descriptions of coronary occlusion and thrombosis in 1980.[6] Large population-based cohort studies, such as the Framingham study,[7] have demonstrated that certain risk factors (eg, smoking, high cholesterol, high blood pressure, diabetes) predispose individuals to developing arterial atherosclerosis. More recently, in a patient-level meta-analysis of more than 250,000 patients in 18 cohort studies, the presence of 1 or more of these risk factors was shown to significantly increase the long-term risk of cardiovascular mortality.[8] The spectrum of ACSs, which include STEMI, non–ST-segment elevation myocardial infarction (NSTEMI), and unstable angina, represent the critical transition of coronary atherosclerosis from a chronic to an acute phase.

In clinical practice, patients who are hospitalized for ACS frequently do not have prior angina or known flow-limiting coronary artery disease. Thus the current model of ACS pathobiology has implicated an acute disruption and thrombosis of coronary plaque as the pathway to coronary artery obstruction, rather than gradual growth of atherosclerotic lesions leading to critical arterial stenosis.[9] The most common mechanism of plaque disruption is rupture of a thin fibrous cap, occurring in up to 75% of fatal coronary events.[10] While episodic plaque rupture or erosion is a precondition for ACS, other thrombotic factors are also required, including high-risk elements of plaque burden and morphology, flow dynamics, and clinical features.[11] All of these factors play an important role in the progression to ACS, and the search for "vulnerable plaque" via noninvasive imaging is an upcoming and exciting area of clinical research.

Following plaque rupture and release of thrombogenic substances, a cascade of events is initiated by activation of clotting factors, most prominently thrombin, with resultant platelet activation and formation of a platelet-rich thrombus. Thrombin also plays a major role in the final pathway of clot development, converting fibrinogen to fibrin and forming a cross-linked fibrin-rich clot. Total thrombotic occlusion of an epicardial artery eventually leads to transmural myonecrosis of the ventricular wall, which is readily diagnosed by persistent ST-segment elevation or new left-bundle branch block on the electrocardiogram. This critical signal leads to rapid activation of time-sensitive STEMI protocols, including urgent percutaneous coronary intervention (PCI) or fibrinolysis to restore arterial patency, coupled with antiplatelet and anticoagulant therapy to prevent the atherothrombotic late effects of STEMI such as impaired coronary microperfusion and stent thrombosis.[12]

ANTICOAGULATION IN PRIMARY PCI

Despite these major improvements in STEMI care, the risk of recurrent ischemic events remains substantial, prompting the development of more effective antiplatelet agents in comparison with clopidogrel.[13] Similarly, new agents that block the coagulation cascade have been studied in recent years. Given the pathogenic role of thrombin, most of the agents used in ACS block thrombin either directly or indirectly. Clinicians can choose between 3 parenteral anticoagulants for STEMI patients undergoing PCI that have earned a Class I recommendation in American College of Cardiology (ACC)/American Heart Association (AHA) guidelines: unfractionated heparin (UFH), enoxaparin, or bivalirudin.[14] Fondaparinux, a factor Xa inhibitor, is acceptable, but an additional anticoagulant with anti–factor IIa activity must also be administered because of the risk of catheter thrombosis when fondaparinux is used alone.[15] These guidelines also recommend glycoprotein IIb/IIa inhibitors (GPIs) for certain patients at the time of PCI (Class IIa),[14] because these agents have been shown to reduce ischemic events and mortality.[16] Ultimately, the ideal anticoagulation regimen should adequately reduce the incidence of recurrent ischemia while limiting iatrogenic bleeding.

BIVALIRUDIN, A DIRECT THROMBIN INHIBITOR

The anticoagulant properties of hirudin were first used by the ancient Egyptians more than 2000 years ago, via the *Hirudo medicinalis* leech.[17] Early studies that evaluated hirudin in ACS populations before the PCI era demonstrated effectiveness compared with UFH, but with an increased risk of bleeding.[18,19] Subsequently, bivalirudin (Angiomax; the Medicines Company, Parsippany, NJ, USA), a synthetic derivative of hirudin, was developed. Bivalirudin binds to thrombin with high affinity and without a cofactor, thereby inhibiting the conversion of fibrinogen to fibrin. It is a 20-amino-acid polypeptide and, because of its small size, can bind not only free thrombin but clot-bound thrombin, in contrast to heparin. Moreover, the observed linear dose response of bivalirudin adds predictability, prolonging the coagulation parameters in a dose-dependent manner, and reducing the need for laboratory monitoring.[20] Other advantages include its short half-life (~25 minutes in patients with normal renal function) and the lack of interaction with platelet factor 4, thus eliminating the problem of heparin-induced thrombocytopenia. More recently, bivalirudin administration was associated with a decrease in both thrombin-induced and collagen-induced platelet activation after PCI, in addition to a decrease in circulatory thrombin concentration.[21]

Given these theoretical advantages over other anticoagulants, a series of randomized controlled trials assessed the safety and efficacy of bivalirudin. While there are noteworthy differences between trials in terms of the population studied, primary end points, and concomitant antiplatelet agents (as shown in **Table 1**), the overall clinical signal has favored bivalirudin. For example, in the Randomized Evaluation in PCI Linking Angiomax to Reduced Clinical Events 2 (REPLACE-2) trial, 6010 patients referred for urgent or elective PCI were randomized to UFH + GPI or bivalirudin monotherapy (with provisional GPI). At 30 days, there was a similar reduction in both arms for the quadruple end point, a composite of death, MI, revascularization, or in-hospital major bleeding (9.2% vs 10.0%, $P = .32$).[22] However, protocol-defined in-hospital major bleeding was significantly reduced in the bivalirudin arm (2.4 vs 4.1%; $P<.001$).[22] Follow-up of this population for 6 months and 1 year showed no difference in mortality or ischemic events between the 2 groups.[23] Another study of patients with predominantly stable angina compared administration of bivalirudin with that of heparin during PCI, and likewise found a reduction in major bleeding with bivalirudin (3.1% vs 4.6%, $P = .008$) versus UFH, with no significant difference in the 30-day ischemic end points or the net clinical benefit.[24]

The Acute Catheterization and Urgent Intervention Triage Strategy (ACUITY) trial enrolled 13,819 patients presenting with ACS and randomized them to 1 of 3 groups: heparin + GPI, bivalirudin + GPI, or bivalirudin monotherapy (with provisional GPI). As demonstrated in the other trials, major bleeding at 30 days occurred significantly less with bivalirudin alone than with heparin + GPI (3.0% vs 5.7%, $P<.001$) while the rate of composite ischemic events (death, MI, or revascularization) was not significantly different between the 2 groups.[25] At 1-year follow-up, there were no significant differences between the 3 groups with regard to mortality or the composite ischemic end point.[26] In Intracoronary Stenting and Antithrombosis Regimen, Rapid Early Action for Coronary Treatment 4 (ISAR REACT-4), 1721 NSTEMI patients who underwent PCI were randomized to UFH + GPI (abciximab) versus bivalirudin. At 30 days, the composite end point of death, recurrent MI, revascularization, or major bleeding was not significantly different between the 2 arms (10.9% vs 11%, $P = .94$).[27] Protocol-defined major bleeding was significantly higher in the UFH + GPI group compared with the bivalirudin group (4.6% vs 2.6%, $P = .02$), as was Thrombolysis in Myocardial Infarction (TIMI) minor bleeding (7.7% vs 4.3%, $P = .003$), but TIMI major bleeding was not significantly different between the 2 arms.[27]

Because of the promising results seen with bivalirudin in ACS patients, the Harmonizing Outcomes with Revascularization and Stents in Acute Myocardial Infarction (HORIZONS-AMI) trial evaluated this agent specifically in STEMI patients. Within 12 hours of symptom onset, 3602 patients were randomized to heparin plus a GPI (abciximab or eptifibatide) or bivalirudin monotherapy (with bailout GPI). At 3 years, patients assigned to the bivalirudin monotherapy arm had lower rates of major bleeding not related to coronary artery bypass grafting (6.9% vs 10.5%, $P = .0001$), all-cause mortality (5.9% vs 7.7%, $P = .03$), and cardiac mortality (2.9% vs 5.1%, $P = .001$).[28] Furthermore, major adverse cardiac events (death, reinfarction, revascularization, or stroke) and net adverse clinical events (death, reinfarction, revascularization, stroke, or major bleeding) were similar in both groups (21.9% vs 21.8%, $P = .95$ and 25.5% vs 27.6%, $P = .09$, respectively).[28]

HAZARDS OF MAJOR BLEEDING

The results of the aforementioned trials demonstrate that while bivalirudin had similar efficacy in reducing ischemic events compared with heparin or heparin plus a GPI, it consistently reduced the risk of hemorrhagic complications. Moreover, bivalirudin adjunct therapy was associated with concordant reductions in short-term and long-term mortality in the highest-risk patients with coronary artery disease, those receiving primary PCI for STEMI. These results are not surprising, given the body of scientific literature that has implicated major bleeding in the causal pathway for adverse clinical outcomes.[29] In terms of pathophysiologic mechanisms, while major bleeding is considered a marker for higher-risk patients,[30] there are related deleterious effects that may actually increase the risk of death. These factors include

Table 1
Bivalirudin phase III trial characteristics

Trial[Ref.]	Publication Year	Population	Total N	Follow-up	Treatment Arm	Control Arm	Thienopyridine Loading Dose	Primary End Point Definition
REPLACE-2[23]	2004	Urgent or elective PCI	6010	30 d, 1 y	Bivalirudin monotherapy (7.2% provisional GPI)	UFH + GPI (abciximab or eptifibatide)	Clopidogrel 300 mg	Composite of death, MI, revascularization, or in-hospital major bleeding
ISAR REACT-3[24]	2008	Stable or unstable angina, PCI	4570	30 d	Bivalirudin monotherapy	UFH monotherapy	Clopidogrel 600 mg	Composite of death, MI, revascularization, or in-hospital major bleeding
ACUITY[67]	2007	NSTE-ACS	13819	30 d, 1 y	Arm 1: bivalirudin monotherapy (9.1% provisional GPI) Arm 2: bivalirudin + GPI (abciximab, eptifibatide, or tirofiban)	UFH or enoxaparin + GPI (abciximab, eptifibatide , or tirofiban)	Clopidogrel 300 mg	Composite of death, MI, revascularization or non-CABG major bleeding
HORIZONS-AMI[28]	2011	STEMI	3602	30 d, 1 y, 3 y	Bivalirudin monotherapy (7.6% provisional GPI)	UFH + GPI (abciximab or eptifibatide)	Clopidogrel 300 or 600 mg	Composite of death, MI, reinfarction, stroke, or major bleeding
ISAR REACT-4[27]	2011	NSTE-ACS, PCI	1721	30 d	Bivalirudin monotherapy	UFH + GPI (abciximab)	Clopidogrel 600 mg	Composite of death, MI, revascularization, or major bleeding

Abbreviations: ACUITY, Acute Catheterization and Urgent Intervention Triage Strategy; CABG, coronary artery bypass grafting; GPI, glycoprotein IIb/IIIa inhibitor; ISAR REACT-3, Intracoronary Stenting and Antithrombosis Regimen, Rapid Early Action for Coronary Treatment 3; ISAR REACT-4, Intracoronary Stenting and Antithrombosis Regimen, Rapid Early Action for Coronary Treatment 4; MI, myocardial infarction; NSTE-ACS, non–ST-segment elevation acute coronary syndrome; PCI, percutaneous coronary intervention; REPLACE-2, Randomized Evaluation in PCI Linking Angiomax to Reduced Clinical Events 2; STEMI, ST-segment elevation myocardial infarction; UFH, unfractionated heparin.

consequent hypotension or shock from a bleeding episode, risk of mortality with intracranial hemorrhage, interruption or discontinuation of cardioprotective agents, and receipt of transfusions of packed red cells with the associated hazards of stored blood.[31,32] The upsurge of inflammatory biomarkers with a major bleed that was observed in a subanalysis of the ACUITY trial might also have prognostic implications.[33]

This link between an early bleeding episode in the setting of ACS and long-term mortality has been relatively consistent in various settings. For example, an analysis of patient-level data from REPLACE-2, ACUITY, and HORIZONS-AMI demonstrated that major bleeding in the first 30 days was significantly associated with increased risk of 1-year mortality across the spectrum of ACS presentations.[34] In this study, the impact of early major bleeding on mortality was found to be different to that of an early MI; the risk of death was more sustained over time, as opposed to a sharp increase within 2 days after an MI that declined quickly and was not as pronounced over time.[35] Likewise, a recent registry analysis of 3148 patients who underwent implantation of a drug-eluting stent demonstrated a higher risk of death with both early and late bleeding events.[36]

The complication of in-hospital major bleeding deserves particular attention. In a post hoc analysis of HORIZONS-AMI, patients who had in-hospital major bleeding (6.9% of all patients) were compared with those who did not. The incidence of major adverse cardiac events and death at 3 years was significantly higher in those patients who had in-hospital bleeding, with an adjusted hazard ratio for 3-year mortality of 2.8 (95% confidence interval 1.89–4.16, $P<.0001$).[37] Lopes and colleagues[38] performed a separate registry analysis of almost 33,000 Medicare patients with NSTEMI, and also found a sustained association over time between in-hospital major bleeding and mortality, from 30 days up to 3 years of follow-up. As mentioned previously, this association is likely related to the bleeding event itself, in addition to other factors such as the reduced likelihood of patients who bleed during their hospitalization being discharged on adequate antiplatelet therapy after ACS.[39]

It is also clear from recent studies that the various types of bleeding differ in their prognostic significance. For example, access-site complications are critical, and have been analyzed in several clinical trials. The largest multicenter trial to date, the Radial Versus Femoral access for coronary intervention (RIVAL) study, compared radial versus femoral access in 7021 ACS patients who underwent PCI. Although the 30-day primary end point of ischemic and major bleeding events was not significantly reduced with radial access, PCI success was similar in both groups, and local bleeding and vascular events were significantly reduced with radial access.[40] Another pooled analysis from REPLACE 2, ACUITY, and HORIZONS-AMI evaluated the impact of access-site and non–access-site bleeding on long-term outcomes. In the combined patient population, the incidence of TIMI major and minor bleeding was 5.3%, and approximately two-thirds of these events were non–access-site bleeds.[41] There was an increased risk of 1-year mortality with both types of hemorrhage (higher with non–access-site bleeding), and bivalirudin reduced both types of major bleeding.[41] Both studies underscore the importance of bleeding avoidance strategies to reduce both access-related and nonaccess-related complications. Of interest, in RIVAL the prespecified subgroups of high-volume radial centers and STEMI patients experienced significantly lower rates of primary end-point events in the radial arm.[40]

A MAJOR LIMITATION OF BIVALIRUDIN: ACUTE STENT THROMBOSIS

One of the main concerns that arose from the HORIZONS-AMI trial was the higher rate of acute stent thrombosis within 24 hours (definite or probable), which occurred in 1.4% in the bivalirudin arm versus 0.3% in the heparin + GPI arm ($P<.001$).[42] These events happened almost entirely within the first 5 hours postprocedure, and 2 patients who had stent thrombosis died, 1 in each randomized group.[43] After 24 hours, the rate of stent thrombosis was lower in the bivalirudin monotherapy group from 24 hours to 3 years post-PCI (4.8% vs 3.1%, $P = .01$), such that the overall rate of stent thrombosis was not significantly different at 3 years (5.1% vs 4.5%, $P = .49$).[12] Consequently it has been hypothesized that the short half-life of bivalirudin was implicated in this early risk of acute stent thrombosis. Its antithrombin effect likely diminishes quickly with drug discontinuation, before maximal inhibition of the $P2Y_{12}$ platelet receptor by clopidogrel, which has a delayed onset of activity.[43]

Of note, the overall incidence of stent thrombosis seen in HORIZONS-AMI was 4% to 5% at 3 years, almost 4 times that seen with elective PCI.[44] Although this is not surprising given that STEMI presentation is associated with a higher risk of stent thrombosis,[45] it is still a cause for concern. There was a similar risk of stent thrombosis in both randomized stent arms in HORIZONS-AMI: 4.8% in the paclitaxel-eluting stent group versus 4.3% in the bare-metal stent group, P = .63.[28] To further investigate this phenomenon, a post hoc analysis of HORIZONS-AMI yielded several independent clinical and angiographic correlates of stent thrombosis, as shown in **Fig. 1**.[46] Strict attention to these risk factors will be crucial to minimize this potentially lethal complication in STEMI patients. Strategies that may reduce early stent thrombosis with bivalirudin include prolonging the bivalirudin infusion after PCI,[47] the use of more potent $P2Y_{12}$ inhibitors, or providing patients with an early preprocedural bolus of UFH (as shown in **Fig. 2**).

Another important analysis of the HORIZONS-AMI data looked at those patients who had received a bolus of UFH before primary PCI and were subsequently randomized to bivalirudin (Switch arm, n = 1178) or UFH + GPI (Control arm, n = 1179). This analysis included 65.4% of all patients in that trial (n = 2357) and should be considered similar to a randomized comparison, given that treatment allocation was stratified according to preprocedural UFH receipt. While acute stent thrombosis (within 24 hours) occurred more often in the Switch group (0.8% vs 0.1%; P = .01), the rate of subacute stent thrombosis (from 24 h to 30 days) was significantly decreased (0.9% vs 1.9%; P = .04), leading to a similar rate of stent thrombosis at 2 years (3.1% vs 4.3%; P = .17).[48] Moreover, patients in the Switch group had lower rates of 2-year net adverse clinical events, cardiac mortality, and major bleeding compared with the Control group, as seen in **Fig. 3**. A sensitivity analysis showed that these findings were not affected by the preprocedural activated clotting times in the Switch group.[48]

SO WHY SHOULD BIVALIRUDIN BE USED IN STEMI?

Based on the foregoing discussion of the large-scale HORIZONS-AMI trial, the use of bivalirudin compared with UFH + GPI was associated with significant reductions in major bleeding, and concordant reductions in cardiac mortality seen early and sustained up to 3 years after the index hospitalization. The higher risk of stent thrombosis in the first 24 hours seen with bivalirudin is concerning; however, it should be interpreted in the context of the accompanying long-term robust mortality benefit. The reduced rate of thrombocytopenia with bivalirudin compared with UFH + GPI, as

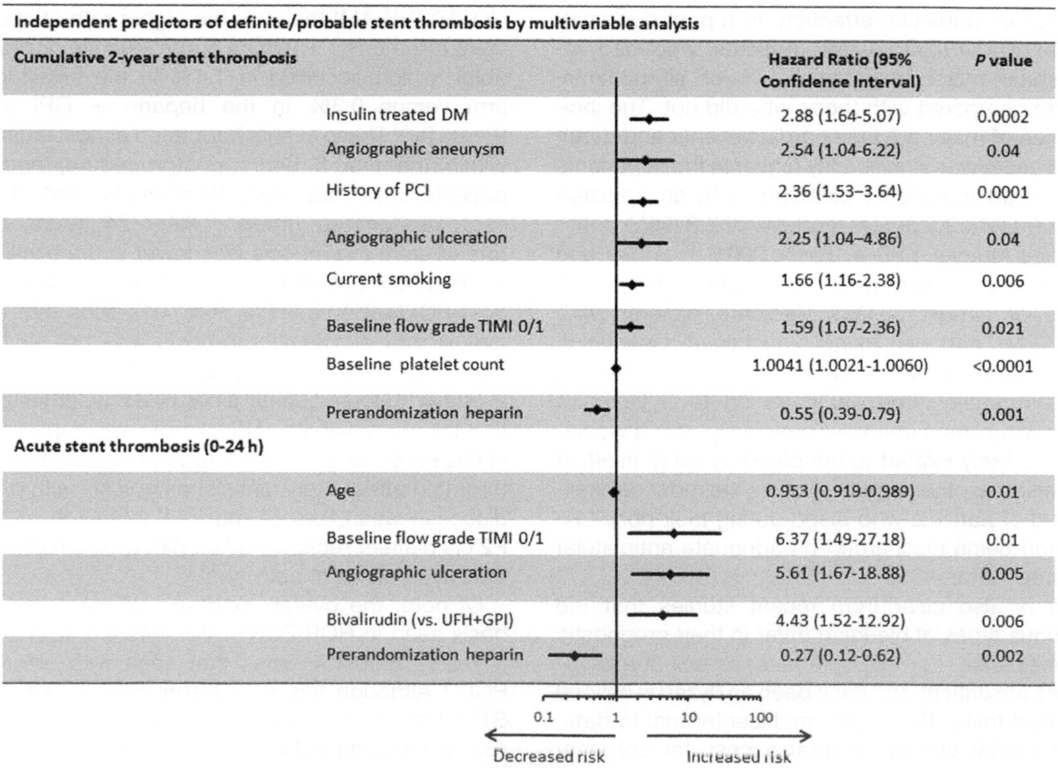

Fig. 1. Correlates of stent thrombosis from HORIZONS-AMI. (*From* Dangas GD, Caixeta A, Mehran R, et al. Frequency and predictors of stent thrombosis after percutaneous coronary intervention in acute myocardial infarction. Circulation 2011;123(16):1745–56; with permission.)

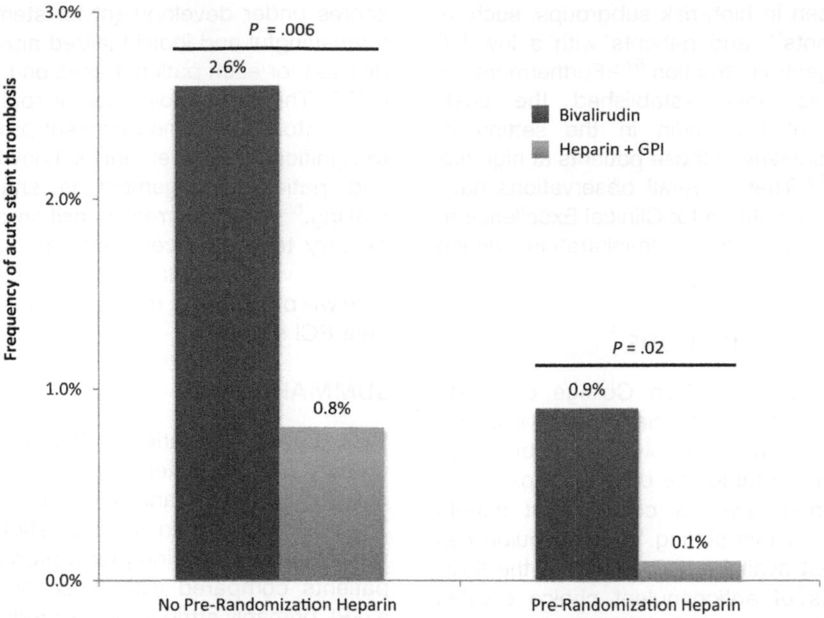

Fig. 2. Impact of prerandomization heparin on acute stent thrombosis (first 24 hours). (*From* Dangas GD, Caixeta A, Mehran R, et al. Frequency and predictors of stent thrombosis after percutaneous coronary intervention in acute myocardial infarction. Circulation 2011;123(16):1745–56; with permission.)

seen in ISAR REACT-4,[24] may also contribute to the mortality benefit given that baseline and acquired thrombocytopenia increase adverse outcomes in ACS.[49,50] Moreover, bivalirudin likely reduces the risk of anemia, which has been shown to predict worse outcomes.[51–53]

Other benefits of bivalirudin in the setting of ACS have been elucidated. In addition to reduction of both thrombin-mediated and collagen-mediated activation of platelets (mentioned previously),[21] bivalirudin administration also significantly reduces platelet aggregation after PCI, in contrast to UFH.[54] Bivalirudin has been shown to decrease monocyte activation after PCI compared with UFH,[55] which may reduce the proinflammatory cytokine release that occurs in STEMI. The benefits of bivalirudin

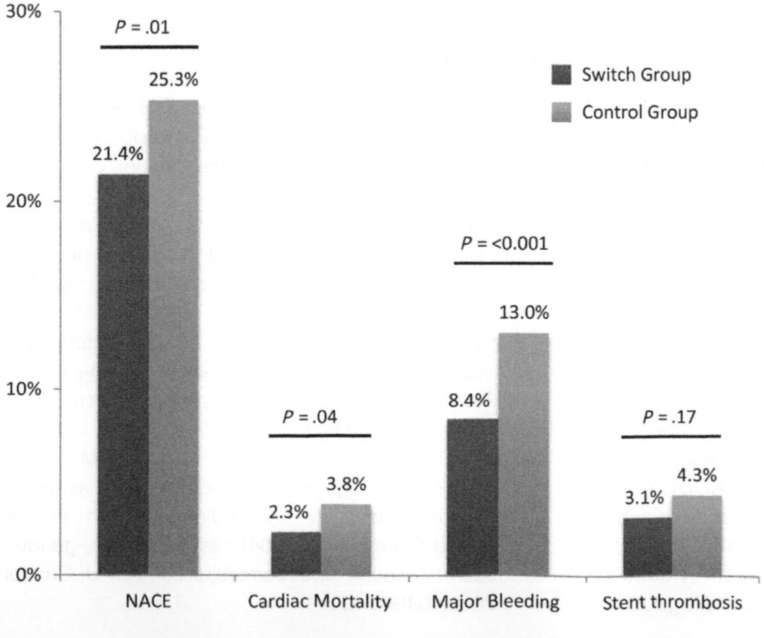

Fig. 3. HORIZONS-AMI Switch analysis, 2-year outcomes. Switch group: patients who received a bolus of heparin prior to randomization to the bivalirudin arm (n = 1178); Control group: patients who received a bolus of heparin prior to randomization to the unfractionated heparin + glycoprotein IIb/IIIa inhibitor arm (n = 1179). NACE, net adverse clinical events (composite of death, reinfarction, revascularization, stroke, or major bleeding). (*From* Dangas GD, Mehran R, Nikolsky E, et al. Effect of switching antithrombin agents for primary angioplasty in acute myocardial infarction: the HORIZONS-SWITCH analysis. J Am Coll Cardiol 2011;57(23): 2309–16; with permission.)

have been seen in high-risk subgroups, such as diabetic patients[56] and patients with a low left ventricular ejection fraction.[57] Furthermore, 3 recent studies have established the cost-effectiveness of bivalirudin in the setting of ACS,[58,59] particularly in those patients at high risk for bleeding.[60] These overall observations have led the National Institute for Clinical Excellence to recommend bivalirudin administration during primary PCI for STEMI.[12]

REAL-WORLD APPLICATIONS

The most current American College of Cardiology/American Heart Association STEMI guidelines favor the use of bivalirudin but also mention the acceptable use of UFH, enoxaparin, and fondaparinux (with a concomitant anti-IIa anticoagulant) in this setting.[14] These guidelines reflect the best available evidence, but the flexibility in terms of anticoagulant choice creates ambiguity and uncertainty for the practicing clinician, with resultant widespread variability in anticoagulant use. This variation was recently demonstrated in an analysis of more than 72,000 patients from the National Cardiovascular Data Registry ACTION-GWTG registry, whereby an estimated 66% of STEMI patients received UFH, 14% received bivalirudin, 8% received low molecular weight heparin, and 6% received no anticoagulation.[61] The remaining 6% of patients received UFH combined with low molecular weight heparin despite the proven risk of combining these 2 agents. Likewise, Marso and colleagues[62] analyzed more than 1.5 million PCI patients in 955 United States hospitals and demonstrated a "risk treatment paradox," whereby the patients at highest risk for bleeding were least likely to receive bivalirudin or vascular closure devices, which mitigate the risk of hemorrhage and vascular complications. Taken together, these data represent a discrepancy between clinical trial results and contemporary real-world practice.

Consequently, there is an evolution in the process of clinical decision making that is occurring in cardiology practice, particularly with respect to PCI. On the one hand, the risk of bleeding in ACS patients has received close attention as exemplified by the multiple risk scores that have been developed in recent years.[63,64] The most recent version was based on a pooled dataset from REPLACE-2, ACUITY, and HORIZONS-AMI, and involved 7 readily available clinical variables that independently predicted TIMI major bleeding within 30 days.[34] Based on these risk scores for bleeding and analogous risk scores under development for stent thrombosis, a meaningful and individualized approach can be devised for each patient based on the risk/benefit of PCI. These data points can be routinely incorporated into the informed consent process, leading to significant improvements in knowledge transfer and patient engagement in shared decision making.[65] In the current transition of health care delivery to patient-centeredness, such tools will become widely available at the bedside, although they will probably be most applicable in the nonurgent PCI setting.

SUMMARY

Patients who experience STEMI and undergo primary PCI with stent implantation are at high risk for ischemic and bleeding complications. The use of bivalirudin has been shown to improve the short-term and long-term prognosis of these patients compared with those on heparin plus a GPI, primarily attributable to a reduction in major bleeding episodes. Balancing the risk of bleeding with the risk of recurrent ischemia (including stent thrombosis) will require accurate assessment of each patient's individual risk profile, complemented by the evolving tools of personalized medicine. The optimal strategy of ischemic efficacy and safety may prove to be a combination of a newer antiplatelet agent with bivalirudin, which has shown early promise[66] and is currently under clinical investigation.

ACKNOWLEDGMENTS

The authors would like to thank Amy Volpert for her editorial support.

REFERENCES

1. Roger VL, Go AS, Lloyd-Jones DM, et al. Heart disease and stroke statistics—2012 update: a report from the American Heart Association. Circulation 2012;125(1):e2–220.
2. Yeh RW, Sidney S, Chandra M, et al. Population trends in the incidence and outcomes of acute myocardial infarction. N Engl J Med 2010;362(23):2155–65.
3. Krumholz HM, Wang Y, Chen J, et al. Reduction in acute myocardial infarction mortality in the United States: risk-standardized mortality rates from 1995-2006. JAMA 2009;302(7):767–73.
4. Movahed MR, John J, Hashemzadeh M, et al. Trends in the age adjusted mortality from acute ST segment elevation myocardial infarction in the United States (1988-2004) based on race, gender, infarct location and comorbidities. Am J Cardiol 2009;104(8):1030–4.

5. Danchin N. Systems of care for ST-segment elevation myocardial infarction: impact of different models on clinical outcomes. JACC Cardiovasc Interv 2009; 2(10):901–8.
6. DeWood MA, Spores J, Notske R, et al. Prevalence of total coronary occlusion during the early hours of transmural myocardial infarction. N Engl J Med 1980;303(16):897–902.
7. Gordon T, Kannel WB. Predisposition to atherosclerosis in the head, heart, and legs. The Framingham study. JAMA 1972;221(7):661–6.
8. Berry JD, Dyer A, Cai X, et al. Lifetime risks of cardiovascular disease. N Engl J Med 2012; 366(4):321–9.
9. Libby P. The vascular biology of atherosclerosis. In: Bonow RO, Zipes DP, et al, editors. Braunwald's heart disease—a textbook of cardiovascular medicine. Philadelphia: Elsevier Saunders; 2011. p. 906–7.
10. Libby P, Theroux P. Pathophysiology of coronary artery disease. Circulation 2005;111(25):3481–8.
11. Sanz G, Fuster V. Polypill and global cardiovascular health strategies. Semin Thorac Cardiovasc Surg 2011;23(1):24–9.
12. Stone GW. Bivalirudin in acute myocardial infarction: NICE guidance. Heart 2012;98(6):435–7.
13. Wallentin L, Becker RC, Budaj A, et al. Ticagrelor versus clopidogrel in patients with acute coronary syndromes. N Engl J Med 2009;361(11):1045–57.
14. Kushner FG, Hand M, Smith SC Jr, et al. 2009 focused updates: ACC/AHA guidelines for the management of patients with ST-elevation myocardial infarction (updating the 2004 guideline and 2007 focused update) and ACC/AHA/SCAI guidelines on percutaneous coronary intervention (updating the 2005 guideline and 2007 focused update): a report of the American College of Cardiology Foundation/American Heart Association Task Force on Practice Guidelines. Circulation 2009;120(22): 2271–306.
15. Yusuf S, Mehta SR, Chrolavicius S, et al. Effects of fondaparinux on mortality and reinfarction in patients with acute ST-segment elevation myocardial infarction: the OASIS-6 randomized trial. JAMA 2006; 295(13):1519–30.
16. De Luca G, Suryapranata H, Stone GW, et al. Abciximab as adjunctive therapy to reperfusion in acute ST-segment elevation myocardial infarction: a meta-analysis of randomized trials. JAMA 2005; 293(14):1759–65.
17. Nikolsky E, Stone GW. Antithrombotic strategies in non-ST elevation acute coronary syndromes: focus on bivalirudin. Future Cardiol 2007;3(4):345–64.
18. Effects of recombinant hirudin (lepirudin) compared with heparin on death, myocardial infarction, refractory angina, and revascularisation procedures in patients with acute myocardial ischaemia without ST elevation: a randomised trial. Organisation to Assess Strategies for Ischemic Syndromes (OASIS-2) investigators. Lancet 1999;353(9151):429–38.
19. Metz BK, White HD, Granger CB, et al. Randomized comparison of direct thrombin inhibition versus heparin in conjunction with fibrinolytic therapy for acute myocardial infarction: results from the GUSTO-IIb Trial. Global Use of Strategies to Open Occluded Coronary Arteries in Acute Coronary Syndromes (GUSTO-IIb) investigators. J Am Coll Cardiol 1998;31(7):1493–8.
20. Abdel-Wahab M, Richardt G. Safety of bivalirudin in patients with coronary artery disease. Expert Opin Drug Saf 2012;11(1):141–50.
21. Kimmelstiel C, Zhang P, Kapur NK, et al. Bivalirudin is a dual inhibitor of thrombin and collagen-dependent platelet activation in patients undergoing percutaneous coronary intervention. Circ Cardiovasc Interv 2011;4(2):171–9.
22. Lincoff AM, Bittl JA, Harrington RA, et al. Bivalirudin and provisional glycoprotein IIb/IIIa blockade compared with heparin and planned glycoprotein IIb/IIIa blockade during percutaneous coronary intervention: REPLACE-2 randomized trial. JAMA 2003;289(7):853–63.
23. Lincoff AM, Kleiman NS, Kereiakes DJ, et al. Long-term efficacy of bivalirudin and provisional glycoprotein IIb/IIIa blockade vs heparin and planned glycoprotein IIb/IIIa blockade during percutaneous coronary revascularization: REPLACE-2 randomized trial. JAMA 2004;292(6):696–703.
24. Kastrati A, Neumann FJ, Mehilli J, et al. Bivalirudin versus unfractionated heparin during percutaneous coronary intervention. N Engl J Med 2008;359(7): 688–96.
25. Stone GW, McLaurin BT, Cox DA, et al. Bivalirudin for patients with acute coronary syndromes. N Engl J Med 2006;355(21):2203–16.
26. Thomas D, Giugliano RP. Day 1 care in patients with non-ST-segment elevation myocardial infarction. Cardiovasc Revasc Med 2010;11(1):41–51.
27. Kastrati A, Neumann FJ, Schulz S, et al. Abciximab and heparin versus bivalirudin for non-ST-elevation myocardial infarction. N Engl J Med 2011;365(21): 1980–9.
28. Stone GW, Witzenbichler B, Guagliumi G, et al. Heparin plus a glycoprotein IIb/IIIa inhibitor versus bivalirudin monotherapy and paclitaxel-eluting stents versus bare-metal stents in acute myocardial infarction (HORIZONS-AMI): final 3-year results from a multicentre, randomised controlled trial. Lancet 2011;377(9784):2193–204.
29. Baber U, Kovacic J, Kini AS, et al. How serious a problem is bleeding in patients with acute coronary syndromes? Curr Cardiol Rep 2011;13(4): 312–9.
30. Spencer FA, Moscucci M, Granger CB, et al. Does comorbidity account for the excess mortality in patients

with major bleeding in acute myocardial infarction? Circulation 2007;116(24):2793–801.
31. White HD. Editorial: do we need another bleeding definition? What does the Bleeding Academic Research Consortium definition have to offer? Curr Opin Cardiol 2011;26(4):275–8.
32. Rao SV, Jollis JG, Harrington RA, et al. Relationship of blood transfusion and clinical outcomes in patients with acute coronary syndromes. JAMA 2004;292(13):1555–62.
33. Campbell CL, Steinhubl SR, Hooper WC, et al. Bleeding events are associated with an increase in markers of inflammation in acute coronary syndromes: an ACUITY trial substudy. J Thromb Thrombolysis 2011;31(2):139–45.
34. Mehran R, et al. Impact of bleeding on mortality after percutaneous coronary intervention results from a patient-level pooled analysis of the REPLACE-2 (randomized evaluation of PCI linking angiomax to reduced clinical events), ACUITY (acute catheterization and urgent intervention triage strategy), and HORIZONS-AMI (harmonizing outcomes with revascularization and stents in acute myocardial infarction) trials. JACC Cardiovasc Interv 2011;4(6):654–64.
35. Mehran R, Pocock S, Nikolsky E, et al. Associations of major bleeding and myocardial infarction with the incidence and timing of mortality in patients presenting with non-ST-elevation acute coronary syndromes: a risk model from the ACUITY trial. Eur Heart J 2009;30(12):1457–66.
36. Kim YH, Lee JY, Ahn JM, et al. Impact of bleeding on subsequent early and late mortality after drug-eluting stent implantation. JACC Cardiovasc Interv 2011;4(4):423–31.
37. Suh JW, Mehran R, Claessen BE, et al. Impact of in-hospital major bleeding on late clinical outcomes after primary percutaneous coronary intervention in acute myocardial infarction the HORIZONS-AMI (Harmonizing Outcomes With Revascularization and Stents in Acute Myocardial Infarction) trial. J Am Coll Cardiol 2011;58(17):1750–6.
38. Lopes RD, Subherwal S, Holmes DS, et al. The association of in-hospital major bleeding with short-, intermediate-, and long-term mortality among older patients with non-ST-segment elevation myocardial infarction. Eur Heart J 2012. [Epub ahead of print].
39. Wang TY, Xiao L, Alexander KP, et al. Antiplatelet therapy use after discharge among acute myocardial infarction patients with in-hospital bleeding. Circulation 2008;118(21):2139–45.
40. Jolly SS, Yusuf S, Cairns J, et al. Radial versus femoral access for coronary angiography and intervention in patients with acute coronary syndromes (RIVAL): a randomised, parallel group, multicentre trial. Lancet 2011;377(9775):1409–20.
41. Verheugt FW, Steinhubl SR, Hamon M, et al. Incidence, prognostic impact, and influence of antithrombotic therapy on access and nonaccess site bleeding in percutaneous coronary intervention. JACC Cardiovasc Interv 2011;4(2):191–7.
42. Stone GW, Witzenbichler B, Guagliumi G, et al. Bivalirudin during primary PCI in acute myocardial infarction. N Engl J Med 2008;358(21):2218–30.
43. Capranzano P, Dangas G. Bivalirudin for primary percutaneous coronary intervention in acute myocardial infarction: the HORIZONS-AMI trial. Expert Rev Cardiovasc Ther 2012;10(4):411–22.
44. Mukherjee D. Antithrombotics and stent type for primary PCI. Lancet 2011;377(9784):2154–6.
45. Lagerqvist B, Carlsson J, Frobert O, et al. Stent thrombosis in Sweden: a report from the Swedish Coronary Angiography and Angioplasty Registry. Circ Cardiovasc Interv 2009;2(5):401–8.
46. Dangas GD, Caixeta A, Mehran R, et al. Frequency and predictors of stent thrombosis after percutaneous coronary intervention in acute myocardial infarction. Circulation 2011;123(16):1745–56.
47. Cortese B, Limbruno U, Severi S, et al. Effect of prolonged Bivalirudin infusion on ST-segment resolution following primary percutaneous coronary intervention (from the PROBI VIRI 2 study). Am J Cardiol 2011;108(9):1220–4.
48. Dangas GD, Mehran R, Nikolsky E, et al. Effect of switching antithrombin agents for primary angioplasty in acute myocardial infarction: the HORIZONS-SWITCH analysis. J Am Coll Cardiol 2011;57(23):2309–16.
49. Wang TY, Ou FS, Roe MT, et al. Incidence and prognostic significance of thrombocytopenia developed during acute coronary syndrome in contemporary clinical practice. Circulation 2009;119(18):2454–62.
50. Hakim DA, Dangas GD, Caixeta A, et al. Impact of baseline thrombocytopenia on the early and late outcomes after ST-elevation myocardial infarction treated with primary angioplasty: analysis from the Harmonizing Outcomes with Revascularization and Stents in Acute Myocardial Infarction (HORIZONS-AMI) trial. Am Heart J 2011;161(2):391–6.
51. Tsujita K, Nikolsky E, Lansky AJ, et al. Impact of anemia on clinical outcomes of patients with ST-segment elevation myocardial infarction in relation to gender and adjunctive antithrombotic therapy (from the HORIZONS-AMI trial). Am J Cardiol 2010;105(10):1385–94.
52. Nikolsky E, Mehran R, Aymong ED, et al. Impact of anemia in patients with acute myocardial infarction undergoing primary percutaneous coronary intervention: analysis from the Controlled Abciximab and Device Investigation to Lower Late Angioplasty Complications (CADILLAC) Trial. J Am Coll Cardiol 2004;44(3):547–53.
53. Bassand JP, Afzal R, Eikelboom J, et al. Relationship between baseline haemoglobin and major bleeding

complications in acute coronary syndromes. Eur Heart J 2010;31(1):50–8.

54. Sibbing D, Busch G, Braun S, et al. Impact of bivalirudin or unfractionated heparin on platelet aggregation in patients pretreated with 600 mg clopidogrel undergoing elective percutaneous coronary intervention. Eur Heart J 2008;29(12): 1504–9.
55. Busch G, Steppich B, Sibbing B, et al. Bivalirudin reduces platelet and monocyte activation after elective percutaneous coronary intervention. Thromb Haemost 2009;101(2):340–4.
56. Witzenbichler B, Mehran R, Guagliumi G, et al. Impact of diabetes mellitus on the safety and effectiveness of bivalirudin in patients with acute myocardial infarction undergoing primary angioplasty: analysis from the HORIZONS-AMI (Harmonizing Outcomes with RevasculariZatiON and Stents in Acute Myocardial Infarction) trial. JACC Cardiovasc Interv 2011;4(7):760–8.
57. Yu J, Dangas G, Baber U, et al. Impact of ejection fraction on mortality in patients undergoing PCI: a patient-level pooled analysis from the REPLACE-2, ACUITY and HORIZONS-AMI trials. Chicago: American College of Cardiology; 2012.
58. Kessler DP, Kroch E, Hlatky MA. The effect of bivalirudin on costs and outcomes of treatment of ST-segment elevation myocardial infarction. Am Heart J 2011;162(3):494–500.e2.
59. Pinto DS, Ogbonnaya A, Sherman SA, et al. Bivalirudin therapy is associated with improved clinical and economic outcomes in ST-elevation myocardial infarction patients undergoing percutaneous coronary intervention: results from an observational database. Circ Cardiovasc Qual Outcomes 2012;5(1): 52–61.
60. Amin AP, Marso SP, Rao SV, et al. Cost-effectiveness of targeting patients undergoing percutaneous coronary intervention for therapy with bivalirudin versus heparin monotherapy according to predicted risk of bleeding. Circ Cardiovasc Qual Outcomes 2010; 3(4):358–65.
61. Kadakia MB, Desai NR, Alexander KP, et al. Use of anticoagulant agents and risk of bleeding among patients admitted with myocardial infarction: a report from the NCDR ACTION Registry-GWTG (National Cardiovascular Data Registry Acute Coronary Treatment and Intervention Outcomes Network Registry-Get With the Guidelines). JACC Cardiovasc Interv 2010;3(11):1166–77.
62. Marso SP, Amin AP, House JA, et al. Association between use of bleeding avoidance strategies and risk of periprocedural bleeding among patients undergoing percutaneous coronary intervention. JAMA 2010;303(21):2156–64.
63. Mehta SK, Frutkin AD, Lindsey JB, et al. Bleeding in patients undergoing percutaneous coronary intervention: the development of a clinical risk algorithm from the National Cardiovascular Data Registry. Circ Cardiovasc Interv 2009;2(3):222–9.
64. Subherwal S, Bach RG, Chen AY, et al. Baseline risk of major bleeding in non-ST-segment-elevation myocardial infarction: the CRUSADE (Can Rapid risk stratification of Unstable angina patients Suppress ADverse outcomes with Early implementation of the ACC/AHA Guidelines) Bleeding Score. Circulation 2009;119(14):1873–82.
65. Spertus J, Bach R, Bethea C, et al. Testing an evidence-based, individualized informed consent form to improve patients' experiences with PCI. Circulation 2011;124(21):2368.
66. Baumbach A, Johnson TW, Oriolo V, et al. Prasugrel and bivalirudin for primary angioplasty: early results on stent thrombosis and bleeding. Int J Cardiol 2011;153(2):222–4.
67. Stone GW, Ware JH, Bertrand ME, et al. Antithrombotic strategies in patients with acute coronary syndromes undergoing early invasive management: one-year results from the ACUITY trial. JAMA 2007; 298(21):2497–506.

Interventions for ST Elevation Myocardial Infarction in Women

Vivian G. Ng, MD, Alexandra J. Lansky, MD*

KEYWORDS

• ST elevation myocardial infarction • Women • Gender • Outcomes

KEY POINTS

- Cardiovascular disease is the leading cause of death in women.
- Women are more likely to present with atypical symptoms and have worse cardiac risk profiles than men.
- Women, especially young women, with ST elevation myocardial infarctions have worse clinical outcomes than men do.
- Although thrombolytic therapy improves outcomes in women, women have high rates of hemorrhagic complications.
- In women, balloon angioplasty improves outcomes compared with thrombolytic therapy because it addresses the underlying stenotic lesion as well as decreases bleeding complications.
- Primary stenting further improves outcomes in women by decreasing rates of acute closure after intervention.

Over the last several decades, the treatment of coronary artery disease (CAD) and ST elevation myocardial infarction (STEMI) has drastically changed from supportive care to thrombolytic therapy and, subsequently, to primary interventional management. CAD remains the leading cause of death in women. However, women present later in life and with different symptoms than men. Furthermore, many studies have suggested that women with STEMI have worse outcomes compared with men. This article reviews the presentation, outcomes, and treatment options for women with STEMI.

EPIDEMIOLOGY AND CLINICAL PRESENTATION

Cardiovascular disease continues to be the leading cause of mortality among women in developed countries.[1,2] Although mortality rates from cardiovascular disease have decreased, the rate of decline in women is slower than that in men.[1] Recent data suggest that the mortality gap is finally starting to narrow between men and women[3]; however, women continue to have higher mortality rates than men and CAD continues to be an underrecognized disease in women.[4] For example, in a survey of 500 primary care physicians, cardiologists, and gynecologists, fewer than 20% of these physicians recognized that more women than men die of cardiovascular disease.[5] Thus, it is of utmost importance to review the presentation of ischemic heart disease in women (**Box 1**) to recognize and direct the treatment of these patients.

Women with CAD present nearly a decade later in life than men.[3,6] The average age of a first myocardial infarction (MI) in men is 65 years old,

Disclosures: The authors have nothing to disclose.
Valve Program, Yale University School of Medicine, Yale University Medical Center, PO Box 208017, New Haven, CT 06520-8017, USA
* Corresponding author.
E-mail address: alexandra.lansky@yale.edu

Intervent Cardiol Clin 1 (2012) 453–465
http://dx.doi.org/10.1016/j.iccl.2012.06.004
2211-7458/12/$ – see front matter

Box 1
The presentation of ischemic heart disease in women compared with men

- Average age of first myocardial infarction (MI)[3]
  - 65 years in men
  - 70 years in women
- Presentation of CAD
  - Women more frequently present with unstable angina or NSTEM
  - Men more frequently present with STEMI
- Symptoms of cardiac ischemia[6–10]
  - Anginal pain the most common initial presentation in women
  - Infarction or sudden death more common initial presentation in men
  - Only 27% of women presented with STEMI in the Global Use of Strategies to Open Occluded Coronary Arteries in Acute Coronary Syndromes IIB (GUSTO IIb) trial[8]
  - 37% of men presented with STEMI in the GUSTO IIB trial[8]
- Among acute MI patients, women are less likely to present with substernal chest pain and are more likely to complain of
  - Atypical chest pain with or without shortness of breath
  - Abdominal pain, nausea or fatigue[11–19]
- Ischemia is often silent in women[20,21]
- MI more often unrecognized in women than men.[22,23]
- Women are more likely to present later after symptom onset than men.[17,24–33]

whereas the average age of a first MI in women is 70 years old.[3] When women seek medical attention for CAD, they present with unstable angina or non-STEMI more frequently than men do and manifest different symptoms of cardiac ischemia than men.[6–10] The Framingham study demonstrated that anginal pain was the most common initial presentation of ischemic heart disease in women (55% of women, 39% of men), whereas infarction or sudden death was more commonly the first presentation in men (36% of women, 53% of men).[6] Similarly, in the Global Use of Strategies to Open Occluded Coronary Arteries in Acute Coronary Syndromes IIb (GUSTO IIb) trial, 37% of men presented with STEMI, whereas only 27% of women presented with STEMI.[8] Among acute MI (AMI) patients, women are less likely to present with substernal chest pain and are more likely to complain of atypical chest pain with or without shortness of breath, abdominal pain, nausea, or fatigue.[11–19] In addition, ischemia is often silent in women[20,21] and MI more often goes unrecognized in women compared with men.[22,23] Because of these differences in symptoms, women may not recognize that their complaints are cardiac in origin and are more likely to present later after symptom onset than men.[17,24–33] In a meta-analysis of 60,000 patients from nine trials, women presented an average of 7 hours after symptom onset compared with 6.2 hours for men.[24] Thus, physicians must be attuned to these differences in symptoms to expedite care once women do present to a medical care setting.

PATHOPHYSIOLOGY OF CAD IN WOMEN

It is thought that women with CAD present a decade later in life than men as a result of the protective effects of estrogen.[3,6,34] Estrogen has been suggested to retard plaque development, stabilize existing plaques, and prevent plaque rupture in women.[34,35] As a result of presenting at an older age, women have higher rates of traditional risk factors such as diabetes, hypertension, and hyperlipidemia at the time of their MI.[8–10,16,27,30,33,36,37] Thus, one would expect women to have more severe CAD when presenting with ischemia; however, angiographically, women have less extensive CAD[38–40] and a higher incidence of nonsignificant CAD compared with men (**Box 2**).[9,14] Furthermore, autopsy studies[41,42] and intravascular ultrasound studies have found less plaque development in women than in men.[43,44] It is remains unclear whether the influence of traditional risk factors on the development of CAD varies between the genders.

Box 2
Pathophysiology of CAD in women

Compared with men, women have

- Less extensive CAD[38–40]
- A higher incidence of nonsignificant CAD[9,14]
- Less plaque development
- Plaque erosion more commonly than plaque rupture, which is more common in men and older patients of both genders

Generally, AMI is caused by rupture of a coronary plaque that has a lipid-rich core covered by a thin fibrous cap. Approximately 75% of fatal MIs are caused by so-called thin-cap fibroatheroma (TCFA) and the remaining 25% are due to plaque erosion rather than rupture. Plaque erosions are rich in smooth muscle cells and proteoglycans, have no apparent injury, and are generally eccentric and nonstenotic with a denuded endothelial lining. Plaque erosions are more common in women, particularly young smokers, whereas plaque rupture is more common in men and older patients of both genders.[45] This finding that may, in part, be hormonally modulated.[46–49] In the PROSPECT (Providing Regional Observations to Study Predictors of Events in the Coronary Tree) trial gender subanalysis, plaque rupture was significantly less common in women versus men (6.6% vs 16.3%; $P = .002$) even after adjusting for comorbidities ($P = .004$).[40] The frequency of other plaque vulnerability phenotypes was similar for men and women including pathologic intimal thickening, TCFA, and thick-cap fibroatheromas; however, among women, the strongest predictor of a major adverse cardiac event (MACE) at 3 years was the presence of a TCFA, which seemed to be a stronger predictor in women than in men. Patients with plaque erosions are more likely to have a longer indolent period of angina compared with patients with plaque ruptures.[50,51] This difference could help explain why women presenting with STEMI are more likely to present later after symptom onset and with anginal symptoms (typical or atypical) than are men who are more likely to present with sudden severe chest pain.[27,52]

COMORBIDITIES AT PRESENTATION

Numerous studies have demonstrated that women with STEMI have worse outcomes compared with men and have more postprocedural complications after intervention.[10,30,36,53–62] For example, in a large registry of 26,035 consecutive STEMI patients (8989 [34.5%] women), Sadowski and colleagues[30] found that women had higher rates of in-hospital death compared with men (11.9% vs 6.9%, $P<.0001$). However, it is unclear whether the gender-based outcome differences are secondary to gender alone or to other confounding factors. Time delays to reperfusion increase mortality and because women tend to seek medical attention later after symptom onset than men they may have decreased amounts of salvageable myocardium once revascularized. Furthermore, women with AMI are older and have worse baseline cardiac risk profiles at presentation, including higher rates of diabetes and hypertension, which are associated with worse outcomes. In addition to clinical characteristics, the coronary anatomy of women may have contributed to their worse outcomes in clinical trials initially. Women are more likely to have smaller vessel diameters, which may or may not be secondary to their smaller body surface areas.[63–65] Smaller vessels are prone to vessel dissection and perforations.[66–68] However, this has been largely overcome with the advent of smaller stents. After adjustment for these clinical characteristics, some studies have found that gender is not a significant predictor of outcomes,[9,15,16,27,33,62,69–75] whereas others have found that female gender remains an independent predictor of worse outcomes.[30,36,53,56,57,60,61,76] In the Sadowski registry, female gender continued to be associated with increased in-hospital mortality rates after a multivariate analysis (odds ratio [OR] 1.13 [1.01–1.26], $P<.03$).[30] Similarly, in another large registry trial containing 16,760 STEMI subjects (3664 [21.9%] women), female gender was an independent predictor of in-hospital mortality after adjustment for baseline clinical characteristics (OR 1.38 [1.16–1.63], $P = .0002$).[36] In contrast, although the GUSTO IIb study found increased 30-day mortality rates in STEMI women compared with men, this result was not statistically significant after a multivariate analysis (OR 1.27 [0.98–1.63], $P = .07$).[8] It remains unclear whether a mortality difference between STEMI women and men truly exists or is the result of unmeasurable confounders.

GENDER AND AGE INTERACTION

Perhaps more significant than other baseline differences between men and women is the gender–age interaction. Young women with STEMI have higher early mortality rates than their male counterparts of the same age when treated medically or with angioplasty.[10,21,72,77–83] A retrospective study of 1025 patients found that women who were less than 75 years old were 49% more likely to die during their hospitalization than men.[77] This difference is accentuated in younger age groups. Women who were less than 50 years old had twice the likelihood of dying in hospital compared with age-matched men. In contrast, after 75 years of age, mortality rates may be equivalent. The National Registry of Myocardial Infarction (NRMI) study containing 384,878 patients (155,565 [40.4%] women) found that the odds of death in women compared with men increased by 7% for every 5 years of decreasing age, even after adjustment for other clinical factors.[79] These differences are not limited to in-hospital and short-term outcomes. In a cohort study of 6826 patients who survived their hospitalization for AMI, younger women suffered from higher long-term mortality rates such that there was a 15.6% relative increase in 2-year mortality risk for every 10-year decrease in age.[78] The Myocardial Infarction Data Acquisition System (MIDAS) study included 49,250 patients with AMI and found that, even after adjustment for covariates, men had a lower 3-year mortality risk compared with women, which was amplified in the younger age group.[83] Why young premenopausal women, who are generally considered to be low-risk patients and who are thought to be protected by estrogen, have worse outcomes compared with age-matched men is unknown. Differences in presenting symptoms may account for decreased disease recognition and worse outcomes, particularly in young women. A recent registry study showed that there is a significant interaction between gender and age on the symptomatology of MI patients. Women are more likely than men with AMI are to present without chest pain and this difference is accentuated in younger patients. For example, AMI women younger than 45 years of age have 30% higher odds of not having chest pain compared with age-matched men (OR 1.30 [1.23, 1.36] for <45 years, and decreases to OR 1.03 [1.02–1.04] in patients older than 75 years). The in-hospital mortality rate of asymptomatic young women with MI is significantly greater than that of asymptomatic young men (OR 1.18 [1.00–1.3]); a difference that is reversed in patients older than 75 years old (OR 0.81 [0.79–0.83]).[21] Furthermore, given the low prevalence of MI in this patient population, it is possible that young women who develop STEMI are predisposed to severe CAD from other risk factors such as a higher prevalence of diabetes, genetic factors, or other pathophysiologic basis of STEMI. The Variation in Recovery: Role of Gender on Outcomes of Young AMI Patients (VIRGO) trial is an ongoing NIH-sponsored study of 3000 AMI patients younger than 55 years old, with 2 to 1 enrollment ratio of women to men. VIRGO will prospectively explore the pathophysiologic basis of gender differences in mortality in patients with premature STEMI.[84]

CORONARY REVASCULARIZATION IN WOMEN

There is increasing research revealing the benefits of reperfusion treatments in women and the guidelines recommend that women receive the same medical and interventional management as men do for STEMI[1,85]; however, women are less likely to have optimized medical regimens[37,76,86–88] or undergo revascularization procedures.[27,32,37,54,83,87–93] The NRMI looked at the rates of guideline-based therapy use in 2,515,106 patients admitted with an MI at 2157 United States' hospitals between 1990 and 2006. Women were significantly less likely to undergo revascularization with either percutaneous coronary intervention (PCI) or coronary artery bypass graft surgery than men were.[94] Furthermore, despite an overall improvement in the use of guideline-based therapies, the gender treatment disparity increased over the study time period.[94] A similar finding was seen in an analysis by the Cooperative Cardiovascular Project, a group which looks at Medicare recipients and determines rates of guideline adherence. Looking at cardiac catheterization rates in 143,444 AMI patients, women were less likely to receive a cardiac catheterization within 60-days of hospitalization than men were (35.7% vs 46.5%, $P<.001$).[95] However, when these data were further broken down, women and men had similar rates of catheterization for strong (44.1% vs 44.6%, $P>.2$) and weak (16.5% vs 18.0%, $P = .096$) indications, but significantly lower rates for equivocal indications (39.4% vs 42.5%, $P<.001$).[95]

Despite the significant rates of STEMI in men and women (4.3% prevalence in men, 2.2% in women),[3] women comprise the minority of patients in large clinical trials.[96,97] Furthermore, there are no trials dedicated to evaluating the optimal treatment strategies in women with STEMI. Most reports compare outcomes between the genders instead of among females by treatment subgroups. Nonetheless, the data provide useful information on how to best treat women with STEMI.

THROMBOLYTIC THERAPY IN WOMEN

Early reperfusion with thrombolytic therapy for STEMI reduces infarct size and heart failure and improves survival. Multiple studies have demonstrated that fibrinolytic therapy increased survival when given acutely to treat AMI. These include the Second International Study of Infarct Survival (ISIS-2), Gruppo Italiano per lo Studio della Streptochinasi nell'Infarto Miocardico, part 1 (ISSI-1), Western Washington Trial, Anglo-Scandinavian

Study of Early Thrombolysis (ASSET), and the Global Utilization of Streptokinase and Tissue Plasminogen Activator for Occluded Coronary Arteries (GUSTO-1).[98–102] For example, in the ISIS-2 trial, 17,070 AMI patients (13,125 [76.9%] men and 3945 [23.1%] women) were randomized to intravenous streptokinase, oral aspirin, both therapies, or neither therapy in a 2-by-2 factorial placebo-controlled trial.[98] A 31% reduction in mortality was observed in women who received streptokinase and aspirin (*P* value not reported for comparison). The GISSI-1 trial, which contained 11,712 AMI patients randomized to streptokinase therapy or conventional therapy, found that men and women had a 10% mortality reduction at 1 year when randomized to streptokinase therapy,[99] establishing the benefit of thrombolytic therapy in women with STEMI.

However, in all of these trials, women had worse mortality rates than men. In ISIS-2, women receiving streptokinase and aspirin had a 12.2% mortality rate, whereas men only had a 6.7% mortality rate.[98] In the GISSI-1 trial, women who received streptokinase had a 28.3% mortality rate, whereas men had a 14.5% mortality rate.[99] Similarly, the ISIS-3 study, which contained 36,080 patients (9600 [26.6%] women) who underwent thrombolytic therapy for AMI, found that women were at increased risk of death at 35-day follow-up even after adjustment for age and other baseline characteristics (OR 1.20 [1.11, 1.29]).[58] It is unclear why women had higher mortality rates. Women presented later in the disease time course, potentially decreasing the extent of salvageable myocardium from thrombolytic administration, which likely translates into higher rates of subsequent cardiac events. There is no current evidence in angiographic studies that reperfusion rates are different between men and women.[38,103,104] In the GUSTO-1 angiographic study, there was no difference in rates of culprit vessel patency 90 minutes after administration of a thrombolytic therapy in women and men (39% vs 38%, $P = .5$). However, although rates of angiographic reocclusion of the culprit artery were higher in women, this difference was not statistically significant (8.7% vs 5.1%, $P = .14$)[103] and does not account for observed differences in outcomes. Most likely, women had decreased survival after MI as a result of bleeding complications and hemorrhagic strokes. In the GUSTO-1 trial, in which 41,021 AMI patients (25.1% women) were randomized to one of four thrombolytic regimens, women had higher rates of death (11.3% vs 5.55, $P<.001$) and serious bleeding events after thrombolytic therapy than men had (15% vs 7%, $P<.001$).[102] Women had a twofold higher stroke rate than men had (2.1% vs 1.2%, $P<.001$), mostly attributable to increased rates of hemorrhagic strokes.

Other studies have identified female gender as an independent predictor of intracranial hemorrhage after thrombolytic therapy for AMI.[105–107] The Cooperative Cardiovascular Project study found that female gender was an independent predictor of hemorrhagic strokes after thrombolytic administration for AMI (OR 1.34 [1.15–1.67], $P = .0007$).[106] The NRMI similarly found that female gender increased the risk of a hemorrhagic stroke by approximately 1.6 times when treated with thrombolysis (OR 1.59 [1.31–1.92]).[107] It is important to emphasize that, despite the higher mortality and bleeding rates in women compared with men, women clearly benefit from thrombolytic therapy when other reperfusion modalities are not available. Thus, when pharmacologic reperfusion is necessary, thrombolytics should not be withheld in women.

PRIMARY ANGIOPLASTY IN WOMEN

Despite the benefit and widespread application of fibrinolytic therapy in the treatment of STEMI, bleeding complications, including devastating hemorrhagic strokes, present a major limitation of this therapy, beyond the substantial proportion (approximately 20%–30%) of patients with failed reperfusion[108–112] and recurrent ischemia.[98,113–115] Although thrombolytics can restore epicardial coronary artery flow, it does not address the underlying unstable plaque and the exposed thrombogenic material thought to cause recurrent ischemic events.

Mechanical reperfusion with primary balloon angioplasty improved reperfusion, recurrent ischemia, and bleeding complication rates.[116–121] The benefit of primary angioplasty compared with thrombolytics is generalizable to women.[122] The Primary Angioplasty in Acute Myocardial Infarction (PAMI) trial included 395 patients (27% women) randomized to either thrombolysis using tissue plasminogen activator or to angioplasty. Women treated with primary angioplasty had a 4% rate of in-hospital mortality compared with 14% for thrombolytic therapy ($P = .07$). Primary angioplasty compared with thrombolytic therapy independently predicted in-hospital survival in women. Nonetheless, as in the thrombolytic trials, women had worse outcomes compared with men. Overall, in-hospital mortality rates were three times higher in women than in men (9.3% vs 2.8%, $P = .005$). However, gender was not an independent predictor of mortality after adjustment for differences in baseline characteristics. Furthermore, when broken down by treatment, mortality rates were significantly higher in women than in men after thrombolytic therapy (14.0% vs 3.5%, $P = .006$), but similar after angioplasty (4.0% vs 2.1%, $P = .46$). Women also had more intracranial hemorrhage events than men had after thrombolysis (5.3% vs 0.7%, $P = .04$); however, intracranial bleeding was completely eliminated in the angioplasty groups.[122] Thus, angioplasty seemed to be a safer treatment modality narrowing the outcomes gap between men and women based on improved reperfusion rates, targeted intervention to the lesion site, and decreased bleeding complications.

However, real-world experiences with these therapies offered conflicting results and suggested that female gender was associated with worse outcomes even after accounting for other confounding variables.[123,124] For example, using the New York State Coronary Angioplasty database, which contained 1044 patients (317 [30.4%] women) who underwent primary angioplasty for AMI in 1995, Vakili and colleagues[123] found that women were older (65 ± 12 years vs 59 ± 12 years, $P<.05$) and had higher rates of hypertension (59% vs 44%, $P<.05$) and diabetes (19% vs 14%, $P<.05$). Furthermore, men were more likely to be treated earlier (within 6 hours) from the time of symptom onset than women (74% vs 63%, $P<.05$). In-hospital mortality rates were higher in women than in men (7.9% vs 2.3%, $P<.05$) in a univariate analysis. This difference persisted even after adjustment for baseline differences such that women had 2.3 times the risk of in-hospital death compared with men after receiving angioplasty (OR 2.3 [1.2, 4.6], $P = .016$). Nonetheless, given the improved mortality rates and decreased rates of bleeding complications, angioplasty became the preferred method of treating STEMI patients, including women.

PRIMARY STENTING IN WOMEN

Although primary angioplasty improves mortality rates compared with thrombolysis, it is associated with higher rates of restenosis.[113,125,126] Although initial studies evaluating primary stenting raised concerns that women may not benefit from stent implantation, subsequent analyses found that women do have improved clinical and angiographic outcomes when treated with stents.

In the Stent PAMI trial, 900 AMI patients (30% women) were randomized to either primary stent placement or balloon angioplasty. Overall, MACE rates were lower in patients undergoing primary stenting compared with balloon angioplasty (17% vs 24%, $P<.01$); however, at 6 months, women had higher mortality rates than men (7.9% vs 2.0%, $P = .0002$) and, although men had improved outcomes after stent placement compared with angioplasty, outcomes in women were not improved.[127]

The Controlled Abciximab and Device Investigation to Lower Late Angioplasty Complications (CADILLAC) trial included 2082 patients (27% women) with AMI and found that patients who underwent primary stent placement with or without glycoprotein IIb/IIIa inhibitors had improved survival rates compared with patients who received balloon angioplasty alone.[125] Among women, MACE (19.1% vs 28.1%, $P = .013$) and ischemic target revascularization (10.8% vs 20.4%, $P = .002$) rates were lower at 1 year with primary stenting compared with balloon angioplasty. Compared with men, women continued to have worse outcomes in terms of a 1-year MACE (23.9% vs 15.4%, $P<.001$) and death (7.6% vs 3.0%, $P<.0001$), and female gender was an independent predictor of a 1-year MACE in a multivariate analysis (OR 1.64 [1.24, 2.17], $P = .04$). Furthermore, procedure-related moderate-to-severe bleeding rates were 2.5 times higher in women, with female gender being an independent predictor of moderate-to-severe bleeding complications. Importantly, female gender was not a predictor of 1-year death.[128]

Women also had improved angiographic outcomes after stenting. A registry study of 1019 AMI patients (230 [22.6%] women) undergoing either balloon angioplasty or stenting evaluated gender outcomes in an unselected STEMI population. Six-month angiographic follow-up data were available in 86.2% of all patients and 83% of women. Women treated with a stent had lower rates of restenosis compared with primary angioplasty (29% vs 52%, $P = .0006$) and female gender was not an independent predictor of angiographic restenosis.[127]

In a contemporary European registry of 16,760 AMI patients (3664 [21.9%] women) treated with stents, women were older (69.7 ± 14.3 years vs 59.3 ± 13.0 years, $P<.0001$), had higher rates of diabetes (19.0% vs 15.6%, $P<.0001$) and cardiogenic shock (6.7% vs 4.0%, $P<.0001$) and had lower procedural success rates (94.7% vs 95.9, $P = .002$) than men. In-hospital mortality was higher in women than in men (9.8% vs 4.3%, $P<.0001$), and women required more transfusions (1.2% vs 0.4%, $P<.0001$). Furthermore, multivariate analysis showed that female gender was associated with higher in-hospital mortality rates,[36] adding to the conflicting long-term mortality results. Bufe and colleagues[129] performed a retrospective analysis of 500 consecutive AMI patients (124 [24.8%]

women) undergoing stenting. Long-term, all-cause mortality rates were similar between women and men (9.7% vs 6.95, $P = .417$) and, in multivariable analysis, gender was not an independent predictor of long-term mortality.

Although the use of a drug-eluting stent (DES) in the setting of primary PCI seems to offer a benefit in terms of prevention of target lesion revascularization, the gender-related differences in long-term benefit remain to be seen. In a subset analysis of AMI patients in the combined Rapamycin-Eluting Stent Evaluated at Rotterdam Cardiology Hospital (RESEARCH) and Taxus-Stent Evaluated at Rotterdam Cardiology Hospital (T-SEARCH) Registries, women continued to have worse outcomes compared with men and had higher rates of MACE despite the routine use of DES (adjusted hazard ratio [HR] 1.7 [1.02, 1.85]).[130] In contrast, in the Korea Acute Myocardial Infarction Registry (KAMIR; 2416 men, 882 women), female gender was not an independent predictor of worse outcomes by multivariable analysis despite higher rates of a 1-year MACE in women compared with men in the univariate analysis (27.8% vs 18.4%, $P<.001$).[131] A post hoc analysis of the Multicentre Evaluation of Single High-Dose Bolus Tirofiban versus Abciximab with Sirolimus-Eluting Stent or Bare-Metal Stent in Acute Myocardial Infarction Study (MULTISTRATEGY) study (N = 745, 24% women), which randomized patients to a sirolimus-eluting stent (SES) versus a bare-metal stent, at 3-year follow-up found that SES use was associated with a significantly lower risk of MACE (adjusted HR 0.62 [0.41 to 0.94], $P = .026$) and target vessel revascularization (adjusted HR 0.35 [0.19 to 0.63], $P<.001$) in men but not in women.[132] Additional studies are needed to further clarify the impact of female gender on STEMI outcomes in the era of the DES.

Primary stenting in women improves outcomes, including mortality, compared with primary angioplasty and should be considered the preferred strategy of reperfusion in treating women with STEMI. Although the gap in gender outcomes has narrowed more recently, women who undergo stenting continue to have worse short-term outcomes compared with men. Additional research is needed to further characterize the cause for this gender difference and ways to optimize outcomes for women with STEMI.

BLEEDING AND VASCULAR COMPLICATIONS

In studies from the 1990s, vascular complications were three to four times more frequent in women than in men. Rates of vascular complications in women have subsequently decreased with the development of less aggressive anticoagulation regimens, weight-adjusted heparin dosing, and the availability of smaller sheath sizes made possible by the smaller profile of newer third- and fourth-generation devices.[85]

Despite improvements, women undergoing PCI (primarily through the femoral artery) continue to have a two-fold increased risk of bleeding and vascular complications compared with men, even after adjusting for differences in baseline and procedural characteristics.[9,133] This gender difference may be even more pronounced in younger women compared with younger men.[134] Women with bleeding complications have ~3-fold increased incidence of stroke, MI, and all-cause death compared with women without bleeding complications and, even after controlling for both clinical and procedural differences, women with bleeding have a 75% increased risk of death, MI, or stroke during their index hospitalization (OR 1.75 [1.23, 2.51]).[133]

The use of the direct thrombin inhibitor bivalirudin during elective PCI lowers the risk of periprocedural ischemic complications and major bleeding in both women and men, although female gender remained associated with an increased risk of 30-day non–CABG-related major bleeding (adjusted HR 1.96, [1.66, 2.32], $P<.0001$) even after adjusting for differences in baseline characteristics (including age, body weight, chronic renal insufficiency, anemia, hypertension, and diabetes) in the Acute Catheterization and Urgent Intervention Triage strategY (ACUITY) trial.[39] Observational data suggest that using a radial access leads to significantly reduced bleeding and vascular complications in both genders and that women experience an even greater benefit because of their increased baseline risk.[135,136] This will be further investigated in women specifically in the ongoing multicenter randomized Study of Access Site for Enhancement of PCI for Women (SAFE PCI for Women) trial. Three thousand women undergoing urgent or elective PCI will be randomized to either transradial or transfemoral PCI. The primary efficacy endpoint is bleeding or vascular complications within 72 hours postprocedure or hospital discharge and the primary feasibility endpoint is procedure failure. Enrollment is currently ongoing and the study is expected to be completed in January 2014.

SUMMARY

Coronary artery disease remains the leading cause of death in women. Symptoms of cardiac ischemia in women presenting with STEMI can be difficult to recognize because women are more likely to present with atypical symptoms. Great advances have been made in the treatment of STEMI starting from the development of thrombolytic therapy and most recently with PCI. Most of the research thus far has focused on the outcome disparities between men and women and has demonstrated that women have worse outcomes than men have even after undergoing reperfusion therapies. However, it is important to note that, despite their high-risk status, women benefit from these therapeutic interventions. Thus, women with STEMI should be treated aggressively and undergo the same treatment algorithms as men undergo. Future research will need to focus on how to improve the diagnosis and treatment of STEMI in women to further improve outcomes.

REFERENCES

1. Stramba-Badiale M, Fox KM, Priori SG, et al. Cardiovascular diseases in women: a statement from the policy conference of the European Society of Cardiology. Eur Heart J 2006;27:994–1005.
2. Heron M. Deaths: leading causes for 2004. Natl Vital Stat Rep 2007;56:1–95.
3. Roger VL, Go AS, Lloyd-Jones DM, et al. Heart disease and stroke statistics–2011 update: a report from the American Heart Association. Circulation 2011;123:e18–209.
4. Rogers WJ, Frederick PD, Stoehr E, et al. Trends in presenting characteristics and hospital mortality among patients with ST elevation and non-ST elevation myocardial infarction in the National Registry of Myocardial Infarction from 1990 to 2006. Am Heart J 2008;156:1026–34.
5. Mosca L, Linfante AH, Benjamin EJ, et al. National study of physician awareness and adherence to cardiovascular disease prevention guidelines. Circulation 2005;111:499–510.
6. Lerner DJ, Kannel WB. Patterns of coronary heart disease morbidity and mortality in the sexes: a 26-year follow-up of the Framingham population. Am Heart J 1986;111:383–90.
7. Kannel WB. The Framingham Study: historical insight on the impact of cardiovascular risk factors in men versus women. J Gend Specif Med 2002;5:27–37.
8. Hochman JS, Tamis JE, Thompson TD, et al. Sex, clinical presentation, and outcome in patients with acute coronary syndromes. Global Use of Strategies to Open Occluded Coronary Arteries in Acute Coronary Syndromes IIb Investigators. N Engl J Med 1999;341:226–32.
9. Akhter N, Milford-Beland S, Roe MT, et al. Gender differences among patients with acute coronary syndromes undergoing percutaneous coronary intervention in the American College of Cardiology-National Cardiovascular Data Registry (ACC-NCDR). Am Heart J 2009;157:141–8.
10. Chang WC, Kaul P, Westerhout CM, et al. Impact of sex on long-term mortality from acute myocardial infarction vs unstable angina. Arch Intern Med 2003;163:2476–84.
11. Douglas PS, Ginsburg GS. The evaluation of chest pain in women. N Engl J Med 1996;334:1311–5.
12. Milner KA, Funk M, Richards S, et al. Gender differences in symptom presentation associated with coronary heart disease. Am J Cardiol 1999;84:396–9.
13. Chen W, Woods SL, Puntillo KA. Gender differences in symptoms associated with acute myocardial infarction: a review of the research. Heart Lung 2005;34:240–7.
14. Dey S, Flather MD, Devlin G, et al. Sex-related differences in the presentation, treatment and outcomes among patients with acute coronary syndromes: the Global Registry of Acute Coronary Events. Heart 2009;95:20–6.
15. Dittrich H, Gilpin E, Nicod P, et al. Acute myocardial infarction in women: influence of gender on mortality and prognostic variables. Am J Cardiol 1988;62:1–7.
16. Fiebach NH, Viscoli CM, Horwitz RI. Differences between women and men in survival after myocardial infarction. Biology or methodology? JAMA 1990;263:1092–6.
17. Meischke H, Larsen MP, Eisenberg MS. Gender differences in reported symptoms for acute myocardial infarction: impact on prehospital delay time interval. Am J Emerg Med 1998;16:363–6.
18. Mosca L, Manson JE, Sutherland SE, et al. Cardiovascular disease in women: a statement for healthcare professionals from the American Heart Association. Writing Group. Circulation 1997;96:2468–82.
19. Milner KA, Vaccarino V, Arnold AL, et al. Gender and age differences in chief complaints of acute myocardial infarction (Worcester Heart Attack Study). Am J Cardiol 2004;93:606–8.
20. Stramba-Badiale M, Bonazzi O, Casadei G, et al. Prevalence of episodes of ST-segment depression among mild-to-moderate hypertensive patients in northern Italy: the Cardioscreening Study. J Hypertens 1998;16:681–8.
21. Canto JG, Rogers WJ, Goldberg RJ, et al. Association of age and sex with myocardial infarction symptom presentation and in-hospital mortality. JAMA 2012;307:813–22.
22. Kannel WB. Silent myocardial ischemia and infarction: insights from the Framingham Study. Cardiol Clin 1986;4:583–91.
23. Kannel WB, Dannenberg AL, Abbott RD. Unrecognized myocardial infarction and hypertension: the Framingham Study. Am Heart J 1985;109:581–5.

24. Indications for fibrinolytic therapy in suspected acute myocardial infarction: collaborative overview of early mortality and major morbidity results from all randomised trials of more than 1000 patients. Fibrinolytic Therapy Trialists' (FTT) Collaborative Group. Lancet 1994;343:311–22.
25. Gibler WB, Armstrong PW, Ohman EM, et al. Persistence of delays in presentation and treatment for patients with acute myocardial infarction: The GUSTO-I and GUSTO-III experience. Ann Emerg Med 2002;39:123–30.
26. Goldberg RJ, Gurwitz JH, Gore JM. Duration of, and temporal trends (1994-1997) in, prehospital delay in patients with acute myocardial infarction: the second National Registry of Myocardial Infarction. Arch Intern Med 1999;159:2141–7.
27. Heer T, Schiele R, Schneider S, et al. Gender differences in acute myocardial infarction in the era of reperfusion (the MITRA registry). Am J Cardiol 2002;89:511–7.
28. Leizorovicz A, Haugh MC, Mercier C, et al. Pre-hospital and hospital time delays in thrombolytic treatment in patients with suspected acute myocardial infarction. Analysis of data from the EMIP study. European Myocardial Infarction Project. Eur Heart J 1997;18:248–53.
29. Sheifer SE, Rathore SS, Gersh BJ, et al. Time to presentation with acute myocardial infarction in the elderly: associations with race, sex, and socioeconomic characteristics. Circulation 2000;102: 1651–6.
30. Sadowski M, Gasior M, Gierlotka M, et al. Gender-related differences in mortality after ST-segment elevation myocardial infarction: a large multicentre national registry. EuroIntervention 2011;6: 1068–72.
31. Bowker TJ, Turner RM, Wood DA, et al. A national Survey of Acute Myocardial Infarction and Ischaemia (SAMII) in the U.K.: characteristics, management and in-hospital outcome in women compared to men in patients under 70 years. Eur Heart J 2000;21:1458–63.
32. Marrugat J, Sala J, Masia R, et al. Mortality differences between men and women following first myocardial infarction. RESCATE Investigators. Recursos Empleados en el Sindrome Coronario Agudo y Tiempo de Espera. JAMA 1998;280:1405–9.
33. Karlson BW, Herlitz J, Hartford M. Prognosis in myocardial infarction in relation to gender. Am Heart J 1994;128:477–83.
34. Williams JK, Adams MR, Klopfenstein HS. Estrogen modulates responses of atherosclerotic coronary arteries. Circulation 1990;81:1680–7.
35. Burke AP, Farb A, Malcom G, et al. Effect of menopause on plaque morphologic characteristics in coronary atherosclerosis. Am Heart J 2001;141: S58–62.
36. Benamer H, Tafflet M, Bataille S, et al. Female gender is an independent predictor of in-hospital mortality after STEMI in the era of primary PCI: insights from the greater Paris area PCI Registry. EuroIntervention 2011;6:1073–9.
37. Jneid H, Fonarow GC, Cannon CP, et al. Sex differences in medical care and early death after acute myocardial infarction. Circulation 2008;118: 2803–10.
38. Lincoff AM, Califf RM, Ellis SG, et al. Thrombolytic therapy for women with myocardial infarction: is there a gender gap? Thrombolysis and Angioplasty in Myocardial Infarction Study Group. J Am Coll Cardiol 1993;22:1780–7.
39. Lansky AJ, Mehran R, Cristea E, et al. Impact of gender and antithrombin strategy on early and late clinical outcomes in patients with non-ST-elevation acute coronary syndromes (from the ACUITY trial). Am J Cardiol 2009;103:1196–203.
40. Lansky AJ, Ng VG, Maehara A, et al. Gender and the extent of coronary atherosclerosis, plaque composition, and clinical outcomes in acute coronary syndromes. JACC Cardiovasc Imaging 2012;5:S62–72.
41. Virmani R, Burke AP, Kolodgie FD, et al. Pathology of the thin-cap fibroatheroma: a type of vulnerable plaque. J Interv Cardiol 2003;16:267–72.
42. Mautner SL, Lin F, Mautner GC, et al. Comparison in women versus men of composition of atherosclerotic plaques in native coronary arteries and in saphenous veins used as aortocoronary conduits. J Am Coll Cardiol 1993;21:1312–8.
43. Kornowski R, Lansky AJ, Mintz GS, et al. Comparison of men versus women in cross-sectional area luminal narrowing, quantity of plaque, presence of calcium in plaque, and lumen location in coronary arteries by intravascular ultrasound in patients with stable angina pectoris. Am J Cardiol 1997;79: 1601–5.
44. Nicholls SJ, Wolski K, Sipahi I, et al. Rate of progression of coronary atherosclerotic plaque in women. J Am Coll Cardiol 2007;49:1546–51.
45. Qian J, Maehara A, Mintz GS, et al. Impact of gender and age on in vivo virtual histology-intravascular ultrasound imaging plaque characterization (from the global Virtual Histology Intravascular Ultrasound [VH-IVUS] registry). Am J Cardiol 2009;103:1210–4.
46. Cheruvu PK, Finn AV, Gardner C, et al. Frequency and distribution of thin-cap fibroatheroma and ruptured plaques in human coronary arteries: a pathologic study. J Am Coll Cardiol 2007;50: 940–9.
47. Farb A, Burke AP, Tang AL, et al. Coronary plaque erosion without rupture into a lipid core. A frequent cause of coronary thrombosis in sudden coronary death. Circulation 1996;93:1354–63.

48. Kramer MC, Rittersma SZ, de Winter RJ, et al. Relationship of thrombus healing to underlying plaque morphology in sudden coronary death. J Am Coll Cardiol 2010;55:122–32.
49. Gurfinkel E, Vigliano C, Janavel JV, et al. Presence of vulnerable coronary plaques in middle-aged individuals who suffered a brain death. Eur Heart J 2009;30:2845–53.
50. Hayashi T, Kiyoshima T, Matsuura M, et al. Plaque erosion in the culprit lesion is prone to develop a smaller myocardial infarction size compared with plaque rupture. Am Heart J 2005;149:284–90.
51. Kojima S, Nonogi H, Miyao Y, et al. Is preinfarction angina related to the presence or absence of coronary plaque rupture? Heart 2000;83:64–8.
52. Murabito JM, Evans JC, Larson MG, et al. Prognosis after the onset of coronary heart disease. An investigation of differences in outcome between the sexes according to initial coronary disease presentation. Circulation 1993;88:2548–55.
53. Greenland P, Reicher-Reiss H, Goldbourt U, et al. In-hospital and 1-year mortality in 1,524 women after myocardial infarction. Comparison with 4,315 men. Circulation 1991;83:484–91.
54. Maynard C, Every NR, Martin JS, et al. Association of gender and survival in patients with acute myocardial infarction. Arch Intern Med 1997;157: 1379–84.
55. Kannel WB, Sorlie P, McNamara PM. Prognosis after initial myocardial infarction: the Framingham study. Am J Cardiol 1979;44:53–9.
56. Puletti M, Sunseri L, Curione M, et al. Acute myocardial infarction: sex-related differences in prognosis. Am Heart J 1984;108:63–6.
57. Tofler GH, Stone PH, Muller JE, et al. Effects of gender and race on prognosis after myocardial infarction: adverse prognosis for women, particularly black women. J Am Coll Cardiol 1987;9:473–82.
58. Malacrida R, Genoni M, Maggioni AP, et al. A comparison of the early outcome of acute myocardial infarction in women and men. The Third International Study of Infarct Survival Collaborative Group. N Engl J Med 1998;338:8–14.
59. Gottlieb S, Harpaz D, Shotan A, et al. Sex differences in management and outcome after acute myocardial infarction in the 1990s: a prospective observational community-based study. Israeli Thrombolytic Survey Group. Circulation 2000;102: 2484–90.
60. Wilkinson P, Laji K, Ranjadayalan K, et al. Acute myocardial infarction in women: survival analysis in first six months. BMJ 1994;309:566–9.
61. Becker RC, Terrin M, Ross R, et al. Comparison of clinical outcomes for women and men after acute myocardial infarction. The Thrombolysis in Myocardial Infarction Investigators. Ann Intern Med 1994; 120:638–45.
62. Goldberg RJ, Gorak EJ, Yarzebski J, et al. A communitywide perspective of sex differences and temporal trends in the incidence and survival rates after acute myocardial infarction and out-of-hospital deaths caused by coronary heart disease. Circulation 1993;87:1947–53.
63. MacAlpin RN, Abbasi AS, Grollman JH Jr, et al. Human coronary artery size during life. A cinearteriographic study. Radiology 1973;108:567–76.
64. Roberts CS, Roberts WC. Cross-sectional area of the proximal portions of the three major epicardial coronary arteries in 98 necropsy patients with different coronary events. Relationship to heart weight, age and sex. Circulation 1980;62:953–9.
65. Dodge JT Jr, Brown BG, Bolson EL, et al. Lumen diameter of normal human coronary arteries. Influence of age, sex, anatomic variation, and left ventricular hypertrophy or dilation. Circulation 1992;86:232–46.
66. Robertson T, Kennard ED, Mehta S, et al. Influence of gender on in-hospital clinical and angiographic outcomes and on one-year follow-up in the New Approaches to Coronary Intervention (NACI) registry. Am J Cardiol 1997;80:26K–39K.
67. Ilia R, Bigham H, Brennan J, et al. Predictors of coronary dissection following percutaneous transluminal coronary balloon angioplasty. Cardiology 1994;85:229–34.
68. Ellis SG, Ajluni S, Arnold AZ, et al. Increased coronary perforation in the new device era. Incidence, classification, management, and outcome. Circulation 1994;90:2725–30.
69. Robinson K, Conroy RM, Mulcahy R, et al. Risk factors and in-hospital course of first episode of myocardial infarction or acute coronary insufficiency in women. J Am Coll Cardiol 1988;11:932–6.
70. Halvorsen S, Eritsland J, Abdelnoor M, et al. Gender differences in management and outcome of acute myocardial infarctions treated in 2006-2007. Cardiology 2009;114:83–8.
71. Vaccarino V, Krumholz HM, Berkman LF, et al. Sex differences in mortality after myocardial infarction. Is there evidence for an increased risk for women? Circulation 1995;91:1861–71.
72. MacIntyre K, Stewart S, Capewell S, et al. Gender and survival: a population-based study of 201,114 men and women following a first acute myocardial infarction. J Am Coll Cardiol 2001;38: 729–35.
73. Kralev S, Hennig O, Lang S, et al. Sex-based differences in clinical and angiographic outcomes in patients with ST-elevation myocardial infarction treated with concomitant use of glycoprotein IIb/IIIa inhibitors. Cardiol J 2010;17:580–6.
74. Sjauw KD, Stegenga NK, Engstrom AE, et al. The influence of gender on short- and long-term outcome after primary PCI and delivered medical

care for ST-segment elevation myocardial infarction. EuroIntervention 2010;5:780–7.

75. Suessenbacher A, Doerler J, Alber H, et al. Gender-related outcome following percutaneous coronary intervention for ST-elevation myocardial infarction: data from the Austrian acute PCI registry. EuroIntervention 2008;4:271–6.
76. Barakat K, Wilkinson P, Suliman A, et al. Acute myocardial infarction in women: contribution of treatment variables to adverse outcome. Am Heart J 2000;140:740–6.
77. Vaccarino V, Horwitz RI, Meehan TP, et al. Sex differences in mortality after myocardial infarction: evidence for a sex-age interaction. Arch Intern Med 1998;158:2054–62.
78. Vaccarino V, Krumholz HM, Yarzebski J, et al. Sex differences in 2-year mortality after hospital discharge for myocardial infarction. Ann Intern Med 2001;134:173–81.
79. Vaccarino V, Parsons L, Every NR, et al. Sex-based differences in early mortality after myocardial infarction. National Registry of Myocardial Infarction 2 Participants. N Engl J Med 1999;341:217–25.
80. Berger JS, Brown DL. Gender-age interaction in early mortality following primary angioplasty for acute myocardial infarction. Am J Cardiol 2006; 98:1140–3.
81. Vaccarino V, Parsons L, Peterson ED, et al. Sex differences in mortality after acute myocardial infarction: changes from 1994 to 2006. Arch Intern Med 2009;169:1767–74.
82. Simon T, Mary-Krause M, Cambou JP, et al. Impact of age and gender on in-hospital and late mortality after acute myocardial infarction: increased early risk in younger women: results from the French nation-wide USIC registries. Eur Heart J 2006;27: 1282–8.
83. Kostis JB, Wilson AC, O'Dowd K, et al. Sex differences in the management and long-term outcome of acute myocardial infarction. A statewide study. MIDAS Study Group. Myocardial Infarction Data Acquisition System. Circulation 1994;90:1715–30.
84. Lichtman JH, Lorenze NP, D'Onofrio G, et al. Variation in recovery: role of gender on outcomes of young AMI patients (VIRGO) study design. Circ Cardiovasc Qual Outcomes 2010;3:684–93.
85. Lansky AJ, Hochman JS, Ward PA, et al. Percutaneous coronary intervention and adjunctive pharmacotherapy in women: a statement for healthcare professionals from the American Heart Association. Circulation 2005;111:940–53.
86. Rathore SS, Berger AK, Weinfurt KP, et al. Race, sex, poverty, and the medical treatment of acute myocardial infarction in the elderly. Circulation 2000;102:642–8.
87. Gan SC, Beaver SK, Houck PM, et al. Treatment of acute myocardial infarction and 30-day mortality among women and men. N Engl J Med 2000;343: 8–15.
88. Chandra NC, Ziegelstein RC, Rogers WJ, et al. Observations of the treatment of women in the United States with myocardial infarction: a report from the National Registry of Myocardial Infarction-I. Arch Intern Med 1998;158:981–8.
89. Maynard C, Litwin PE, Martin JS, et al. Gender differences in the treatment and outcome of acute myocardial infarction. Results from the Myocardial Infarction Triage and Intervention Registry. Arch Intern Med 1992;152:972–6.
90. Kudenchuk PJ, Maynard C, Martin JS, et al. Comparison of presentation, treatment, and outcome of acute myocardial infarction in men versus women (the Myocardial Infarction Triage and Intervention Registry). Am J Cardiol 1996;78:9–14.
91. Udvarhelyi IS, Gatsonis C, Epstein AM, et al. Acute myocardial infarction in the Medicare population. Process of care and clinical outcomes. JAMA 1992;268:2530–6.
92. Weitzman S, Cooper L, Chambless L, et al. Gender, racial, and geographic differences in the performance of cardiac diagnostic and therapeutic procedures for hospitalized acute myocardial infarction in four states. Am J Cardiol 1997;79: 722–6.
93. Fang J, Alderman MH. Gender differences of revascularization in patients with acute myocardial infarction. Am J Cardiol 2006;97:1722–6.
94. Peterson ED, Shah BR, Parsons L, et al. Trends in quality of care for patients with acute myocardial infarction in the National Registry of Myocardial Infarction from 1990 to 2006. Am Heart J 2008; 156:1045–55.
95. Rathore SS, Wang Y, Radford MJ, et al. Sex differences in cardiac catheterization after acute myocardial infarction: the role of procedure appropriateness. Ann Intern Med 2002;137:487–93.
96. Gurwitz JH, Col NF, Avorn J. The exclusion of the elderly and women from clinical trials in acute myocardial infarction. JAMA 1992;268:1417–22.
97. Lee PY, Alexander KP, Hammill BG, et al. Representation of elderly persons and women in published randomized trials of acute coronary syndromes. JAMA 2001;286:708–13.
98. Randomized trial of intravenous streptokinase, oral aspirin, both, or neither among 17,187 cases of suspected acute myocardial infarction: ISIS-2.ISIS-2 (Second International Study of Infarct Survival) Collaborative Group. J Am Coll Cardiol 1988;12:3A–13A.
99. Long-term effects of intravenous thrombolysis in acute myocardial infarction: final report of the GISSI study. Gruppo Italiano per lo Studio della Streptochi-nasi nell'Infarto Miocardico (GISSI). Lancet 1987;2:871–4.

100. Wilcox RG, von der Lippe G, Olsson CG, et al. Trial of tissue plasminogen activator for mortality reduction in acute myocardial infarction. Anglo-Scandinavian Study of Early Thrombolysis (ASSET). Lancet 1988;2:525–30.
101. Kennedy JW, Ritchie JL, Davis KB, et al. The western Washington randomized trial of intracoronary streptokinase in acute myocardial infarction. A 12-month follow-up report. N Engl J Med 1985; 312:1073–8.
102. Weaver WD, White HD, Wilcox RG, et al. Comparisons of characteristics and outcomes among women and men with acute myocardial infarction treated with thrombolytic therapy. GUSTO-I investigators. JAMA 1996;275:777–82.
103. Woodfield SL, Lundergan CF, Reiner JS, et al. Gender and acute myocardial infarction: is there a different response to thrombolysis? J Am Coll Cardiol 1997;29:35–42.
104. Murphy SA, Chen C, Cannon CP, et al. Impact of gender on angiographic and clinical outcomes after fibrinolytic therapy in acute myocardial infarction. Am J Cardiol 2002;90:766–70.
105. White HD, Barbash GI, Modan M, et al. After correcting for worse baseline characteristics, women treated with thrombolytic therapy for acute myocardial infarction have the same mortality and morbidity as men except for a higher incidence of hemorrhagic stroke. The Investigators of the International Tissue Plasminogen Activator/Streptokinase Mortality Study. Circulation 1993;88:2097–103.
106. Brass LM, Lichtman JH, Wang Y, et al. Intracranial hemorrhage associated with thrombolytic therapy for elderly patients with acute myocardial infarction: results from the Cooperative Cardiovascular Project. Stroke 2000;31:1802–11.
107. Gurwitz JH, Gore JM, Goldberg RJ, et al. Risk for intracranial hemorrhage after tissue plasminogen activator treatment for acute myocardial infarction. Participants in the National Registry of Myocardial Infarction 2. Ann Intern Med 1998;129:597–604.
108. Topol EJ, Califf RM, George BS, et al. A randomized trial of immediate versus delayed elective angioplasty after intravenous tissue plasminogen activator in acute myocardial infarction. N Engl J Med 1987;317:581–8.
109. Grines CL, Nissen SE, Booth DC, et al. A prospective, randomized trial comparing combination half-dose tissue-type plasminogen activator and streptokinase with full-dose tissue-type plasminogen activator. Kentucky Acute Myocardial Infarction Trial (KAMIT) Group. Circulation 1991;84:540–9.
110. Carney RJ, Murphy GA, Brandt TR, et al. Randomized angiographic trial of recombinant tissue-type plasminogen activator (alteplase) in myocardial infarction. RAAMI Study Investigators. J Am Coll Cardiol 1992;20:17–23.
111. Zijlstra F, de Boer MJ, Hoorntje JC, et al. A comparison of immediate coronary angioplasty with intravenous streptokinase in acute myocardial infarction. N Engl J Med 1993;328:680–4.
112. The effects of tissue plasminogen activator, streptokinase, or both on coronary-artery patency, ventricular function, and survival after acute myocardial infarction. The GUSTO Angiographic Investigators. N Engl J Med 1993;329:1615–22.
113. Stone GW, Grines CL, Browne KF, et al. Implications of recurrent ischemia after reperfusion therapy in acute myocardial infarction: a comparison of thrombolytic therapy and primary angioplasty. J Am Coll Cardiol 1995;26:66–72.
114. Simoons ML, Serruys PW, van den Brand M, et al. Early thrombolysis in acute myocardial infarction: limitation of infarct size and improved survival. J Am Coll Cardiol 1986;7:717–28.
115. Schroder R, Neuhaus KL, Leizorovicz A, et al. A prospective placebo-controlled double-blind multicenter trial of intravenous streptokinase in acute myocardial infarction (ISAM): long-term mortality and morbidity. J Am Coll Cardiol 1987;9: 197–203.
116. Grines CL, Browne KF, Marco J, et al. A comparison of immediate angioplasty with thrombolytic therapy for acute myocardial infarction. The Primary Angioplasty in Myocardial Infarction Study Group. N Engl J Med 1993;328:673–9.
117. Zijlstra F, Hoorntje JC, de Boer MJ, et al. Long-term benefit of primary angioplasty as compared with thrombolytic therapy for acute myocardial infarction. N Engl J Med 1999;341:1413–9.
118. Rogers WJ, Baim DS, Gore JM, et al. Comparison of immediate invasive, delayed invasive, and conservative strategies after tissue-type plasminogen activator. Results of the Thrombolysis in Myocardial Infarction (TIMI) Phase II-A trial. Circulation 1990;81:1457–76.
119. O'Neill W, Timmis GC, Bourdillon PD, et al. A prospective randomized clinical trial of intracoronary streptokinase versus coronary angioplasty for acute myocardial infarction. N Engl J Med 1986; 314:812–8.
120. Weaver WD, Simes RJ, Betriu A, et al. Comparison of primary coronary angioplasty and intravenous thrombolytic therapy for acute myocardial infarction: a quantitative review. JAMA 1997;278:2093–8.
121. Andersen HR, Nielsen TT, Rasmussen K, et al. A comparison of coronary angioplasty with fibrinolytic therapy in acute myocardial infarction. N Engl J Med 2003;349:733–42.
122. Stone GW, Grines CL, Browne KF, et al. Comparison of in-hospital outcome in men versus women treated by either thrombolytic therapy or primary coronary angioplasty for acute myocardial infarction. Am J Cardiol 1995;75:987–92.

123. Vakili BA, Kaplan RC, Brown DL. Sex-based differences in early mortality of patients undergoing primary angioplasty for first acute myocardial infarction. Circulation 2001;104:3034–8.
124. Azar RR, Waters DD, McKay RG, et al. Short- and medium-term outcome differences in women and men after primary percutaneous transluminal mechanical revascularization for acute myocardial infarction. Am J Cardiol 2000;85:675–9.
125. Stone GW, Grines CL, Cox DA, et al. Comparison of angioplasty with stenting, with or without abciximab, in acute myocardial infarction. N Engl J Med 2002;346:957–66.
126. Keeley EC, Boura JA, Grines CL. Primary angioplasty versus intravenous thrombolytic therapy for acute myocardial infarction: a quantitative review of 23 randomised trials. Lancet 2003;361:13–20.
127. Antoniucci D, Valenti R, Moschi G, et al. Sex-based differences in clinical and angiographic outcomes after primary angioplasty or stenting for acute myocardial infarction. Am J Cardiol 2001;87: 289–93.
128. Lansky AJ, Pietras C, Costa RA, et al. Gender differences in outcomes after primary angioplasty versus primary stenting with and without abciximab for acute myocardial infarction: results of the Controlled Abciximab and Device Investigation to Lower Late Angioplasty Complications (CADILLAC) trial. Circulation 2005;111:1611–8.
129. Bufe A, Wolfertz J, Dinh W, et al. Gender-based differences in long-term outcome after ST-elevation myocardial infarction in patients treated with percutaneous coronary intervention. J Womens Health (Larchmt) 2010;19:471–5.
130. Onuma Y, Kukreja N, Daemen J, et al. Impact of sex on 3-year outcome after percutaneous coronary intervention using bare-metal and drug-eluting stents in previously untreated coronary artery disease: insights from the RESEARCH (Rapamycin-Eluting Stent Evaluated at Rotterdam Cardiology Hospital) and T-SEARCH (Taxus-Stent Evaluated at Rotterdam Cardiology Hospital) Registries. JACC Cardiovasc Interv 2009;2: 603–10.
131. Woo JS, Kim W, Ha SJ, et al. Impact of gender differences on long-term outcomes after successful percutaneous coronary intervention in patients with acute myocardial infarction. Int J Cardiol 2010;145:516–8.
132. Ferrante G, Presbitero P, Corrada E, et al. Sex-specific benefits of sirolimus-eluting stent on long-term outcomes in patients with ST-elevation myocardial infarction undergoing primary percutaneous coronary intervention: insights from the Multicenter Evaluation of Single High-Dose Bolus Tirofiban Versus Abciximab With Sirolimus-Eluting Stent or Bare-Metal Stent in Acute Myocardial Infarction Study trial. Am Heart J 2012;163:104–11.
133. Ahmed B, Piper WD, Malenka D, et al. Significantly improved vascular complications among women undergoing percutaneous coronary intervention: a report from the Northern New England Percutaneous Coronary Intervention Registry. Circ Cardiovasc Interv 2009;2:423–9.
134. Argulian E, Patel AD, Abramson JL, et al. Gender differences in short-term cardiovascular outcomes after percutaneous coronary interventions. Am J Cardiol 2006;98:48–53.
135. Pristipino C, Pelliccia F, Granatelli A, et al. Comparison of access-related bleeding complications in women versus men undergoing percutaneous coronary catheterization using the radial versus femoral artery. Am J Cardiol 2007;99:1216–21.
136. Rao SV, Ou FS, Wang TY, et al. Trends in the prevalence and outcomes of radial and femoral approaches to percutaneous coronary intervention: a report from the National Cardiovascular Data Registry. JACC Cardiovasc Interv 2008;1:379–86.

STEMI Interventions via the Radial Route

Tejas Patel, MD, DM, FESC, FSCAI[a,b,*], Sanjay Shah, MD, DM[a,b],
Samir Pancholy, MD, FACC, FSCAI[c]

KEYWORDS

• Transradial approach • STEMI • Coronary intervention

KEY POINTS

- Bleeding complications during percutaneous coronary intervention (PCI) are associated with an increased risk for myocardial infarction (MI), stent thrombosis, stroke, and death, as well as increased costs.
- A large proportion of bleeding complications in patients undergoing PCI is related to vascular access site.
- Patients undergoing ST-elevation myocardial infarction (STEMI) interventions are at the highest risk of bleeding for many reasons, including generous use of anticoagulants, antiplatelets, thrombolytics, and glycoprotein-2b3a-inhibitors.
- A body of literature supports the role of the transradial approach (TRA) for STEMI interventions in reducing bleeding and vascular complications without sacrificing procedural success.
- TRA is likely to offer patients with STEMI exponential benefits, ie, reduction in bleeding and related complications, better quality of life for patients and support staff, as well as cost benefits for the hospital management.

INTRODUCTION AND HISTORICAL PERSPECTIVE

In 1989, Lucien Campeau[1] published his successful series of 100 coronary angiographies performed via the radial route with minimal complications. Subsequently, in 1993 Kiemeneij and Laarman[2] described and published the use of the radial route for percutaneous coronary interventions (PCIs) using 6-F guide catheters in a time when most interventional procedures were performed with larger 8-F guide catheters. Since then, the transradial approach (TRA) for PCI has emerged as an effective alternative to the transfemoral approach (TFA) for practically all subsets of PCI, including multivessel lesions, left main coronary artery (LMCA) lesions, bifurcation lesions, chronic total occlusions (CTO), calcified lesions, and acute coronary syndromes (ACS), including acute ST-elevation myocardial infarction (STEMI).[3–9] Initially, TRA continued to gain popularity in some regions of Europe, Canada, South America, Japan, and South Asia; however, the United States was the last to adopt transradial intervention (TRI).[10–13] Ochiai and colleagues[14] performed the first observational pilot study on TRA for acute myocardial infarction (AMI) interventions. In the past decade,

[a] Department of Cardiovascular Sciences, Apex Heart Institute, Mondeal Business Park, Block G-K Thaltej, S.G. Highway, Ahmedabad, Gujarat 380054, India; [b] Department of Cardiovascular Sciences, Sheth K.M. School of Post Graduate Medicine and Research, Smt. NHL Municipal Medical College, Sheth V.S. General Hospital, Gujarat University, Ellisbridge, Ahmedabad, Gujarat 380001, India; [c] Department of Cardiovascular Sciences, The Commonwealth Medical College, The Wright Center for Graduate Medical Education, 501 Madison Avenue, Scranton, PA 18510, USA

* Corresponding author. Department of Cardiovascular Sciences, Apex Heart Institute, Mondeal Business Park, Block G-K Thaltej, S.G. Highway, Ahmedabad, Gujarat 380054.

E-mail address: tejaspatel@tcvsgroup.org

Intervent Cardiol Clin 1 (2012) 467–477
http://dx.doi.org/10.1016/j.iccl.2012.06.011
2211-7458/12/$ – see front matter

interventional.theclinics.com

several studies on TRA for AMI interventions and its randomized comparison with TFA have been published.[4,14–23] This has led to transradial access being considered an equivalent, and likely superior, alternative access site to transfemoral access for primary PCI.

Bleeding as an Independent Predictor of Adverse Outcomes

PCI is one of the most commonly performed cardiac procedures. Since its introduction more than 3 decades ago, a steady evolution has occurred in both devices and pharmacotherapy. Data from large registries have confirmed that periprocedural adverse events have decreased over time.[11–13,24–26] Several studies have shown that bleeding complications during treatment for coronary artery disease are associated with an increased risk for death, AMI, stroke, stent thrombosis, and increased costs.[11–13,24–26] Studies also indicate that a large proportion of bleeding complications in patients undergoing PCI is related to the vascular access site.[12,13] Therefore, strategies that address this issue may potentially reduce bleeding and vascular complications and improve PCI outcomes. Hence, bleeding, blood transfusions, and related complications have become clinical priority. A summary of evidence is described in the remainder of this section.

The National Heart, Lung and Blood Institute Dynamic Registry evaluated the relationship between access-site hematomas requiring blood transfusions and in-hospital and 1-year mortality.[10] This included data on 6656 patients and captured 120 hematomas requiring transfusion with an incidence of 1.8%; 97% of the patients with hematomas had femoral artery access. In-hospital mortality was about 9 times higher in those with hematomas requiring blood transfusions than in those without (9.9% vs 1.2%). Similarly, at 1 year, mortality among those who developed hematoma requiring transfusion was approximately 4.5 times higher than those who had not (18.8% vs 9.9%). After adjustment for demographic, clinical, angiographic, and procedural variables, hematomas requiring transfusion remained an independent predictor of death both within the hospital (odds ratio [OR] = 3.59, 95%, confidence interval [CI] = 1.66–7.77) and at 1 year (hazard ratio [HR] = 1.65, 95% CI 1.01–2.70).

The Acute Catheterization and Urgent Intervention Triage strategY (ACUITY) trial showed a 30-day analysis of the impact of major bleeding on mortality and clinical outcomes.[11] In this study, major bleeding was an independent predictor of 30-day mortality with an OR of 7.55 (95% CI 4.68–12.18, *P*<.0001). Those patients with major bleeding had a higher 30-day mortality (7.3% vs 1.2%, *P*<0.0001) than patients without major bleeding. In addition, at 30 days those with major bleeding had higher rates of composite ischemia, defined as death, MI, or unplanned revascularization for ischemia (23.1% versus 6.8%, *P*<0.0001), as well as stent thrombosis (3.4% vs 0.6%, *P*<0.0001).

The MORTAL (Mortality benefit Of Reduced Transfusion after percutaneous coronary intervention via the Arm or Leg) study by Chase and colleagues[12] reported on reductions in mortality, likely mediated through reduced transfusions after PCIs performed through TRA when compared with TFA. The study evaluated 38,872 PCI procedures in 32,822 patients in British Columbia. TFA was used in 79.5% of PCI and TRA in 20.5%. In the TFA group, 2.8% of procedures were complicated by the need for periprocedural transfusions, whereas in the TRA group only 1.4% of the procedures were associated with a transfusion. Thus, the transfusion rate was 50% lower in the TRA group. The reduced transfusion rate was associated with a significant reduction in mortality at 30 days and 1 year. The death rates at 30 days of the transfused group versus the nontransfused group were 12.6% and 1.3% respectively. At 1 year, the death rates were 22.9% and 3.2%. The adjusted OR for death at 30 days in the transfused group versus the nontransfused group was 4.01 (95% CI 3.08–5.22) and at 1 year was 3.58 (95% CI 2.94–4.36). The number of transfusions that must be avoided to prevent 1 death (number needed to treat) calculated to be approximately 15 transfusions.

Rao and colleagues[13] retrospectively analyzed data from 593,094 procedures in the National Cardiovascular Data Registry (606 sites; 2004–2007). They evaluated trends in use and outcomes of TRA to PCI. TRA was associated with a procedural success rate similar to TFA and with significantly lower rates of bleeding and vascular complications, even among high-risk groups, such as elderly patients, women, and patients with ACS. Compared with the femoral approach, the radial approach had a significantly lower risk of bleeding (OR = 0.42, 95% CI 0.31–0.56).

A meta-analysis comparing TRA versus TFA for PCI performed by Agostoni and colleagues[24] identified 12 studies that met their criteria for inclusion. The primary outcomes evaluated were major adverse cardiac events (MACE), access site complications, including bleeding, and procedural success. The MACE rate in the TRA and TFA groups was not significantly different, at 2.4% and 2.1% respectively. However, there were significantly fewer access-site complications in the TRA group (0.3%) compared with the TFA group (2.8%) with an OR of 0.20 (95% CI 0.09–0.42, $P<.0001$).

Jolly and colleagues[25] evaluated 23 randomized trials comparing TRA to TFA and analyzed its impact on major bleeding and ischemic events. There was a 73% reduction in major bleeding in the TRA group (0.05% vs 2.3%, OR = 0.27, 95% CI 0.16–0.45). Also noted was a nonstatistically significant reduction in the rates of death, myocardial infarction, and stroke.

Eikelboom and colleagues[26] evaluated the impact of bleeding on prognosis in 34,146 patients with acute coronary syndrome by combining patient data from the Organization to Assess Strategies in Acute Ischemic Syndromes (OASIS) Registry, OASIS-2 trial, and Clopidogrel in Unstable Angina to prevent Recurrent Events (CURE) trial. A total of 667 (2%) patients developed major bleeding. Those with major bleeding were 5 times more likely to die within the first 30 days (12.8% vs 2.5%; $P< 0.0001$) and 1.5 times more likely to die between 30 days and 6 months (4.6% vs 2.9%; $P< 0.002$).

In a nutshell, periprocedural bleeding after PCI remains a significant complication, having an adverse impact on short-term and long-term outcomes. It is also noteworthy that patients with AMI are at the highest risk for bleeding for multiple reasons, but particularly related to anticoagulation/antiplatelet/thrombolytic status and the emergent nature of their procedures. It is also troublesome that bleeding complications in this patient subset are more likely to be associated with repeat ischemia, as well as short-term and long-term adverse cardiac events, including mortality. TRA for PCI has repeatedly shown reduction in bleeding complications and improvement in clinical outcomes, including mortality.

TRA FOR STEMI INTERVENTIONS: WHAT IS THE EVIDENCE?

Kelley and colleagues,[15] in their quantitative review of 23 randomized trials, demonstrated that earlier treatment of STEMI with primary PCI improved outcomes compared with treatment with thrombolysis.

Ochiai and colleagues[14] were the first to perform an observational pilot study to determine if risk-stratified patients with AMI could experience reduced bleeding complications and earlier mobilization with TRI and primary stenting. Fifty-six patients with Killip Class I or II were subjected to TRA for AMI interventions with 100% success in stent deployment and 97% success in normalization of distal coronary blood flow. No major vascular complications occurred in this experience.

Phillippe and colleagues[16] showed similar results in their series of 119 consecutive patients with AMI having primary PCI via the radial (64 patients) or femoral (55 patients) approach with adjunctive abciximab therapy. Hospital length of stay was higher in the TFI group compared with the TRI group (5.9 vs 4.5 days respectively, $P = 0.05$). There were no vascular complications in the TRI group, compared with 3 (5.5%) in the TFI group ($P = 0.04$). They did observe longer radiation exposure times in the TRI cohort.

Cruden and associates[17] published their registry observations in 287 patients having rescue PCI in patients with unsuccessful thrombolysis for AMI. In this retrospective analysis, procedural success was similar for TRI and TFI (98% vs 93%, $P = 0.3$); however, vascular complication rate (0% vs 13%, $P<0.01$) and length of stay (7.0 vs 7.9 days, $P<0.005$) favored TRI over TFI.

The TEMPURA (test for myocardial infarction by prospective unicenter randomization for access sites) study by Saito and colleagues[18] randomized 149 patients with AMI less than 12 hours from onset, to TRI (n = 77) or TFI (n = 72). Procedural success (TRI of 96.1% vs TFI of 97.1%, P = NS) and adverse cardiac events (TRI of 5.2% vs TFI of 8.3%, P = NS) were similar between these groups. Severe bleeding was seen in 3% patients with TFI and none with TRI. Procedural time was slightly shorter with TRI as compared with TFI in this series.

Cantor and colleagues,[19] in the forearm artery (RADIAL) AMI pilot study, randomized 50 patients having primary or rescue PCI to TRI or TFI approaches. No major bleeding or transfusion was required in either group. Procedural time slightly favored TFI over TRI. Final TIMI flow, contrast, and fluoroscopy time were similar for TRI and TFI.

Yan and colleagues[20] compared TRA with TFA in elderly (age ≥65 years) Chinese patients undergoing AMI interventions. There was no statistically significant difference between the 2 groups for success rate, puncture time, cannulation time, reperfusion time, and total procedural time. However, hospital stay was longer with TFA as compared with TRA (10.1 ± 4.6 days vs 7.2 ± 2.6 days, $P<0.01$), and vascular access site–related complications were higher in the TFA group (13.1% vs 1.8%, $P<0.05$).

De Carlo and colleagues[21] published results of a prospective registry enrolling patients presenting with an ACS, either STEMI or high-risk non-ST-segment elevation acute coronary syndromes (NSTEACS) treated with either abciximab or tirofiban in addition to standard medical therapy, who underwent urgent/emergency PCI through the TRI in a span of 2 years. All possible high-risk subsets, including patients older than 80 years, patients undergoing rescue PCI after failed thrombolysis, and patients with cardiogenic shock were enrolled. The results of this study demonstrated that TRA allows for near-abolition of vascular access bleeding and blood transfusion rates without any negative impact on procedural success rate, procedural duration, or 1-year clinical outcome.

Weaver and colleagues[22] compared TRA versus TFA for time to intervention for patients presenting with AMI. Of 240 total patients, 205 underwent successful PCI (124 in the TRA group, 116 in the TFA group). No significant difference was observed in pre-catheterization laboratory times. Mean case start times for the TRA group was significantly longer (12.5 ± 5.4 minutes for TRA vs 10.5 ± 5.7 minutes for TFA, $P = 0.005$) owing to patient preparation. Once arterial access was obtained, balloon inflation occurred faster in the TRA group (18.3 vs 24.1 minutes, $P<0.001$). Total time from patient arrival to the catheterization laboratory to PCI was reduced in the TRA group as compared with the TFA group (28.4 vs 32.7 minutes, $P = 0.01$). There was a small but statistically significant difference in door-to-balloon time (TRA group: 76.4 minutes versus the TFA group: 86.5 minutes, $P<0.008$) favoring TRA. The TRA group also had shorter fluoroscopy times as compared with the TFA group (12.5 ± 7.9 minutes vs 15.2 ± 10.1 minutes, $P = 0.02$).

Pancholy and colleagues[23] compared door-to-balloon times for primary PCI using TRA versus TFA. A total of 313 consecutive patients with STEMI undergoing primary PCI were divided into 2 groups, group 1 (n = 204) undergoing PCI using TFA and group 2 (n = 109) undergoing PCI using TRA. Door-to-balloon time was 72 ± 14 minutes in group I compared with 70 ± 17 minutes in group II; the difference was not statistically significant ($P>.27$). Group II patients had significantly fewer access site complications compared with group I ($P<.05$). Demographics, predischarge adverse events, and MACE at 1-year follow-up were comparable between the 2 groups.

Siudak and colleagues[27] gathered and analyzed consecutive data on patients with STEMI transferred for primary PCI in hospital STEMI networks between November 2005 and January 2007 from 7 countries in Europe (EUROTRANSFER registry). A total of 1650 patients were studied. Abciximab was administered in 1086 patients (66%), 169 patients were assigned to TRA, whereas 917 were assigned to TFA. Puncture site hematomas were more frequent in the TFA group (1.2 vs 9.4% $P<.001$). Major bleedings requiring blood transfusion occurred similarly in both groups.

Vin and colleagues[28] examined the feasibility of routine TRA in primary PCI for STEMI in 2209 procedures done between January 2001 and December 2008 in a single high-volume center. In 84 patients (3.8%), access site crossover was needed. Crossover rates decreased from 5.9% in 2001 to 2002 to 1.5% in 2007 to 2008 ($P = .001$). The procedural success rate was 94.1%, which remained stable over the years. Despite an increased complexity of primary PCI, total procedural duration decreased from 38 minutes (interquartile range [IQR] 28–50) in 2001 to 2002, to 24 minutes (IQR 18–33) in 2007 to 2008 ($P<.001$). The study demonstrated that systematic use of TRA in primary PCI yields low access site crossover, high procedural success rates, and excellent procedural performances. Hence, TRA can represent the primary access site in the vast majority of patients with STEMI.

The harmonizing outcomes with revascularization and stents in acute myocardial infarction (HORIZONS-AMI) study investigators did a post hoc analysis of 3340 patients who underwent primary PCI for STEMI.[29] They analyzed the TRA group (n = 200) versus the TFA group (n = 3134) with respect to end points, including the 30-day and 1-year rates of major adverse cardiovascular events (MACE: death, reinfarction, stroke, or target vessel revascularization), non–coronary artery bypass graft (CABG)-related major bleeding, and net adverse clinical events (NACE: MACE or major bleeding). TRA compared with TFA was associated with significantly lower 30-day rates of composite death or reinfarction (1% vs 4.3%, $P = .02$) non–CABG-related major bleeding (3.5% vs 7.6%, $P = .03$), MACE (2% vs 5.6%, $P = .02$) and NACE (5% versus 11.6%, $P = .01$). At 1 year, the TRA group still had significantly reduced rates of death or reinfarction (4.0% vs 7.8%, $P = .05$), non–CABG-related major bleeding (3.5% vs 8.1%, $P = .02$), MACE (6% vs 12.4%, $P<.01$), and NACE (8.5% vs 7.8%, $P<.001$) by multivariable analysis. TRA was an independent predictor of freedom from MACE and NACE at 30 days and 1 year.

Radial versus femoral access for coronary angiography and intervention in patients with acute coronary syndromes (RIVAL) study investigators enrolled 7021 patients with acute coronary syndrome from 158 hospitals in 32 countries; 3507 patients were randomly assigned to the TRA group and 3514 to the TFA group.[30] Although the study concluded that both TRA and TFA are safe and effective for PCI, local vascular complication rate was significantly lower in the TRA group (n = 42 for the TRA group versus n = 106 for the TFA group, $P<.001$). Investigators also observed statistically significant (40%) relative reduction in the risk of death, MI, stroke or non–CABG-related major bleeding and a significant (61%) relative reduction in the risk of death among patients with STEMI treated via the radial route. They also reported a significant reduction in the risk of the primary outcome (51%) among PCI centers that performed the highest volume of radial procedures. The absence of a significant difference in the primary end point in the overall cohort may have been a result of an unusually low access site complication rate in the transfemoral group, underpowering this study for the alternate hypothesis.

The radial versus femoral randomized investigation in ST-elevation acute coronary syndrom (RIFLE-STEACS) study, which was presented at transcatheter cardiovascular therapeutics (TCT) 2011, was a prospective randomized parallel group multicenter trial to evaluate TRA versus TFA for primary PCI.[31] A total of 1001 patients were enrolled and randomized between TRA and TFA. At 30 days, the rate of NACE was significantly lower in the TRA group versus the TFA group (13.6% vs 21%). The lower rate was evidenced by a reduction of both the major adverse cardiac and cerebrovascular evens (7.2% vs 11.4%) and of bleeding (7.8% vs 12.2%). The rate of cardiac death at 30 days was 9.2% in the femoral group and 5.2% in the radial group.

All these studies have shown that TRA for AMI is safe, effective, and reproducible, and has fewer vascular access–related complications as compared with TFA, particularly in the hands of experienced operators and support staff. RIVAL and RIFLE-STEACS have shown a mortality benefit in patients with STEMI undergoing primary PCI via the radial route, compared with the femoral route.

RATIONALE OF USING TRA FOR STEMI INTERVENTIONS

An interventionalist needs a good reason to learn and switch to a new and less-tested technique from a well-established time-tested technique. It took almost 2 decades for TRA to gain universal acceptance. It has proven its superiority over TFA in different technique-related issues, including reduction in local vascular complication rates (minor and major), increase in patient and support staff comfort levels, and reduction in the cost for hospital management.[24,25,32–34] These benefits were achieved in average risk interventions, as well as in difficult and demanding subsets including complex and calcified lesions, LMCA lesions, bifurcation lesions, and so forth.[3–9]

Table 1
Baseline characteristics of patients undergoing TR AMI interventions

Age	64.3 ± 27.0 y
Males	79%
Smokers	34%
Hypertension	35%
Diabetes mellitus	46%
Dyslipidemia	32%
Family history	43%
Infarct Territory	
AWMI	67%
IWMI	24%
LWMI	5%
PWMI	4%
Killip Class at presentation	
Class I	18%
Class II	39%
Class III	34%
Class IV	9%
Mean LVEF	34.6% ± 24%

Abbreviations: AWMI, anterior wall myocardial infarction; IWMI, inferior wall myocardial infarction; LWMI, lateral wall myocardial infarction; PWMI, posterior wall myocardial infarction; LVEF, left ventricular ejection fraction.

TRA and Quality-of-Life and Economic Benefits

Early ambulation has the potential to reduce cost by expediting room turnover/increasing throughput (both in the catheterization laboratory and the recovery unit), decreasing the intensity of care required by nursing and support staff, shortening length of stay, and enhancing the ability to perform same day PCI.[34] It has the additional potential economic benefit of providing a more rapid return to productivity for working patients.

Table 2
Procedural characteristics

Right radial approach	92%
Radial artery cannulation time	1.86 ± 0.44 min
Procedure time (time from sheath insertion to guide catheter removal)	18.3 ± 10.5 min
Fluoroscopy time	6.46 ± 4.3 min
Direct stenting	38%

Table 3
Technical details

Transradial failure	0%
Cross-over to contralateral TRA	0.8%
Cross-over to TFA	0%
Multiple guide catheter exchanges	3.3%
Use of IABP	14%
Use of GP2b3a-inhibitors	
• Abciximab bolus only	21%
• Abciximab bolus followed by infusion	9%
• Eptifibatide bolus followed by infusion	12%

Abbreviations: GP, glycoprotein; IABP, intra-aortic balloon pump; TFA, transfemoral approach; TRA, transradial approach.

AMI intervention is prone to higher bleeding and access site–related complications, particularly through TFA.[12,13,24,25] Large groin hematoma and retroperitoneal hematoma can lead to need for several additional investigations (ie, femoral vascular ultrasound, computed tomography of abdomen/pelvis, laboratory investigations), blood transfusions, and longer hospital stay.[34] This additional cost of treating the complications and prolonged hospital stay can be minimized or eliminated using TRA for AMI interventions.

Cooper and colleagues[32] studied and compared quality-of-life parameters of patients undergoing TFA and TRA. Of patients who have had both TFA and TRA, 80% had a strong preference for TRA, 18% were undecided, and only 2% had a strong preference for TFA. Preference for TRA was related to more favorable rankings of back and body pain, social functioning, mental health, the ability to use the bathroom, and the ability to ambulate.

Amoroso and colleagues[33] quantified the workload for both catheterization laboratory and recovery area nurses following 260 consecutive TRA (n = 208) and TFA (n = 52) procedures. The workload was significantly reduced for TRA procedures (TRA = 86 minutes vs TFA = 174 minutes,

Table 4
In-hospital follow-up

Reinfarction	1.9%
Target vessel revascularization	0.9%
Subacute stent thrombosis	0.9%
Stroke	0.6%
Congestive heart failure	13%
Death	2.8%

Table 5
Radial access related minor vascular complications

Puncture failure	1%
Pain /spasm	9%
Hematoma	7%

$P<0.001$) and for TRA recovery time (TRA = 386 minutes vs TFA = 720 minutes). The workload and time savings were related to less time spent for sheath removal, early patient mobility, shorter recovery time, and shorter time to ambulation. This benefit should be profound in complex and more demanding situations of AMI interventions, particularly using TRA.

Early ambulation and a secure access site may allow for an earlier return to productivity. It is also rational to expect that those patients experiencing access site complications, significantly more frequent with TFA, would be delayed in returning to work by an extended recovery. Although early ambulation is possible with use of femoral vascular closure devices, there is no reduction in bleeding and vascular complication rates and approximately 5 times the closure cost of a radial hemostasis device.[32,33]

So, improved quality of life for the patients, relatively shorter and relaxed periprocedural care for the nursing and supportive staff, and significant cost savings for the hospital management are good reasons to use TRA for AMI interventions.

DEVELOPING A TRANSRADIAL ACUTE MYOCARDIAL INFARCTION PROGRAM

Of 37,810 transradial (TR) procedures done by us between December 2001 and December 2011, 9830 (26%) were PCIs. Of them, 883 (9.0%) patients with STEMI were offered TR PCI. Baseline characteristics, procedural characteristics, technical details, in-hospital follow-up, and 1-year follow-up and radial access–related major and minor vascular complications are shown in Tables **Tables 1–7**.

Table 6
Radial access related major vascular complications

Hand ischemia	0%
Transfusion (owing to bleeding from puncture site)	0%
Vascular surgery	0%

Table 7
One-year follow-up

TLR	8.7%
MI	3.8%
CABG	1.7%
Death	2.8%
Composite MACE	17%

Abbreviations: CABG, coronary artery bypass graft; MACE, major adverse cardiac events; MI, myocardial infarction; TLR, target lesion revascularization.

As of now, no formalized guidelines exist regarding development of a TR AMI program; however, it is reasonable to assume that this should be an important off-shoot of a standard elective TRI program. On the basis of available literature combined with our own vast experience in this area, we give the following recommendations for establishment of a new TR AMI program.

1. Before embarking on using TRA for STEMI, the operator and supportive staff should have experience of managing well-selected, stable, and noncomplex lesions in an elective setting to develop skill and experience with this approach. This elective experience should be gradually expanded to more complex areas, including bifurcations, LMCA lesions, calcified and/or tortuous segments, radial loops, and subclavian loops. This will allow the operator to become more accustomed to technique modification and device choices that are suited for these situations in a more controlled environment before encountering these circumstances in patients who are less stable and when time to perfusion is critical. Although it is not a routine practice in regular cases, we strongly recommend injecting contrast through the puncture canula to define the vascular anatomy before introducing the sheath. If anatomy is unfavorable or very difficult, immediate switchover to femoral access will save important time. With increasing experience of an operator, the number of crossovers will decrease remarkably. **Fig. 1** shows an example of a complex radio-brachial loop. Although they are uncommon, beginners should switch over to contralateral radial or TFA. Experienced operators should be able to work through these loops without wasting time. **Fig. 2** is an example of working through arteria lusoria and complex subclavian anatomy to address left anterior descending stenosis in a patient with acute anterior wall MI. **Fig. 3** demonstrates an example of balloon-assisted tracking of a catheter through a difficult radial anatomy.
2. The number of cases to develop a stable ongoing TR AMI program will depend on various factors, including operator experience, operator skills, number of operators in a group, overall number of procedures in a program, and number of supportive staff, including catheterization laboratory/intensive care unit nurses/technicians. The previously mentioned factors combined with determination and perseverance of the team will develop a good TR AMI program. However, there is no magic number at which one suddenly becomes a TR AMI expert; the more you perform, the better you will become.[35] We recommend performing at least 250 coronary angiograms and 75 PCI through TRA in stable cases before indulging into a TR AMI program. These numbers will enable an operator to handle an adequate number of anatomic variations at radio-brachial and subclavian regions and increase comfort levels while performing AMI interventions.[36–40] It

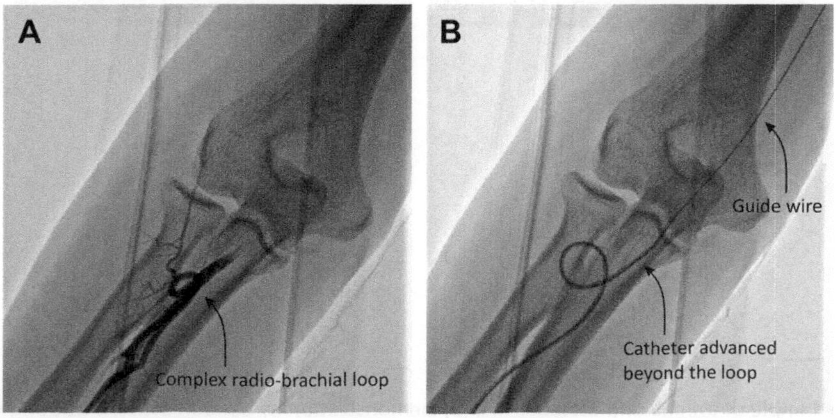

Fig. 1. (*A*) An example of a complex radiobrachial loop. (*B*) A 6-F guide catheter was advanced beyond the loop.

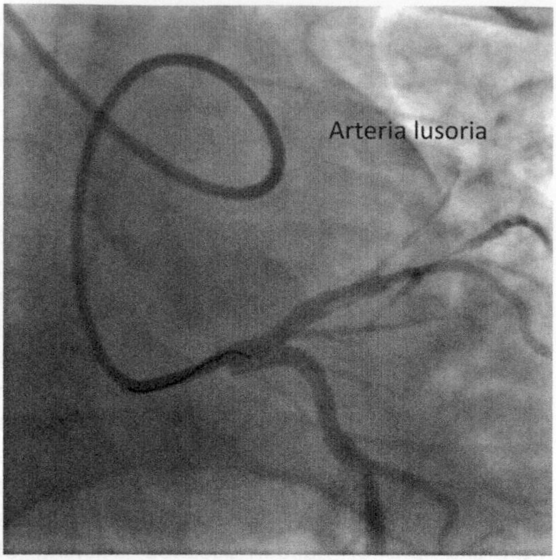

Fig. 2. The LCA cannulation with a 6-F guide catheter was done through the arteria lusoria.

is important to select at least 25 hemodynamically stable AMI cases in the initial stage of a TR AMI program, to overcome a "new" learning curve without delay in reperfusion.

3. Catheterization laboratory preparation and patient setup are important for a TR AMI program. Arm board for the access site should be placed close to the femoral position to mimic the TFA. Many operators shift a standard femoral window drape so the right femoral window is over the right radial (for right TRA) and left femoral window is overlying the right femoral artery (for femoral crossover or intra-aortic balloon pump (IABP)/hemodynamic support device placement). This method works well for nonobese patients. An alternative method is to use towel drapes for the desired radial access site and standard femoral window drapes for the legs. Although the preparation time is slightly prolonged to prepare provisional femoral access, it is typically justified to minimize this activity when femoral access is needed during the procedure. This delay may be offset by the ability to access the radial without needing fluoroscopic guidance (ie, while the staff is completing room setup).[41]
4. Diagnostic angiography should be performed in the noninfarct vascular distribution, followed by angiography with a guide catheter for infarct-related distribution (choice of guide catheter should be as per operator practice or discretion). Guide catheter anchoring support, deep seating or other augmentation may be used as needed. A 5-F guide catheter should be used very sparingly and by an experienced operator. Thrombectomy, percutaneous tranluminal coronary angioplasty (PTCA), or direct stenting can then be performed and PCI completed in the usual fashion. Vascular hemostasis can be achieved in the typical transradial fashion using a radial closure device (per the discretion of the operator).

LIMITATIONS

TRA for STEMI interventions, despite having certain definite advantages, has a relatively slow adoption because of certain procedure-related issues.

A "new" learning curve is slightly more difficult because of unstable cardiac status and mental pressure on the operator for early reperfusion; however, after achieving certain experience in TRA, these issues are minimized.[38,41,42] Prolonged puncture time and procedural time are other issues.[18–23] However, Saito and colleagues[18] and Weaver and colleagues[22] showed shorter timings

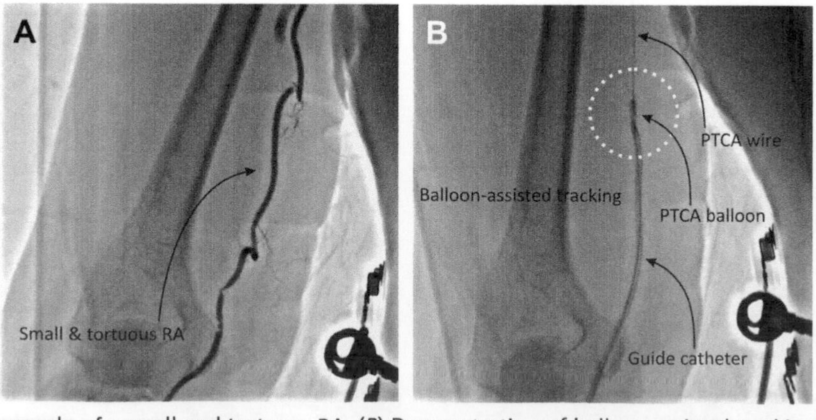

Fig. 3. (*A*) An example of a small and tortuous RA. (*B*) Demonstration of balloon-assisted tracking of a 6-F guide catheter through the difficult RA anatomy.

with TRA compared with TFA. The puncture and procedural times become shorter with increasing experience. Selecting relatively stable AMI cases for interventions and defining vascular anatomy by injecting contrast through a canula before introducing the sheath in initial cases, will increase the comfort level of a beginner with this technique. Comfortable use of bulky devices, including a thrombectomy device, a distal protection device, or kissing balloons is possible with TRA because most devices are 6-F guide catheter compatible and most radials can accommodate 7-F guide catheters.[40,42] There is an argument against using TRA in AMI intervention when IABP support is required. However, puncturing one groin for IABP insertion and PCI through TRA for AMI intervention will spare another groin. So, logically, groin-related vascular complications should be reduced to half. Certain studies have shown increased radiation exposure and fluoroscopy time with TRA as compared with TFA.[16,43–46] This is believed to be because of a relatively longer procedural time and proximity of the operator to the x-ray tube during the procedure.[35] Keeping the arm board for access site parallel and close to the femoral position instead of perpendicular, should resolve this issue to a great extent. Increasing experience, smart application of certain procedure-related tricks, and miniaturization of hardware should help an operator overcoming "so-called" limitations.

SUMMARY

STEMI intervention is one of the commonly performed subsets of PCI. Since its introduction more than 15 years ago, there has been a steady evolution in both devices and pharmacotherapy. Data from large registries have confirmed that periprocedural adverse events have decreased over time.[47] This trend mirrors that seen with ACS and has made bleeding complications a clinical priority.[48–50] Several studies have confirmed that bleeding complications during PCI are associated with an increased risk for MI, stent thrombosis, stroke, death, and increased costs.[11,26,34] Studies also indicate that a large proportion of bleeding complications in patients undergoing PCI is related to vascular access site.[12,13,24,25] Therefore, strategies that address this issue should potentially reduce bleeding and vascular complications and improve PCI outcomes. Moreover, a body of literature now supports the role of TRA in reducing bleeding and vascular complications without sacrificing procedural success. As patients undergoing STEMI interventions are at the highest risk of bleeding for multiple reasons, including generous use of anticoagulants, antiplatelets, thrombolytics, and glycoprotein-2b3a-inhibitors, TRA is likely to offer them exponential benefits, ie, reduction in bleeding and related complications, better quality of life for patients and support staff, and cost benefits for the hospital management.

ACKNOWLEDGMENTS

The authors express their sincere thanks to Mr Yash Soni and Mr Chidambaram Iyer for the help extended during preparation of this manuscript.

REFERENCES

1. Campeau L. Percutaneous radial artery approach for coronary angiography. Cathet Cardiovasc Diagn 1989;16(1):3–7.
2. Kiemeneij F, Laarman GJ. Percutaneous transradial artery approach for coronary stent implantation. Cathet Cardiovasc Diagn 1993;30(2):173–8.
3. Cheng CI, Wu CJ, Fang CY, et al. Feasibility and safety of transradial stenting for unprotected left main coronary artery stenosis. Circ J 2007;71:855–61.
4. Ranjan A, Patel TM, Shah SC, et al. Transradial primary angioplasty and stenting in Indian patients with acute myocardial infarction: acute results and 6-month follow-up. Indian Heart J 2005;57:681–7.
5. Yip HK, Chung SY, Chai HT, et al. Safety and efficacy of transradial vs transfemoral arterial primary coronary angioplasty for acute myocardial infarction: single-center experience. Circ J 2009;73: 2050–5.
6. Rathore S, Hakeem A, Pauriah M, et al. A comparison of the transradial and the transfemoral approach in chronic total occlusion percutaneous coronary intervention. Catheter Cardiovasc Interv 2009;73:883–7.
7. Yang YJ, Xu B, Chen JL, et al. Comparison of immediate and follow-up results between transradial and transfemoral approach for percutaneous coronary intervention in true bifurcational lesions. Chin Med J (Engl) 2007;120:539–44.
8. Ziakas A, Klinke P, Mildenberger R, et al. A comparison of the radial and the femoral approach in vein graft PCI. A retrospective study. Int J Cardiovasc Intervent 2005;7:93–6.
9. Ziakas A, Klinke P, Mildenberger R, et al. Comparison of the radial and femoral approaches in left main PCI: a retrospective study. J Invasive Cardiol 2004;16:129–32.
10. Yatskar L, Selzer F, Feit F, et al. Access site hematoma requiring blood transfusion predicts mortality in patients undergoing percutaneous coronary intervention: data from the National Heart, Lung and Blood Institute dynamic registry. Catheter Cardiovasc Interv 2007;69:961–6.

11. Manoukian SV, Feit F, Mehran R, et al. Impact of major bleeding on 30-day mortality and clinical outcomes in patients with acute coronary syndromes, an analysis from the ACUITY trial. J Am Coll Cardiol 2007;49:1362–8.
12. Chase AJ, Fretz EB, Warbutton WP, et al. Association of the arterial access site at angioplasty with transfusion and mortality, the M.O.R.T.A.L. study (Mortality benefit Of Reduced Transfusion after percutaneous coronary intervention via the Arm or Leg). Heart 2008;94:1019–25.
13. Rao SV, Ou FS, Wang TY, et al. Trends in the prevalence and outcomes of radial and femoral approaches to percutaneous coronary intervention: a report from the national cardiovascular data registry. JACC Cardiovasc Interv 2008;1:379–86.
14. Ochiai M, Isshiki T, Toyoizumi H, et al. Efficacy of transradial primary stenting in patients with acute myocardial infarction. Am J Cardiol 1999;83:966–8 A910.
15. Kelley EC, Boura JA, Grines CL. Primary angioplasty versus intravenous thrombolytic therapy for acute myocardial infarction: a quantitative review of 23 randomised trials. Lancet 2003;361:13–20.
16. Phillippe F, Larrazer F, Meziane T, et al. Comparison of transradial vs transfemoral approach in the treatment of acute myocardial infarction with primary angioplasty and abciximab. Catheter Cardiovasc Interv 2004;61:67–73.
17. Cruden NL, The CH, Starkey IR, et al. Reduced vascular complications and length of stay with transradial rescue angioplasty for acute myocardial infarction. Catheter Cardiovasc Interv 2007;70:670–5.
18. Saito S, Tanaka S, Hiroe Y, et al. Comparative study on transradial approach vs. transfemoral approach in primary stent implantation for patients with acute myocardial infarction: results of the test for myocardial infarction by prospective unicenter randomization for access sites (TEMPURA) trial. Catheter Cardiovasc Interv 2003;59:26–33.
19. Cantor WJ, Puley G, Natarajan MK, et al. Radial versus femoral access for emergent percutaneous coronary intervention with adjunct glycoprotein IIb/IIIa inhibition in acute myocardial infarction—the RADIAL-AMI pilot randomized trial. Am Heart J 2005;1560:543–9.
20. Yan Z, Zhou Y, Zhao Y, et al. Safety and feasibility of transradial approach for primary percutaneous coronary intervention in elderly patients with acute myocardial infarction. Chin Med J 2008;121(19):782–6.
21. De Carlo M, Borelli G, Gistri R, et al. Effectiveness of the transradial approach to reduce bleedings in patients undergoing urgent coronary angioplasty with GP IIb/IIIa inhibitors for acute coronary syndromes. Catheter Cardiovasc Interv 2009;74:408–15.
22. Weaver AN, Henderson RA, Gilchrist IC, et al. Arterial access and door-to-balloon times for primary percutaneous coronary intervention in patients presenting with acute ST-elevation myocardial infarction. Catheter Cardiovasc Interv 2010;75:695–9.
23. Pancholy S, Patel T, Sanghvi K, et al. Comparison of door-to-balloon times for primary PCI using transradial versus transfemoral approach. Catheter Cardiovasc Interv 2010;75(7):991–5.
24. Agostoni P, Biondi-Zoccai GG, de Benedictis ML, et al. Radial versus femoral approach for percutaneous coronary diagnostic and interventional procedures; systematic overview and meta-analysis of randomized trials. J Am Coll Cardiol 2004;44:349–56.
25. Jolly SS, Amlani S, Hamon M, et al. Radial versus femoral access for coronary angiography or intervention and the impact on major bleeding and ischemic events: a systematic review and meta-analysis of randomized trials. Am Heart J 2009;157(1):132–40.
26. Eikelboom JW, Mehta SR, Anand SS, et al. Adverse impact of bleeding on prognosis in patients with acute coronary syndromes. Circulation 2006;114:774–82.
27. Siudak Z, Zawislak B, Dziewierz A, et al. Transradial approach in patients with ST-elevation myocardial infarction treated with abciximab results in fewer bleeding complications: data from EUROTRANSFER registry. Coron Artery Dis 2010;21(5):292–7.
28. Vin MA, Amoroso G, Dirksen MT, et al. Routine use of the transradial approach in primary percutaneous coronary intervention: procedural aspects and outcomes in 2209 patients treated in a single high-volume centre. Heart 2011;97(23):1938–42.
29. Genereux P, Mehran R, Palmerini T, et al. Radial access in patients with ST-segment elevation myocardial infarction undergoing primary angioplasty in acute myocardial infarction: the HORIZONS-AMI trial. EuroIntervention 2011;7:905–16.
30. Jolly SS, Yusuf S, Cairns J, et al. Radial versus femoral access for coronary angiography and intervention in patients with acute coronary syndromes (RIVAL): a randomized, parallel group, multicentre trial. Lancet 2011;377:1409–20.
31. Romagnoli E, Sciahbasi A, Pendenza G, et al. Radial versus femoral randomized investigation in ST elevation acute coronary syndrome: the RIFLE STEACS study. J Am Coll Cardiol 2011;13(20 Suppl B):58.
32. Cooper CJ, El-Shiekh RA, Cohen DJ, et al. Effect of transradial access on quality-of-life and cost of cardiac catheterization: a randomized comparison. Am Heart J 1999;138(3 Pt 1):430–6.
33. Amoroso G, Sarti M, Bellucci R, et al. Clinical and procedural predictors of nurse workload during and after invasive coronary procedures: the potential benefit of a systematic radial access. Eur J Cardiovasc Nurs 2005;4:234–41.

34. Caputo R. Transradial arterial access: economical considerations. J Invasive Cardiol 2009;21(Suppl A): 18A–20A.
35. Trammel J. Launching a successful transradial program. J Invasive Cardiol 2009;21(Suppl A):3A–8A.
36. Patel T, Shah S, Ranjan A. Patel's atlas of transradial intervention: the basics. Chap 6-11, 40–154. Seattle, Washington, DC: Sea Script Company; 2007.
37. Louvard Y, Lefevre T. Loops and transradial approach in coronary diagnosis and intervention. Catheter Cardiovasc Interv 2000;51:250–2.
38. Gilchrist IC. Transradial technical tips. Catheter Cardiovasc Interv 2000;49(3):353–4.
39. Barbeau GR. Radial loop and extreme vessel tortuosity in the transradial approach: advantage of hydrophilic-coated guidewires and catheters. Catheter Cardiovasc Interv 2003;59(4):442–50.
40. Hamon M, McFadden E. Transradial approach for cardiovascular interventions. Caen, France: Europa Stethoscope Media; 2003.
41. Thompson CA. Transradial approach for percutaneous intervention in acute myocardial infarction. J Invasive Cardiol 2009;21(Suppl A):25A–7A.
42. Patel T, Shah S, Ranjan A. Patel's atlas of transradial intervention: the basics. Appendix1; 191–196. Seattle, Washington, DC: Sea Script Company; 2007.
43. Mehta SR, Bassand JP, Chrolavicius S, et al. Design and rationale of CURRENT-OASIS 7: a randomized, 2 x 2 factorial trial evaluating optimal dosing strategies for clopidogrel and aspirin in patients with ST and non-ST-elevation acute coronary syndromes managed with an early invasive strategy. Am Heart J 2008;156:1080–1088. e1.
44. Feit F, Voeltz MD, Attubato MJ, et al. Predictors and impact of major hemorrhage on mortality following percutaneous coronary intervention from the REPLACE-2 trial. Am J Cardiol 2007;100:1364–9.
45. Lange HW, von Boetticher H. Randomized comparison of operator radiation exposure during coronary angiography and intervention by radial or femoral approach. Catheter Cardiovasc Interv 2006;67:12–6.
46. Brasseler C, Blanpain T, Tassan-Mangina S, et al. Comparison of operator radiation exposure with optimized radiation protection devices during coronary angiograms and ad hoc percutaneous coronary interventions by radial and femoral routes. Eur Heart J 2008;29:63–70.
47. Singh M, Rihal CS, Gersh BJ, et al. Twenty-five-year trends in in-hospital and long-term outcome after percutaneous coronary intervention: a single-institution experience. Circulation 2007;115:2835–41.
48. Fox KA, Steg PG, Eagle KA, et al. Decline in rates of death and heart failure in acute coronary syndromes, 1999-2006. JAMA 2007;297:1892–900.
49. Rao SV, Eikelboom JA, Granger CB, et al. Bleeding and blood transfusion issues in patients with non-ST-segment elevation acute coronary syndromes. Eur Heart J 2007;28:1193–204.
50. Doyle BJ, Rihal CS, Gastineau DA, et al. Bleeding, blood transfusion, and increased mortality after percutaneous coronary intervention: implications for contemporary practice. J Am Coll Cardiol 2009; 53:2019–27.

Global Acute Myocardial Infarction Perspectives
Beyond Door-to-Balloon Interventions

Sameer Mehta, MD, MBA[a,b,e,*], Jennifer C. Kostela, MS, MD[c,d], Estefania Oliveros, MD[e], Camilo Pena, MD[e], Rebecca Rowen, BS[d], Kevin Treto, BS[f], Ana Isabel Flores, MD[e], Salomon Cohen, MD[g], Tracy Zhang, BS[e]

KEYWORDS

• STEMI • PPCI • Acute myocardial infarction • Global AMI care

KEY POINTS

- Currently, the three main constraints in ST elevation myocardial infarction (STEMI) intervention in North America are delayed patient presentation, excessive rates of self-transportation, and legislative barriers.
- Enhanced patient education and legislative solutions will propel the United States to be foremost among nations in providing STEMI care.
- Globally, acute myocardial infarction (AMI) care must undergo four phases of development, guided by population-based programs of AMI management.
- Adherence to North American and European guidelines globally remains an unrealistic goal given unparalleled cultural, demographic, and fiscal dynamics.
- Globally, a pharmacoinvasive approach to STEMI care must be based upon socioeconomic impedance.

Dramatic progress has been made, most notably in the United States, in door-to-balloon (D2B) interventions.[1,2] As a result, D2B times that were dismally low are now improving in the United States. Specifically, D2B times ranged from 4% to 10% a decade ago and now exceed 90%.[3] This increase has resulted in unprecedented reductions in mortality from acute myocardial infarction (AMI).[4,5] Several centers now achieve high volumes of D2B interventions, with mortalities ranging from 2% to 3%. Parallel to this decrease in mortality is an even more powerful reduction in morbidity associated with AMI.[6–8]

EUROPE AND CANADA

Most of the progress that the United States achieved was initially learned from the experience

Disclosure: Sameer Mehta is Chief Medical Officer, Asia Pacific, for the Medicines Company. The rest of the authors report no conflict of interest regarding the content herein.

[a] Miller School of Medicine, University of Miami, 1400 Northwest 12th Avenue, Miami, FL 33136, USA; [b] Mercy Medical Center, 3663 South Miami Avenue, Miami, FL 33133, USA; [c] Internal Medicine, New York Hospital Queens, 56-45 Main Street, Flushing, NY 11355, USA; [d] Ross University School of Medicine, 630 US Highway 1, North Brunswick, NJ 08902, USA; [e] Lumen Foundation, 55 Pinta Road, Miami, FL 33133, USA; [f] Ross University School of Medicine, 786 Seneca Meadows Road, Winter Springs, FL 32708, USA; [g] Departamento de Neurocirugia, Instituto Mexicano del Seguro Social, Avenida Club de Golf#3 Torre A Dep. 1501, Lomas Country, Huixquilucan Edo de Mexico, 52779, Mexico
* Corresponding author. 185 Shore Drive South, Miami, FL 33133.
E-mail address: mehtas@bellsouth.net

Intervent Cardiol Clin 1 (2012) 479–484
http://dx.doi.org/10.1016/j.iccl.2012.06.001
2211-7458/12/$ – see front matter

of primary percutaneous coronary intervention (PPCI) in Europe and Canada.[9,10] In particular, uniform success across the continent of Europe was highly inspiring. Although most early PPCI was performed in the United States, the true population-based benefits were noticed in Europe, initially in the Czech Republic, Denmark, and the Netherlands.[9,11–13] This work was notable for showing that patients who were transferred for PPCI did better than those treated with thrombolytic therapy, despite the added transfer times.[14–16] However, Europe comprises several countries that are relatively small and have very sophisticated ambulance services, and patient awareness remains significantly higher in Europe than in the United States.[17] Therefore, Europe succeeded in creating superb AMI care. Further progress in Europe clearly will be slow because of the near-total penetration of excellent ST elevation myocardial infarction (STEMI) care in the continent. Nonetheless, outstanding public educational campaigns, such as STENT for LIFE,[9] are adding new dimensions of care across the spectrum of prehospital presentation, STEMI care, and post–myocardial infarction management. The STENT for LIFE program has made numerous additional contributions, such as improving the overall care of patients presenting with an AMI. Very few patients now miss care altogether, and those that receive thrombolytic therapy are obtaining the treatment earlier. Europe has also advanced innovative prehospital management of patients with AMI treated with thrombolytic therapy and with PPCI.

Despite the massive size of the country, the progress in Canada was similar to that in Europe. However, this occurred in a nation where almost 90% of the population is populated in large urban areas close to the United States border. In Canada, several excellent population-based PPCI programs have been created, particularly in Ontario.[10,18]

AMAZING STEMI PROGRESS IN THE UNITED STATES

The progress in the United States was expected to occur through the creation of a national STEMI policy, akin to trauma care. In this model, patients would be preferentially transported to an STEMI center in a manner similar to trauma patients. It was also anticipated that, similar to a level 1 national trauma program, patients with AMI would obtain clinical triage and transfer to a center performing 24/7 PCI. However, none of these innovations occurred, being hindered by legislative challenges. Nevertheless, some amazing and unprecedented progress was made through collaborative actions of American Heart Association (AHA) and America College of Cardiology (ACC). Leadership within these organizations conceptualized an STEMI system-of-care approach.[19] Its genius was not only this remarkable joint educational endeavor but also the urgent incorporation of an STEMI systems of care mandate as a Class I recommendation in the current AHA/ACC guidelines.[20] With such an STEMI system-of-care methodology, every hospital in this vast nation is mandated to pronounce itself as either a PCI or a non-PCI facility. Transfer protocols have been formed to create unambiguous pathways of transfer from a non-PCI to a PCI facility. This monstrously difficult task has been achieved almost single-handedly by AHA's Mission Lifeline.[21]

Clear navigational pathways of patient care have facilitated the STEMI process that appeared chaotic and simply impossible to achieve.

Phenomenal advancements in the ambulance services have occurred, including remarkable penetration of information technology into ambulances,[22] development of innovative guidelines for prehospital alert[23] and triage, and establishment of a somewhat controversial but colossal mandate permitting STEMI interventions to be performed without surgical stand-by.[24]

It is a tribute to the United States' collaborating organizations and the brilliance of some individual cardiologists (Dr Timothy Henry, Dr Ivan Rokos, Dr Christopher Granger, Dr James Jollis, Dr Henry Ting, Dr Cindy Grines, Dr Alice Jacobs, Dr Elizabeth Bradley, Dr Harlan Krumholz, and Dr Brahmajee Nallamothu) that have enabled this unprecedented breakthrough.

CHALLENGES IN U.S. STEMI INITIATIVES

Deficiencies, however, still exist in the management of AMI in the United States, particularly in STEMI interventions. These limitations currently exist in three large areas: delayed patient presentation, excessive rates of self-transportation, and legislative barriers. With regard to legislative issues, two disruptive practices prevail. With the first one, patients with STEMI being transported by ambulance are not always taken to an STEMI institution first. An equally distributed second set of circumstances legislatively impairs the prompt transfer of patients with STEMI from a non-PCI to a PCI institution.[25–27] These three challenges are reviewed in detail.

In addition to these three mega-challenges, several smaller deficiencies are also seen, including some philosophic disagreements. Are D2B times excellent scientific parameters or a fuzzy metric prone to manipulation? Are physicians not better off measuring true ischemic times? Physicians performing STEMI interventions do not seem to have adequate volumes. Specific STEMI interventional training is lacking altogether and thrombus management for STEMI lesions is clearly inadequate. Controversies exist as to whether bare metal or drug-eluting stents are superior. Thrombectomy devices, at best, are crude. Mostly, achieving D2B times on weekends and off-hours remains challenging.[28] Finally, several patients are uninsured, placing deep burden on hospitals and attending physicians.

Returning to the three major constraints in present STEMI care, the authors discern lack of patient education as the most critical flaw. Making a difference in this crucial deficit will not be easy. Lack of patient education often results from a myriad of causes that include cultural and educational dissimilarities. Educating patients about the need and availability of STEMI interventions is a formidable task. Patients must be educated to promptly recognize the symptoms of a heart attack without referring their clinical state to a primary physician and, even worse, relatives.[29] Women in particular demonstrate atypical symptoms, the recognition of which must be a major component of patient education.[28] Similarly, elderly patients manifest presentations that are more difficult to recognize because they live alone. Early recognition of heart attack will require a multifaceted approach and the earnest efforts of a broad segment of stakeholders, including patients, family physicians, internists, cardiologists, hospital administrators, insurers, medical societies, community organizations, and other philanthropic organizations. Ultimately, patients must educate themselves and learn to recognize their presenting clinical symptoms that may represent a heart attack. The role of media can never be overemphasized.

For the United States to continue its unprecedented success in combating heart attacks, patient education must remain paramount.

Legislation represents the next major impasse. D2B times in STEMI interventions are still the low hanging fruit in AMI care. Without education and prudent legislation, further progress in AMI care can only be limited. Legislation must be enacted in two specific areas. First, a patient who is identified as having a heart attack must be safely and urgently transported to a PCI center and bypass the nearest facility.[22,30–33] The secondary particular anomaly pertains to appropriate transfer of a patient with STEMI from a non-PCI to a PCI institution. Disturbingly, these non-PCI institutions are conflicted by financial reasons and they often delay transportation that is urgently needed for these patients. Disparate management is also encountered at these non-PCI institutions based on the patient's insurance status and the ability to pay.

The authors firmly believe that enhanced patient education and legislative solutions will propel the United States to be foremost among nations in providing STEMI care.

GLOBAL STEMI CARE

Unfortunately, approximately 7.5 million patients still continue to die from an imminently treatable entity that costs more than $400 billion in health care resources.[34] As tremendous as the gains of AMI care are in the Western World, so are the desolate conditions prevailing in developing countries in caring for patients with heart attacks. Trained interventional cardiologists are easily able to perform STEMI interventions in developed and in developing countries. It is not the STEMI procedure but the STEMI process that is lacking in most countries. Although an STEMI intervention procedure is not terribly complicated, it does entail immediate availability and moderate skills. A much larger problem pertains to the process and the gross unavailability of adequate resources required for caring for a patient with STEMI. Ambulance services are often qualitatively and quantitatively lacking, and financial constraints prevent STEMI interventions from being performed in several developing countries. These countries struggle to provide basic cardiac catheterization services even in major metropolitan areas. Developing sophisticated 24/7 STEMI teams is clearly not possible, nor does there seem to be a realistic chance of its happening for decades. Poorer countries have very meager financial resources, making allocation of funds and services for the care of patients with heart attack extremely difficult. Based on these deep financial constraints, it is unrealistic to expect STEMI interventions to become a dominant form of AMI management in these developing countries.

Based on the authors' extensive global work, they confidently predict a phased global progress in AMI care. With this proposed methodology, developing countries will go through the scenario depicted in **Table 1**. Basic thrombolytic therapy must be universally available as a first stage. Further development of infrastructure and ambulance services can lead to a mid-stage pharmacoinvasive management. Only after decades of deep financial resource allocation and governmental commitment can one expect progress to the final phase of population-based, pragmatic D2B management for patients with STEMI. The authors believe that most countries will progress

Table 1
Phases of development: population-based programs of AMI management

	Stage 1	Stage 2	Stage 3	Stage 4
Stage target goal	Immediate availability of appropriate lytic agent nationwide	Access to reliable ambulance service nationwide	Pharmacoinvasive strategy	Primary PCI nationwide D2B <90 min
Role of ambulatory services	Rudimentary ambulance system	Moderate ambulance system	Ambulance system with wireless transmission of 12-lead electrocardiogram prehospital triage transfer protocols	Emergency medical services transport with ambulance as STEMI management center bypass emergency department
Strategy	First-generation lytics	Tenecteplase pharmacoinvasive management	D2B-dominant strategy	Nationwide STEMI system
Duration	1–3 y	10 y	10 y	Unknown
Lives saved	Millions	Millions	Millions	Millions
Funding	Financial constraints	Private and public funding	Adequate funding	Adequate funding
Mortality	12%	8%–10%	<5%	<2%

to D2B interventions only after ascending through these stages. However rapid ascent up the ladder of STEMI phases is possible and can occur through injection of a financial and infrastructure bolus. In smaller nations, patient education and physician commitment can provide this fertile environment; however, large nations with massive populations, such as China and India, will struggle to ascend the nomenclature enlisted in **Table 1**. The authors do not, however, restrict their

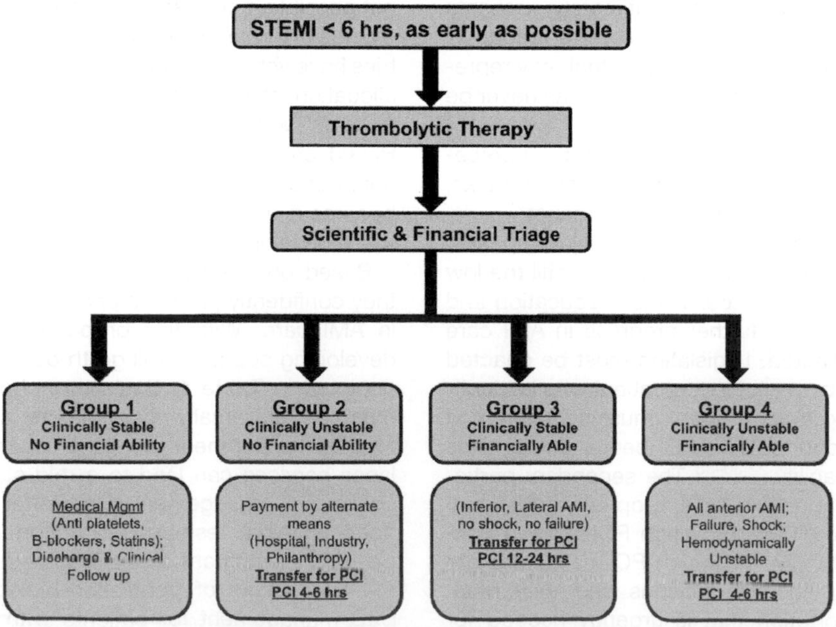

Fig. 1. Transfer AMI: pragmatic model.

predictions to having a single stage of development at a single time. For example, the possibility definitely exists that in particular countries, several stages of care be delivered simultaneously. With this methodology, several metropolitan cities will provide D2B interventions, and rural areas will deliver basic thrombolytic therapy. Good medical management remains an integral part of the proposed management strategies.

Regarding pharmacoinvasive management, it seems transparent to the authors that science cannot remain the sole guidance for care of patients with AMI. Specially, the authors allude to pharmacoinvasive management and United States and European guidelines that mandate PCI strategy universally for patients who receive thrombolytic therapy (**Fig. 1**).[14–16,33]

SUMMARY

The authors sincerely believe that scientific recommendations must be balanced with fiscal prudence. With earnest conviction, they propose a strategy that balances medicine and financial realities. This financial balance will be needed to deliver appropriate care to the millions of people in developing countries who are vulnerable to a heart attack.

REFERENCES

1. Herrin J, Miller LE, Turkmani DF, et al. National performance on door-in to door-out time among patients transferred for primary percutaneous coronary intervention. Arch Intern Med 2011;171(21):1879–86.
2. Nallamothu BK, Bates ER, Wang Y, et al. Driving times and distances to hospitals with percutaneous coronary intervention in the United States: implications for prehospital triage of patients with ST-elevation myocardial infarction. Circulation 2006;113(9):1189–95.
3. Krumholz HM, Herrin J, Miller LE, et al. Improvements in door-to-balloon time in the United States, 2005 to 2010. Circulation 2011;124(9):1038–45.
4. Nallamothu B, Bates ER. Percutaneous coronary intervention versus fibrinolytic therapy in acute myocardial infarction: is timing (almost) everything? Am J Cardiol 2003;92:824–6.
5. Keeley EC, Boura JA, Grines CL. Primary angioplasty versus intravenous thrombolytic therapy for acute myocardial infarction: a quantitative review of 23 randomised trials. Lancet 2003;361(9351):13–20.
6. Stenestrand U, Lindback J, Wallentin L. Long-term outcome of primary percutaneous coronary intervention vs prehospital and in-hospital thrombolysis for patients with ST-elevation myocardial infarction. JAMA 2006;296(14):1749–56.
7. Shavelle DM, Rasouli ML, Frederick P, et al. Outcome in patients transferred for percutaneous coronary intervention (a national registry of myocardial infarction 2/3/4 analysis). Am J Cardiol 2005;96(9):1227–32.
8. Brodie BR, Stuckey TD, Hansen C, et al. Benefit of coronary reperfusion before intervention on outcomes after primary angioplasty for acute myocardial infarction. Am J Cardiol 2000;85(1):13–8.
9. Widimsky P, Wijns W, Fajadet J, et al. Reperfusion therapy for ST elevation acute myocardial infarction in Europe: description of the current situation in 30 countries. Eur Heart J 2010;31(8):943–57.
10. Le May M. Code STEMI: implementation of a city-wide program for rapid assessment and management of myocardial infarction. CMAJ 2009;181(8):E136–7.
11. Andersen H, Nielsen TT, Rasmussen K, et al. DANAMI-2. A comparison of coronary angioplasty with fibrinolytic therapy in acute myocardial infarction. N Engl J Med 2003;349(8):733–42.
12. Widimsky P, Budesinsky T, Vorac D, et al. Long distance transport for primary angioplasty vs immediate thrombolysis in acute myocardial infarction. Final results of the randomized national multicentre trial–PRAGUE-2. Eur Heart J 2003;24(1):94–104.
13. Widimsky P, Groch L, Zelizko M, et al. Multicentre randomized trial comparing transport to primary angioplasty vs immediate thrombolysis vs combined strategy for patients with acute myocardial infarction presenting to a community hospital without a catheterization laboratory. The PRAGUE study. Eur Heart J 2000;21(10):823–31.
14. Larson DM, Duval S, Sharkey SW, et al. Safety and efficacy of a pharmaco-invasive reperfusion strategy in rural ST-elevation myocardial infarction patients with expected delays due to long-distance transfers. Eur Heart J 2012;33(10):1232–40.
15. D'Souza SP, Mamas MA, Fraser DG, et al. Routine early coronary angioplasty versus ischaemia-guided angioplasty after thrombolysis in acute ST-elevation myocardial infarction: a meta-analysis. Eur Heart J 2011;32(8):972–82.
16. Bohmer E, Hoffmann P, Abdelnoor M, et al. Efficacy and safety of immediate angioplasty versus ischemia-guided management after thrombolysis in acute myocardial infarction in areas with very long transfer distances results of the NORDISTEMI (NORwegian study on DIstrict treatment of ST-elevation myocardial infarction). J Am Coll Cardiol 2010;55(2):102–10.
17. Lee RS, Kaushal R, Bholat T, et al. Patient differences by mode of hospital arrival for ST-elevation myocardial infarction treated with primary PCI. Available at: http://www.tctmd.com/txshow.aspx?tid=2640&id=110728&trid=2. Accessed March 26, 2012.

18. So DY, Ha AC, Turek MA, et al. Comparison of mortality patterns in patients with ST-elevation myocardial infarction arriving by emergency medical services versus self-transport (from the prospective Ottawa Hospital STEMI Registry). Am J Cardiol 2006;97(4):458–61.
19. Jacobs AK, Antman EM, Ellrodt G, et al. Recommendation to develop strategies to increase the number of ST-segment-elevation myocardial infarction patients with timely access to primary percutaneous coronary intervention. Circulation 2006; 113(17):2152–63.
20. Wright RS, Anderson JL, Adams CD, et al. 2011 ACCF/AHA focused update incorporated into the ACC/AHA 2007 Guidelines for the Management of Patients with Unstable Angina/Non-ST-Elevation Myocardial Infarction: a report of the American College of Cardiology Foundation/American Heart Association Task Force on Practice Guidelines developed in collaboration with the American Academy of Family Physicians, Society for Cardiovascular Angiography and Interventions, and the Society of Thoracic Surgeons. J Am Coll Cardiol 2011;57(19):e215–367.
21. American Heart Association. Mission: Lifeline. Available at: http://missionlifelinecommunity.americanheart.org/home. Accessed March 1, 2012.
22. Sanchez-Ross M, Oghlakian G, Maher J, et al. The STAT-MI (ST-Segment Analysis Using Wireless Technology in Acute Myocardial Infarction) trial improves outcomes. JACC Cardiovasc Interv 2011;4(2): 222–7.
23. Diercks DB, Kontos MC, Chen AY, et al. Utilization and impact of pre-hospital electrocardiograms for patients with acute ST-segment elevation myocardial infarction: data from the NCDR (National Cardiovascular Data Registry) ACTION (Acute Coronary Treatment and Intervention Outcomes Network) Registry. J Am Coll Cardiol 2009;53(2):161–6.
24. Dehmer GJ, Kutcher MA, Dey SK, et al. Frequency of percutaneous coronary interventions at facilities without on-site cardiac surgical backup—a report from the American College of Cardiology-National Cardiovascular Data Registry (ACC-NCDR). J Am Coll Cardiol 2007;99(3):329–32.
25. Harjai K, Orshaw P, Boura J, et al. Reperfusion delay in patients with ST-elevation myocardial infarction presenting to hospitals without angioplasty capability: should 'door-to-ambulance' time be the new quality parameter for non-PCI hospitals? 2012. Available at: http://www.tctmd.com/txshow.aspx?tid=2640&id=110743&trid=2. Accessed March 26, 2012.
26. Wang TY, Nallamothu BK, Krumholz HM, et al. Association of door-in to door-out time with reperfusion delays and outcomes among patients transferred for primary percutaneous coronary intervention. JAMA 2011;305(24):2540–7.
27. Miedema MD, Newell MC, Duval S, et al. Causes of delay and associated mortality in patients transferred with ST-segment-elevation myocardial infarction. Circulation 2011;124(15):1636–44.
28. Concannon TW, Nelson J, Goetz J, et al. A percutaneous coronary intervention lab in every hospital? Circ Cardiovasc Qual Outcomes 2012; 5(1):14–20.
29. Hand MM. "Act in Time to Heart Attack Signs" action plan: a patient-based critical pathway. Crit Pathw Cardiol 2002;1(1):61–5.
30. Ting HH, Rihal CS, Gersh BJ, et al. Regional systems of care to optimize timeliness of reperfusion therapy for ST-elevation myocardial infarction: the Mayo Clinic STEMI Protocol. Circulation 2007; 116(7):729–36.
31. Ting HH, Krumholz HM, Bradley EH, et al. Implementation and integration of prehospital ECGs into systems of care for acute coronary syndrome: a scientific statement from the American Heart Association Interdisciplinary Council on Quality of Care and Outcomes Research, Emergency Cardiovascular Care Committee, Council on Cardiovascular Nursing, and Council on Clinical Cardiology. Circulation 2008;118(10):1066–79.
32. Concannon TW, Kent DM, Normand SL, et al. Comparative effectiveness of ST-segment-elevation myocardial infarction regionalization strategies. Circ Cardiovasc Qual Outcomes 2010;3(5):506–13.
33. Rokos IC, French WJ, Mattu A, et al. Appropriate cardiac cath lab activation: optimizing electrocardiogram interpretation and clinical decision-making for acute ST-elevation myocardial infarction. Am Heart J 2010;160(6):995–1003.e1–8.
34. Bradley E, Roumanis S, Radford M, et al. Achieving door-to-balloon times that meet quality guidelines: how do successful hospitals do it? J Am Coll Cardiol 2005;46(7):1236–41.

Compulsive Thrombus Management in STEMI Interventions

Sameer Mehta, MD, MBA[a,b,e,*], Jennifer C. Kostela, MS, MD[c,d], Estefania Oliveros, MD[e], Ana Isabel Flores, MD[e], Camilo Pena, MD[e], Salomon Cohen, MD[f], Rebecca Rowen, BS[d], Kevin Treto, BS[g]

KEYWORDS

• STEMI • Acute myocardial infarction • D2B time • Pharmacoinvasive • Thrombus management

KEY POINTS

- The Mehta strategy is a selective strategy for thrombus management in STEMI interventions based on the thrombus grade, with direct stenting recommended for low-grade thrombus, thromboaspiration for moderate thrombus, and rheolytic thrombectomy for high-grade thrombus (depending on suitable anatomy).
- Thrombus grade must be determined before thrombectomy by crossing the entire lesion with a guide wire for optimal grading.
- To reach this point of optimal thrombectomy, we advocate making successive passes until the last pass makes no further progress in debulking.
- Thromboaspiration is the default strategy for thrombus management, because aspiration thrombectomy devices are user-friendly, relatively inexpensive, and take no more than a balloon catheter to prepare and deploy.

INTRODUCTION

Thrombus is central to the pathophysiology of ST-elevated myocardial infarction (STEMI); its identification and compulsive management constitute absolute essentials in optimal door-to-balloon (D2B) STEMI interventions. Even in elective percutaneous coronary interventions (PCI), management of thrombus is especially challenging. Not only is thrombus associated with increased abrupt vessel closure, lower procedural success, and increased major in-hospital complications, including death and myocardial infarction (MI) but it is also associated with increased incidence of emergency bypass surgery.[1–4] Several mechanical adjunctive

Disclosure: Sameer Mehta is Chief Medical Officer, Asia Pacific, for the Medicines Company. The rest of the authors report no conflict of interest regarding the content herein.

[a] Miller School of Medicine, University of Miami, 1400 Northwest 12th Avenue, Miami, FL 33136, USA; [b] Mercy Medical Center, 3663 South Miami Avenue, FL 33133, USA; [c] Internal Medicine, New York Hospital Queens, 56-45 Main Street, Flushing, NY 11355, USA; [d] Ross University School of Medicine, 630 US Highway 1, North Brunswick, NJ 08902, USA; [e] Lumen Foundation, 55 Pinta Road, Miami, FL 33133, USA; [f] Departamento de Neurocirugia, Instituto Mexicano del Seguro Social, Avenida Club de Golf #3 Torre A Dep. 1501, Lomas Country, Huixquilucan Edo de Mexico, 52779, Mexico; [g] Ross University School of Medicine, 786 Seneca Meadows Road, Winter Springs, FL 32708, USA

* Corresponding author. 185 Shore Drive South, Miami, FL 33133.

E-mail address: mehtas@bellsouth.net

Intervent Cardiol Clin 1 (2012) 485–505
http://dx.doi.org/10.1016/j.iccl.2012.06.006

devices and pharmacologic options have shown diverse benefits in managing thrombus.[5,6]

In our structured approach to D2B STEMI interventions that are particularly challenged by the constraints of a clicking clock, identification of the culprit lesion and compulsive management of thrombus remain the critical determinant of procedural success. Our compulsive methodology for thrombus management in STEMI interventions has been developed from our extensive work with the SINCERE (Single Individual Community Experience Registry) database, which has included 1034 short D2B interventions. The Mehta strategy for selective thrombus management has recently been published in *Clinics of America*[7] and we anticipate that the simplicity of our quantitatively based strategy makes it an attractive management option.

PATHOPHYSIOLOGY OF THROMBUS

Atherosclerosis is the chronic inflammatory process that is fundamental to intimal plaque development in human vasculature, including the coronary vessels. Several risk factors, including advanced age, male sex, genetics, hyperlipidemia, hypertension, tobacco use, and diabetes mellitus, predispose to endothelial injury. Atherogenesis, or plaque formation, involves a dynamic interplay of endothelial injury and inflammatory element recruitment (eg, lipoproteins, macrophages, platelets, smooth muscle cells, collagen) and deposition.[8]

In addition to locally produced mediators, products of blood coagulation and thrombosis likely contribute to atheroma evolution and complication. This involvement justifies the use of the term atherothrombosis to convey the inextricable links between atherosclerosis and thrombosis.[8] Plaque is subjected to a variety of intrinsic and extrinsic stressors, which lead to an acute plaque change.[9] The rupture, fissuring, erosion, or ulceration of plaque initiates the thrombosis cascade in one of 2 pathways.[8] The first pathway involves exposed collagen of the vessel wall. The exposed collagen of disrupted endothelium interacts with platelet glycoproteins. Specifically, platelet glycoprotein VI binds with the collagen of the exposed vessel, whereas platelet glycoprotein Ib-V-IX interacts with the collagen-bound von Willebrand factor. This process not only secures the adherence of platelets to the vessel wall but also initiates platelet activation and granule release, independent of thrombin.[10] This pathway leads to the formation of the white thrombi consisting of varying amounts of cellular debris, fibrin, and platelets and a limited number of erythrocytes. Succeeding the white thrombi, the second pathway leads to formation of a red thrombi, an erythrocyte-rich and thrombin-rich complex.[11]

A membrane protein–tissue factor mediates the second pathway. Among its functions, tissue factor initiates the extrinsic coagulation cascade. It binds to the activated factor VII, which then activates factor IX, leading to the cascade that generates thrombin. The thrombin then cleaves protease-activated receptor 4 on the platelet surface. This cleavage in turn activates platelets, causing the release of adenosine diphosphate, serotonin, and thromboxane A_2, all of which are agonists in the activation of other platelets.[10] Depending on the initial size of plaque, both pathways can occlude the lumen of the coronary vessel, leading to an MI.[12–16] The timing and intrinsic ability of the second pathway to stabilize, enlarge, and increase the density of the primary white thrombi[11] contribute to the complexity of management of thrombus, especially in the setting of D2B time constraints.

THROMBUS BURDEN

Clinical experience recommends against the use of balloon angioplasty in thrombus burden (TB), because they cause distal embolization and myocardial necrosis, TB has been shown to

Table 1
TIMI thrombus grade

0	No cineangiographic characteristics of thrombus present
1	Possible thrombus present. Angiography shows characteristics such as reduced contrast density, haziness, irregular lesion contour, or a smooth convex meniscus at the site of total occlusion suggestive but not diagnostic of thrombus
2	Thrombus present, small size: definite thrombus with greatest dimensions less than or equal to half vessel diameter
3	Thrombus present, moderate size: definite thrombus but with greatest linear dimension greater than half but less than 2 vessel diameters
4	Thrombus present, large size: as in grade 3 but with the largest dimension greater than or equal to 2 vessel diameters
5	Total occlusion

Data from The TIMI-IIIA Investigators. Early effects of tissue-type plasminogen activator added to conventional therapy on the culprit coronary lesion in patients presenting with ischemic cardiac pain at rest. Circulation 1993;87:38–52; and van't Hof AW, Liem A, Suryapranata H, et al. Angiographic assessment of myocardial reperfusion in patients treated with primary angioplasty for acute myocardial infarction: myocardial blush grade. Zwolle Myocardial Infarction Study Group. Circulation 1998;97:2302–6.

adversely affect clinical outcomes in both cerebrovascular accidents and acute coronary syndromes.[17–20] Barreto and colleagues undertook a retrospective review of patients with stroke and correlated the clinical outcomes to the angiographic TB, using the same classification scheme outlined in **Table 1**. Compared with the patients with thrombus grades 0 to 3, patients with thrombus grade 4 required longer treatment times and experienced increased mechanical clot disruption, poor outcomes, and mortality.[21] Using the same classification scheme, Sianos and colleagues reported in their landmark work the importance of TB in clinical outcomes in acute

Table 2
Trials of thrombus aspiration

Study	Thrombectomy Device	Primary and Clinical End Points
Aspiration Thrombectomy		
Ciszewski et al,[23] 2011	Rescue/Diver CE	(+) Myocardial salvage, (=) In-hospital mortality
TOTAL[24] 2010	Export	Ongoing
INFUSE AMI[25] 2011	Atrium ClearWay	Ongoing
TASTE[26] 2010	Export	Ongoing
EXPIRA[27,28] 2009	Export	(+) MBG >2, (+) STR, (+) IS, (+) 2-y CD, (+) 2-y MACE
Liistro et al,[29] 2009	Export	(+) STR, (=) 6-mo MACE
Lipiecki et al,[30] 2009	Export	(=) IS
TAPAS[31] 2008	Export	(+) MBG 0-1, (+) STR, (+) 1-y mortality, (+) 1-y CD
EXPORT[32]	Export	(+) MBG 3, (+) STR, (=) 30-d MACCE
VAMPIRE[33] 2008	TVAC	(+ trend) SR/NR, (+) 8-month MACE
Chao et al,[34] 2008	Export	(+) TIMI flow, (+) MBG
PIHRATE[35] 2008	Diver CE	(=) STSR, (=) 6-mo mortality
Andersen et al,[36] 2007	Rescue	(+) Left ventricular function
Kaltoft et al,[37] 2006	Rescue	(-) Myocardial salvage, (=) 30-d MACE
DEAR-MI[38] 2006	Pronto	(+) MBG 3, (+) STR, (=) 30-d MACE
De Luca et al,[39] 2006	Diver CE	(+) TIMI flow, (+) MBG 3, (+) 30-d MACE
REMEDIA[40] 2005	Diver CE	(+) STR, (+) MBG $\geq$2
Mechanical Thrombectomy		
SMART-PCI[41] 2011	AngioJet	Ongoing
JETSTENT[42] 2010	AngioJet	(+) STR, (=) IS, (+) 1-y MACE
AIMI[43] 2006	AngioJet	(+) IS, (–) TIMI flow, (–) MBG, (–) STR, (–) 30-d MACE
X-AMINE ST[44] 2005	X-Sizer	(–) IS, (–) TIMI flow, (–) 30-d MACE
Antoniucci et al,[45] 2004	AngioJet	(+) STR, (–) 30-d MACE
Napodano et al,[46] 2003	X-Sizer	(+) MBG 3, (=) 30-d MACE
Beran et al,[47] 2002	X-Sizer	(+) STR, (=) 30-d MACE

Abbreviations: (+), improved end point; (=), neutral effect on end point; (–), worsened end point; AIMI, AngioJet Rheolytic Thrombectomy in Patients Undergoing Primary Angioplasty for Acute Myocardial Infarction; CD, cardiac death; DEAR-MI, Dethrombosis to Enhance Acute Reperfusion in Myocardial Infarction; EXPIRA, Thrombectomy with Export Catheter in Infarct-Related Artery During Primary Percutaneous Coronary Intervention; EXPORT, Prospective, Multicentre, Randomized Study of the Export Aspiration Catheter; IS, infarct size; JETSTENT, Comparison of AngioJet Rheolytic Thrombectomy Before Direct Infarct Artery Stenting with Direct Stenting Alone in Patients with Acute Myocardial Infarction; MACCE, major adverse cardiac and cerebral events; MBG, myocardial blush grade; NR, no-reflow; PIHRATE, Polish-Italian-Hungarian Randomized Thrombectomy Trial; REMEDIA, Randomized Evaluation of the Effect of Mechanical Reduction of Distal Embolization by Thrombus Aspiration in Primary and Rescue Angioplasty; SMART-PCI, Comparison of Manual Aspiration with Rheolytic Thrombectomy in Patients Undergoing Primary PCI; SR, slow-reflow; STSR, ST-segment resolution; TAPAS, Thrombus Aspiration During Percutaneous Coronary Intervention in Acute Myocardial Infarction Study; TASTE, Thrombus Aspiration in ST-Elevation Myocardial Infarction in Scandinavia; TIMI, thrombolysis in myocardial infarction flow grade; TOTAL, Trial of Routine Aspiration Thrombectomy with Percutaneous Coronary Intervention (PCI) Versus PCI Alone in Patients With ST-Segment Elevation Myocardial Infarction Undergoing Primary PCI; VAMPIRE, Vacuum Aspiration Thrombus Removal; X-AMINE ST, X-Sizer in AMI for Negligible Embolization and Optimal ST Resolution; TVAC, Thrombus Vacuum Aspiration Catheter.

Table 3
Strategy based on thrombus grade for management of the STEMI lesion: Mehta classification

Grade	Thrombus Definition	Angiographic Examples			Mehta Classification	Technical Tips of Use: Aspiration catheter	Technical Tips of Use: AngioJet
0	No cineangiographic characteristics of thrombus present	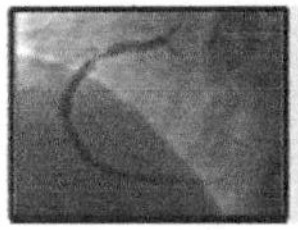	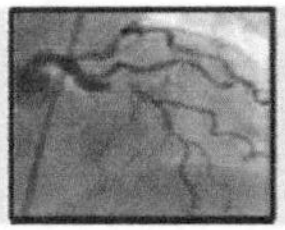	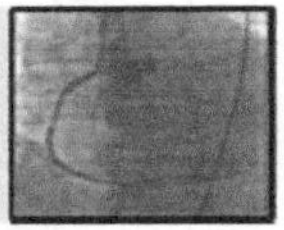	Direct stent ± predilatation	Most effective with fresh clot; organized thrombus is more resistant to debulking Have different profiles, different pushability, tractability, and aspiration rates	Can be used from the radial route. Although LAD (left anterior descending) and some LCX (left circumflex) may not need a TPM (temporary pacemaker), we place TPMs in all AngioJet procedures
1	Possible thrombus present. Angiography shows reduced contrast density, haziness, irregular lesion contour, or a smooth convex meniscus at the site of total occlusion, suggestive but not diagnostic of thrombus	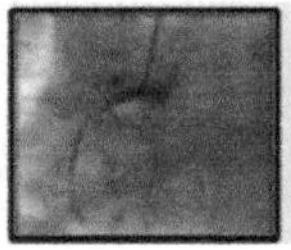	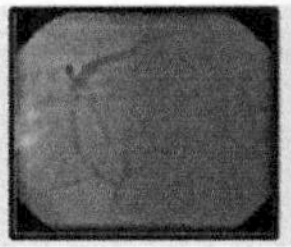	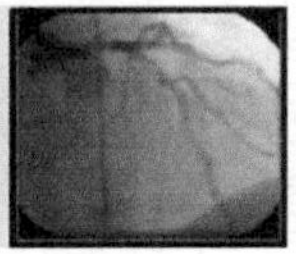		All are 6-Fr compatible; it is useful to stock and be familiar with the use of at least one	Often, multiple passes are required. Try to pause after every 2–3 passes to enable hemodynamics to be restored, to optimize guide wire and guiding catheter support, and to evaluate the results
2	Thrombus present, small size: definite thrombus with greatest dimensions less than or equal to half vessel diameter	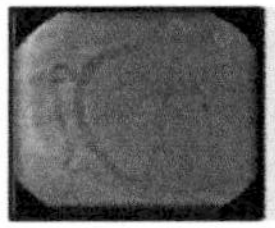	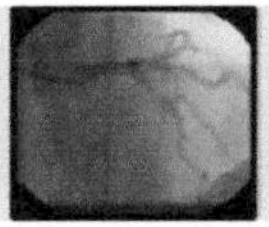	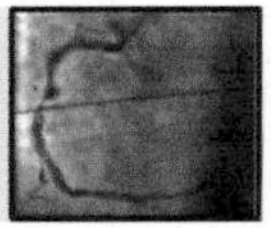	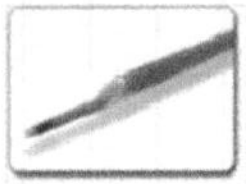 Aspiration thrombectomy	Flush catheter lumen well before use because it facilitates better tracking over the wire	
3	Thrombus present, moderate size; definite thrombus but with greatest linear dimension greater than half but less than 2 vessel diameters	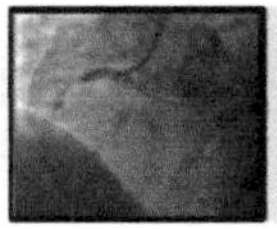	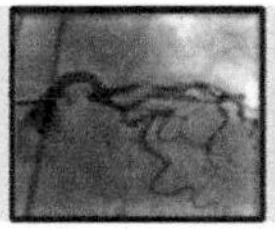	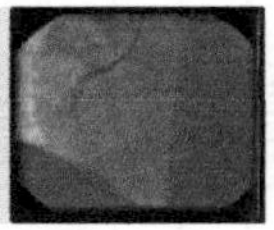		Avoid kinking the catheter: advance slowly over the initial, softer portion of the catheter	Often, just the first passage restores adequate flow Resistant and stubborn thrombus requires more distal advancement that must be performed more carefully
4	Thrombus present, large size; as in grade 3, but with the largest dimension ≥2 vessel diameters	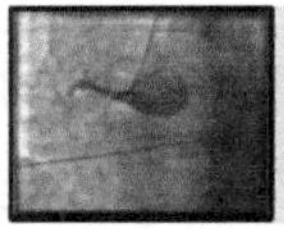	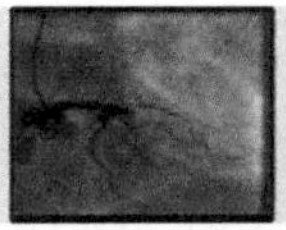	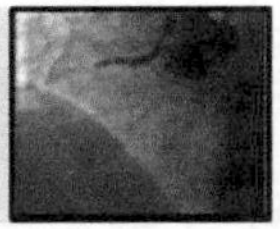	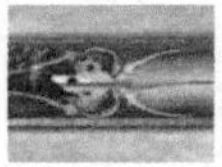 AngioJet	Monitor distal tip of the guide wire as the aspiration catheter is advanced; it is not uncommon for the guide wire to advance during this maneuver	Avoid advancing in severe tortuosity and in vessels <2 mm
5	Total occlusion					Advance the aspiration catheter through the length of occlusive disease	Because the AngioJet is used for large TB and high thrombus grade, consider abciximab as adjunctive therapy

coronary syndromes.[22] Compared with small TB (grades 0–3), these investigators found that large intracoronary TB (grade 4) was an independent predictor of mortality and major adverse cardiovascular event (MACE). Evidently, clinical outcome is dependent on TB.

Thrombus removal before STEMI intervention has proved superior to standard PCI alone as shown by randomized controlled trials and retrospectives studies as outlined in **Table 2**.

Despite the positive clinical outcome of the TAPAS (Thrombus Aspiration During Percutaneous Coronary Intervention in Acute Myocardial Infarction Study) trial,[48] we strongly believe that this study is constrained by having a single strategy for all-comers without volumetric adjustments for TB. Although philosophically we remain in complete agreement with the intent to aspirate thrombus, as is clearly demonstrable in the TAPAS trial, we believe that this sole aspiration strategy

Table 4
Thrombectomy devices

Device	Unique Characteristics
Aspiration Thrombectomy	
Diver CE 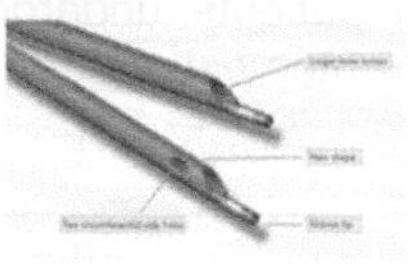	Available in 2 versions: aspiration lumen with side holes (for fresh thrombus removal, 2–6 h after symptom onset) and aspiration lumen without side holes (for organized thrombus removal, 6–24 h after symptom onset) Ultraflexible shaft from increased trackability
Export 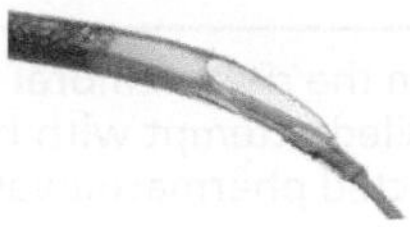	Optimal kink resistance and deliverability as a result of full wall variable braiding technology: The distal end is flexible with high-density variable braiding The proximal end has low-density variable braiding for support and pushability
Pronto 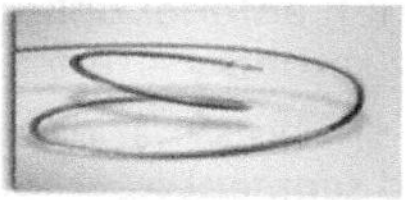	Embedded longitudinal wire enhances deliverability and kink resistance Patented Silva distal tip provides vessel protection
QuickCat 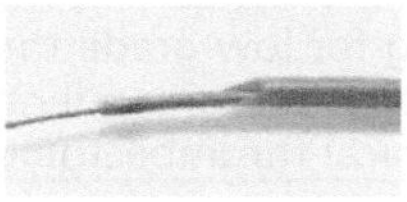	6F aspiration catheter with a low-profile moderate suction ability, kinks easily, and could perform better with more tensile strength of catheter
Mechanical Thrombectomy	
AngioJet 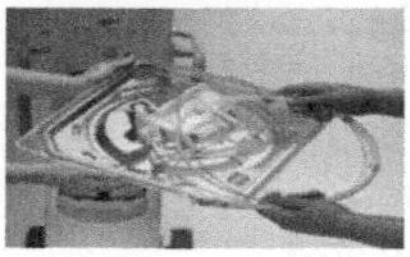	Rheolytic thrombectomy system that uses high-velocity saline jets at the distal catheter tip. The jets create a negative pressure to collect the thrombus Only thrombectomy device indicated for native coronary arteries and synthetic grafts
X-Sizer 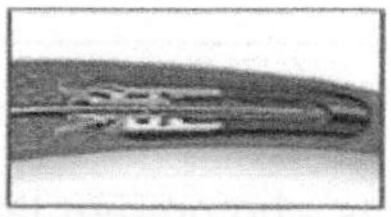	Uses a helix cutter at the distal tip of the catheter The Archimedes screw is designed to grab thrombus on contact, quickly drawing it in, shearing, and removing it

does not suffice for all thrombus grades and it particularly fails to effectively treat dense, organized thrombus that is commonly seen in delayed presentations. Dense, organized thrombus in late-presenting anterior MI (AMI) is the commonest presentation in developing countries that lack sophisticated ambulance systems and STEMI systems of care. In such situations, it is infrequent to find the easy-to-treat, white thrombus with aspiration thrombectomy, as was shown in the TAPAS trial. Dense, organized thrombus, which is present often in these infarct-related vessels, is simply too complex to manage with simple, presently available, aspiration catheters. Based on our work, we strongly consider that such lesions are better managed by mechanical devices, such as the AngioJet (Possis Medical, Minneapolis, MN), provided the anatomy is favorable (avoid severe tortuosity and vessels <2.5 mm). Although there is little evidence of benefit for such use, we also believe that the excimer laser coronary angioplasty (ELCA) may prove effective in ablating such dense, thrombotic lesions. The speed of laser angioplasty (single pass with appropriately sized catheter) makes the use of ELCA particularly attractive for such applications.

Concerning clinical support for our selective thrombus management strategy, the drawback of using a single-aspiration thrombectomy strategy has been partially corrected in the JETSTENT (AngioJet Thrombectomy and Stenting for Treatment of Acute Myocardial Infarction) trial, which uses angiography to grade the TB before thrombus aspiration and subsequent PCI intervention.[45] Yet, despite using a selective strategy for thrombus intervention, the overall results of the trial provide little advance. For almost the same reasons of lacking a selective strategy, we have some reluctance about the design for the new intracoronary abciximab infusion and aspiration thrombectomy in patients undergoing percutaneous coronary intervention for anterior ST

Table 5
Step-by-step technique for STEMI interventions

Step	Technique	Comments
1	Obtain a clean, 6F arterial access	Routinely from the right femoral route (radial route for failed attempt with both groins, and for selected pharmacoinvasive, transfer patients)
2	Cineangiography with 6F diagnostic catheter of the noninfarct-related vessel	Two orthogonal views for left coronary artery and a single left anterior oblique projection for the right coronary artery
3	6F guiding catheter for culprit vessel cannulation	Obtaining set-up shots that precisely define the occluded segment
4	Hydrophilic 0.36-mm (0.014-in) guide wire	Particularly useful for crossing thrombotic lesions
5	Accurately assessing thrombus grade and using a selective thrombectomy strategy	Direct stenting for low-grade thrombus, thromboaspiration for moderate thrombus, and mechanical thrombectomy for large TB
6	Abciximab for large TB	Preferably via intracoronary use
7	Stenting	Drug-eluting stent for left anterior descending, diabetic, long lesions, and small vessels
8	Liberal intracoronary nitroprusside	After confirming satisfactory stent result and removing the guide wire
9	Left ventriculography	In right anterior oblique projection
10	Sheath removal	With closure device
Prefer rheolytic mechanical thrombectomy		
A	For thrombus grade 4 and 5	
B	In large vessels with voluminous thrombus	
C	Saphenous vein graft (SVG) STEMI interventions	
D	For treating dense, organized thrombus, in particular, in patients who present late	
E	Failure to treat thrombotic lesions with aspiration thrombectomy	

segment elevation myocardial infarction (INFUSE AMI) trial.[25] This disparity notwithstanding, we emphatically agree with the strategy in the INFUSE AMI trial about the use of bivalirudin as a foundation anticoagulant for STEMI interventions.

Because TB or grade can be quickly assessed angiographically, a thrombus-grade approach is practical. This is the major advantage of the Mehta classification (**Table 3**), because it provides a selective strategy for thrombus management, based on the thrombus grade. This methodology contradicts the notion that thrombus can be managed by a single modality, as proposed by the TAPAS trial, which used thromboaspiration as an effective strategy, irrespective of the thrombus grade.[48] In this article, and in the article on illustrated cases by Mehta and colleagues elsewhere in this issue, we present numerous cases that support our rationale for a selective, thrombus-grade–based strategy. Specifically, we cite numerous procedures in which dense, organized thrombus could not be effectively managed by thromboaspiration, instead requiring a change to mechanical thrombectomy. **Table 4** outlines available thrombectomy devices (within the United States). In **Table 5**, we have identified 5 distinct situations in which the use of mechanical thrombectomy seems mandatory. Some of the most memorable successes in the SINCERE database used these tenets. The situation with organized, dense thrombus in late-presenting patients with STEMI is the most noteworthy of these cases. These can be difficult cases, and their management (from crossing the impenetrable lesions to debulking them) requires considerable skills, and often, mechanical thrombectomy. The technical

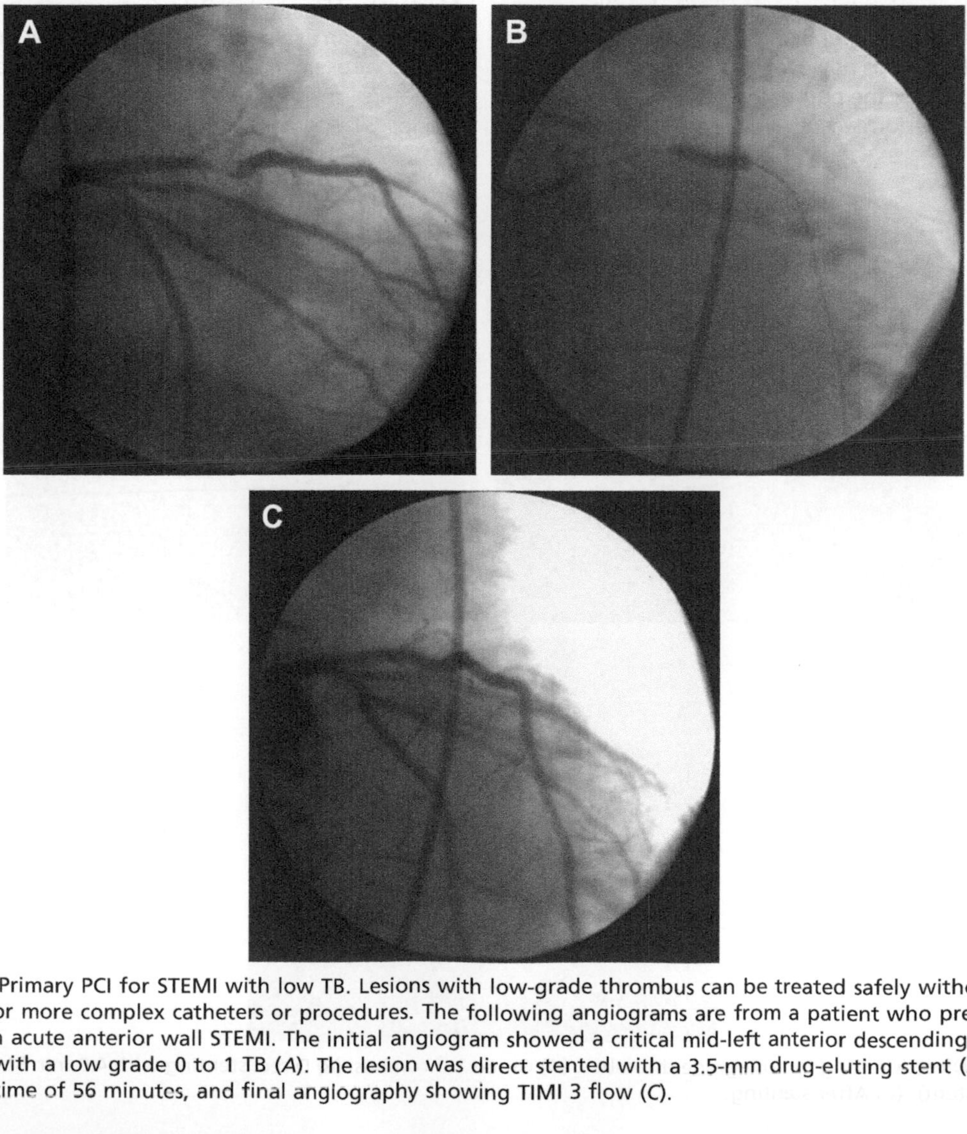

Fig. 1. Primary PCI for STEMI with low TB. Lesions with low-grade thrombus can be treated safely without the need for more complex catheters or procedures. The following angiograms are from a patient who presented with an acute anterior wall STEMI. The initial angiogram showed a critical mid-left anterior descending culprit lesion with a low grade 0 to 1 TB (*A*). The lesion was direct stented with a 3.5-mm drug-eluting stent (*B*) with a D2B time of 56 minutes, and final angiography showing TIMI 3 flow (*C*).

tips and teaching highlights for performing these specific cases are described in detail in the comments after the illustrated cases, and we hope that they show our clinically based strategy to guide STEMI interventions.

MEHTA STRATEGY FOR THROMBUS MANAGEMENT

The TIMI (thrombolysis in myocardial infarction) flow grade classifies the thrombus based on angiography (see **Table 1**) and is the basis for the Mehta strategy for thrombus management (see **Table 3**). The pioneering work by Sianos and colleagues[22] led to this classification, which has now been routinely practiced in more than 1034 short D2B STEMI interventions in the SINCERE database.[49] **Table 4** presents a formulation of the stepwise technique of performing the entire STEMI procedure using this standardized algorithm.

Optimal angiographic visualization of thrombus is the first step; however, thrombus is labile and its grading for the purpose of further management is better performed after crossing the thrombotic STEMI lesion with the guide wire. Balloon catheters are not recommended because they cause distal embolization and myocardial necrosis. We recommend their use for only 3 rare situations: (1) uncertainty as to whether the guide wire is in the true lumen, after it has crossed a thrombotically occluded segment; in this situation, a small 2.0-mm balloon can be rapidly inflated; (2) for a patient with overwhelming ischemia and massive ST segment elevation; the role of the balloon is to achieve some TIMI flow rapidly; however, even this may result in thrombus migration and this strategy must be used with discretion; and (3) unavailable thrombectomy catheters or devices.

Often, there is no change in thrombus grade, but thrombus grade 5 most commonly is downsized after wire passage. If the extent of thrombus is small (thrombus grade 0–1), direct angioplasty and stenting may be sufficient (**Figs. 1–4**). Moderate TB, grades 2 to 3, warrants pretreatment with an aspiration catheter. Several randomized controlled trials have shown that aspiration catheters result in superior myocardial blush grade, ST-segment resolution, improved clinical

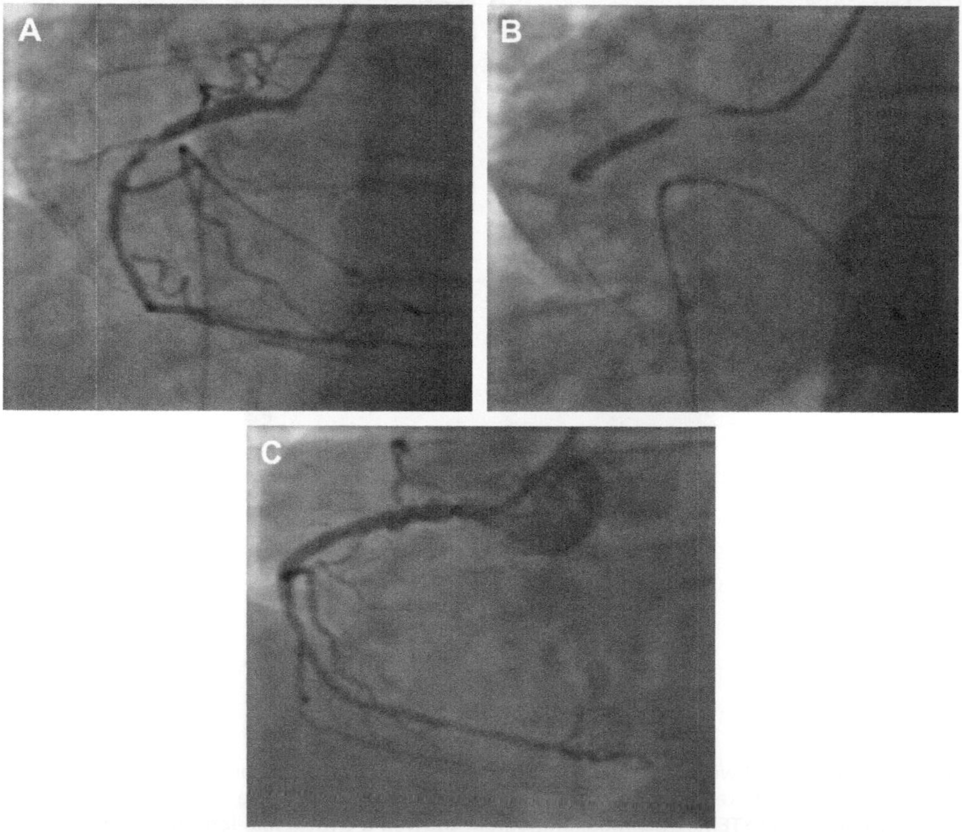

Fig. 2. Direct stenting for low-grade thrombus. (*A*) Grade 1 thrombus. (*B*) Direct stenting with 4.0-mm BMS (bare metal stent). (*C*) After stenting.

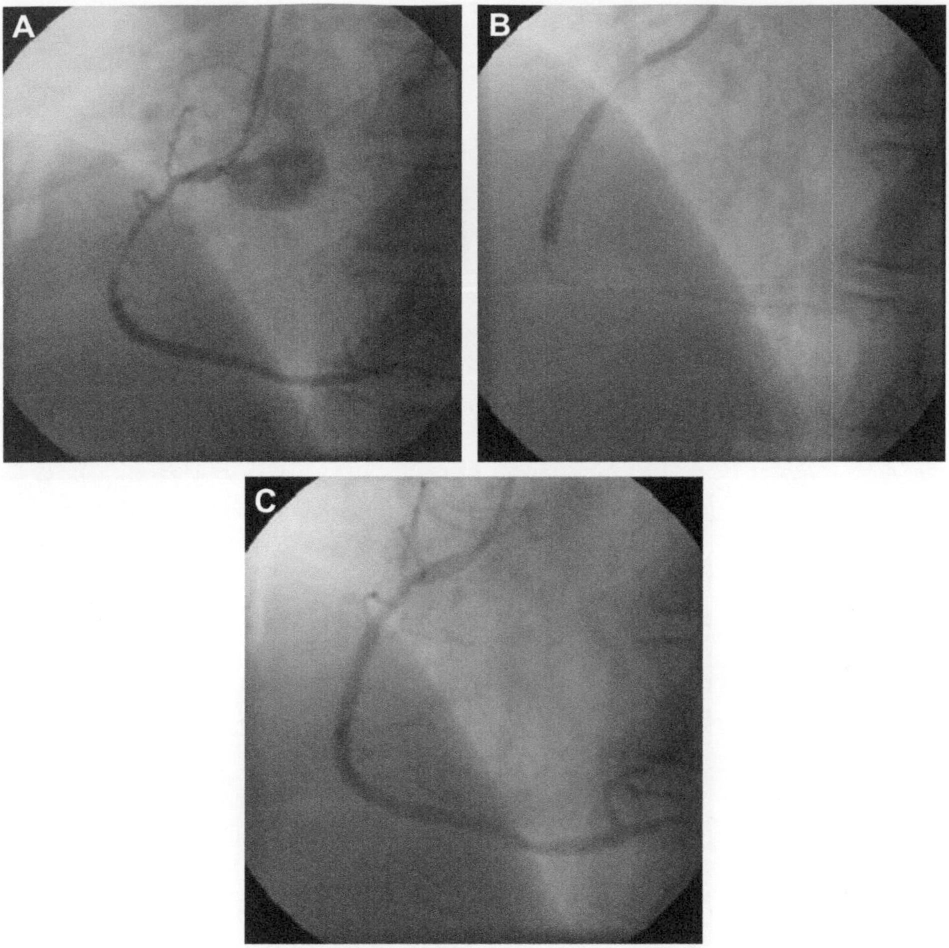

Fig. 3. Direct stenting for low-grade thrombus. (*A*) Grade 1 thrombus. (*B*) Direct stenting with 4.0-mm BMS. (*C*) After stenting.

outcome, rates of TIMI 3 flow rates, and decreased angiographic evidence of distal embolization.[45,48,49] **Figs. 5–8** show aspiration pretreatment in a STEMI with moderate TB.

GRADE 0 TO 1

With low thrombus grades, direct stenting is an acceptable strategy and we advocate it over the use of predilatation, which carries its individual risk of distal embolization. Clearly, we complement this strategy, as with all STEMI interventions, with the use of intracoronary vasodilators. Although various pharmacologic agents can be used for this purpose (adenosine, verapamil, diltiazem, nicardipine, clevidipine), our preferred agent as an intracoronary vasodilator is nitroprusside. Our technique of using intracoronary nitroprusside has been highlighted in other articles elsewhere in this issue.

GRADE 2 TO 3

Moderate TB management with aspiration catheters can be augmented with some practical techniques. Passes with the aspiration catheters should be made until there is no angiographic evidence of thrombus; often just 2 passes are sufficient. It is important to advance the catheter throughout the length of thrombus. Despite their ease of use and effectiveness, the aspiration catheters are not perfect monorail devices, and attention should be paid to the tip of the guide wire as these catheters are advanced. Reducing the imaging magnification and monitoring the distal end of the guide wire as the aspiration catheter is advanced are practical techniques in preventing adverse results. Thrombus often clogs the aspiration holes of these catheters, halting aspiration. Before abandoning them as unsuccessful, it is important to remove the catheter, flush it profusely, and reuse. In rare situations, the

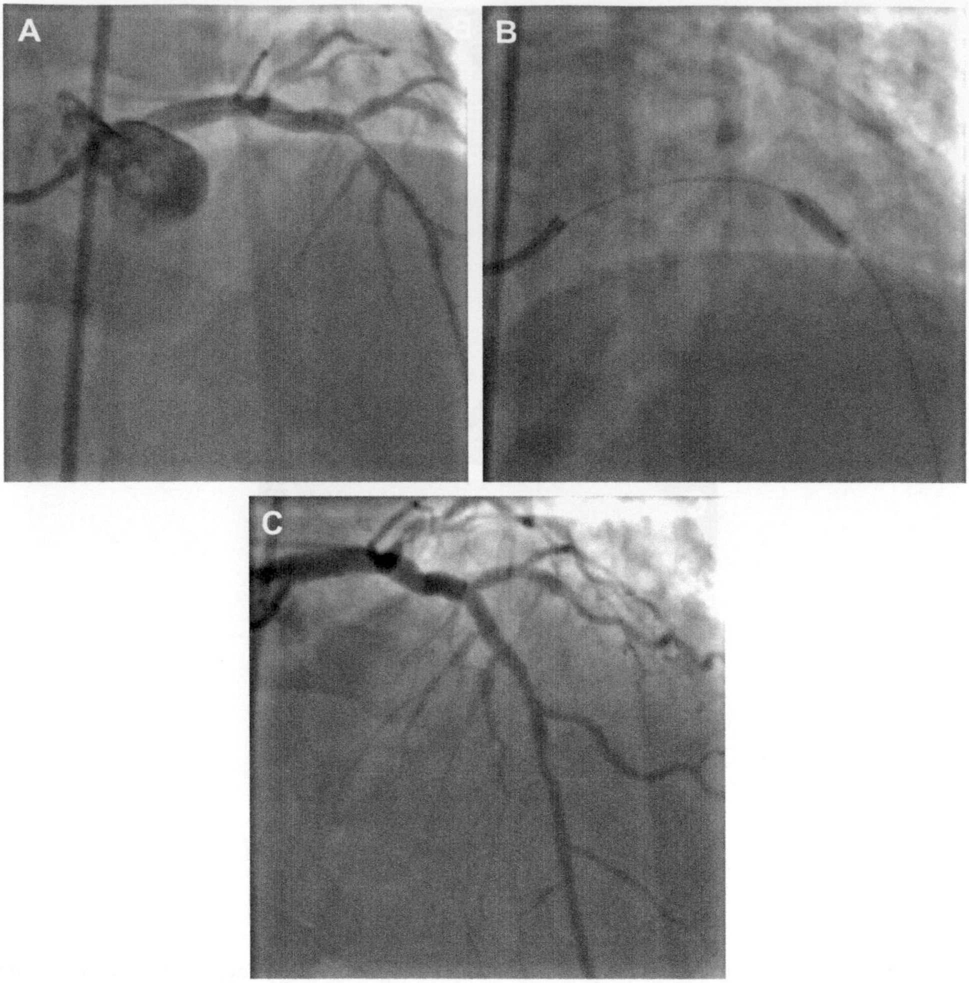

Fig. 4. Direct stenting for low-grade thrombus. (*A*) Grade 1 thrombus. (*B*) Direct stenting with 4.0-mm BMS. (*C*) After stenting.

aspiration catheter drags the tail of a long thread thrombus which may get dislodged. In 1 clinical case documented in the SINCERE database, a thrombus was dragged from the obtuse marginal branch and lodged at the bifurcation of the left circumflex; this was managed by suctioning with the AngioJet. The newer, aspiration catheters are easy to use and their use has now become the default strategy for managing thrombus for most lesions, except for those with very large TB, in whom mechanical thrombectomy is invaluable.

Grade 4 to 5

Larger TB (grades 4–5) presents more challenges. As shown in **Figs. 9–12**, aspiration may be insufficient in patients with grade 4 to 5 thrombus. In such patients, thrombectomy may be justified. The AngioJet catheter is an effective device for debulking such voluminous thrombi. Thrombus is aspirated and extracted after high-velocity water jets create a vacuum in this catheter-based system.[50] Compared with stenting alone, trials have found the AngioJet to be successful in improving epicardial flow, frame count, myocardial blush grade, and infarct size.[45,51] The VeGAS (Vein Graft AngioJet Study) 2 trial found that the AngioJet catheter system was superior to intracoronary urokinase administration in improving device and procedural success, with lower major adverse effects, bleeding, and vascular complications.[52]

Some practical techniques in using the AngioJet thrombectomy device improve clinical outcomes. The new Spiroflex AngioJet device is quick to set up; the speed of set-up is vital to maintain the goals of achieving short D2B times. The new catheters, including the 4F thrombectomy catheter,

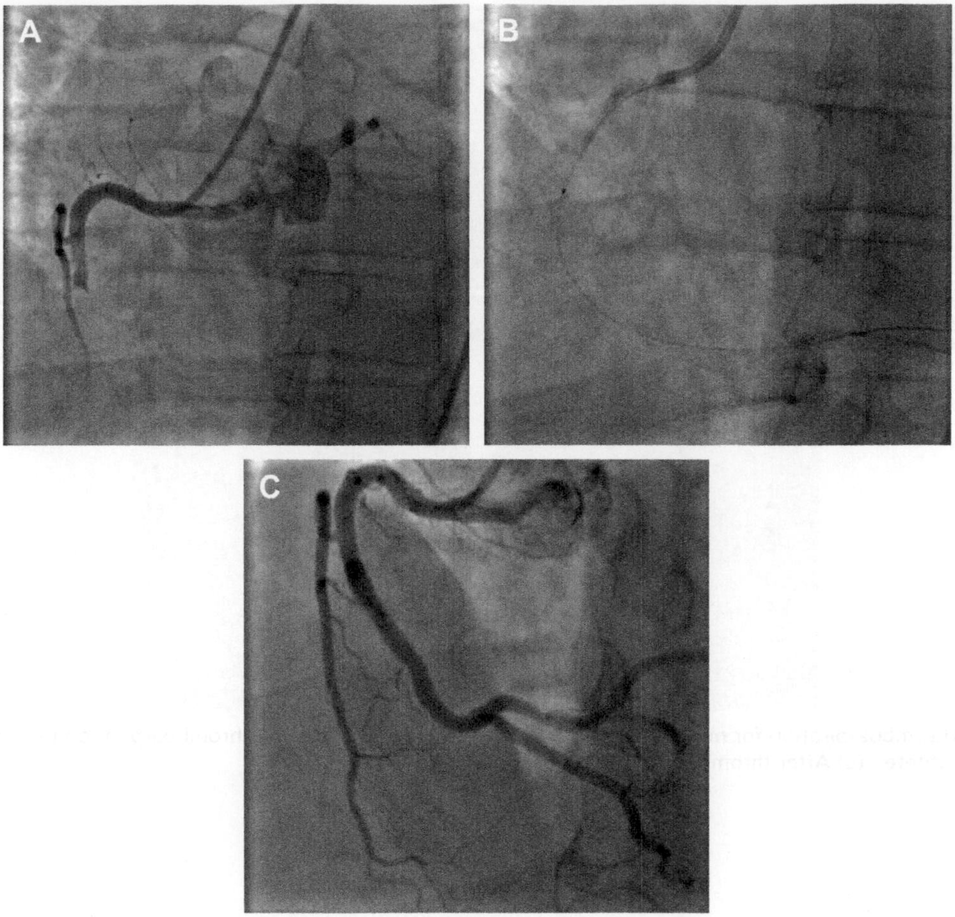

Fig. 5. Primary PCI for STEMI with moderate TB. Lesions with moderate-grade thrombus are best treated with aspiration thrombectomy devices, before definitive treatment and stenting. The next angiogram shows a moderate thrombus (grade 3) in a patient with ST-elevation in leads D to V. The first angiogram shows a discerning mid-right coronary artery culprit lesion with a moderate-grade thrombus (*A*). The lesion was treated then with an aspiration catheter (*B*) followed by angioplasty and stenting with a 4.0-mm bare-metal stent with a D2B time of 61 minutes with great results (*C*).

track well. Thrombectomy should be performed through the length of thrombus; the most frequent error with this device is inadequate passes and not ablating through the complete length of the thrombotic segment. In addition to being a critical device for removing large and bulky thrombus, the AngioJet is invaluable in managing organized thrombus in late-presenting patients. The SINCERE database includes several successful AngioJet procedures in which aspiration thrombectomy catheters were unsuccessful in aspirating such dense, organized thrombus. Temporary pacing is recommended for all AngioJet procedures. The pacing wire can be removed after the procedure, even although pacing is rare.

We offer another valuable tip for using both the aspiration and mechanical catheters: when is thrombectomy deemed adequate? To reach this point of optimal thrombectomy, we advocate making successive passes until the last pass makes no further progress in debulking. Sometimes, this goal can be difficult to assess by angiography, but this broad strategy provides a philosophic approach to approaching these thrombotic lesions with thrombectomy devices.

The Mehta strategy is offered as "a selective strategy for thrombus management in STEMI interventions based on the thrombus grade, with direct stenting recommended for low-grade thrombus, thromboaspiration for moderate thrombus, and rheolytic thrombectomy for high-grade thrombus (depending on suitable anatomy). For unsuitable anatomy or unavailability of rheolytic thrombectomy, a strategy of de thrombosis with intracoronary abciximab via the ClearWay catheter is an acceptable approach."

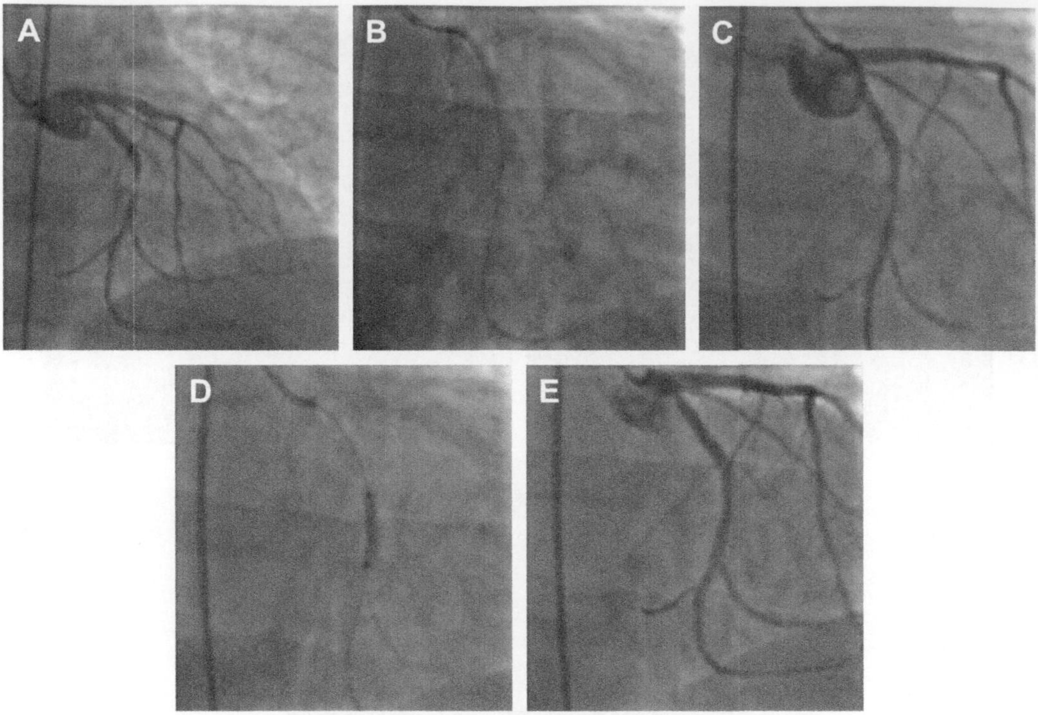

Fig. 6. Thromboaspiration for moderate thrombus. (*A*) Grade 2 thrombus. (*B*) Thromboaspiration performed by export catheter. (*C*) After thrombectomy. (*D*) 3.5-mm BMS. (*E*) After stenting.

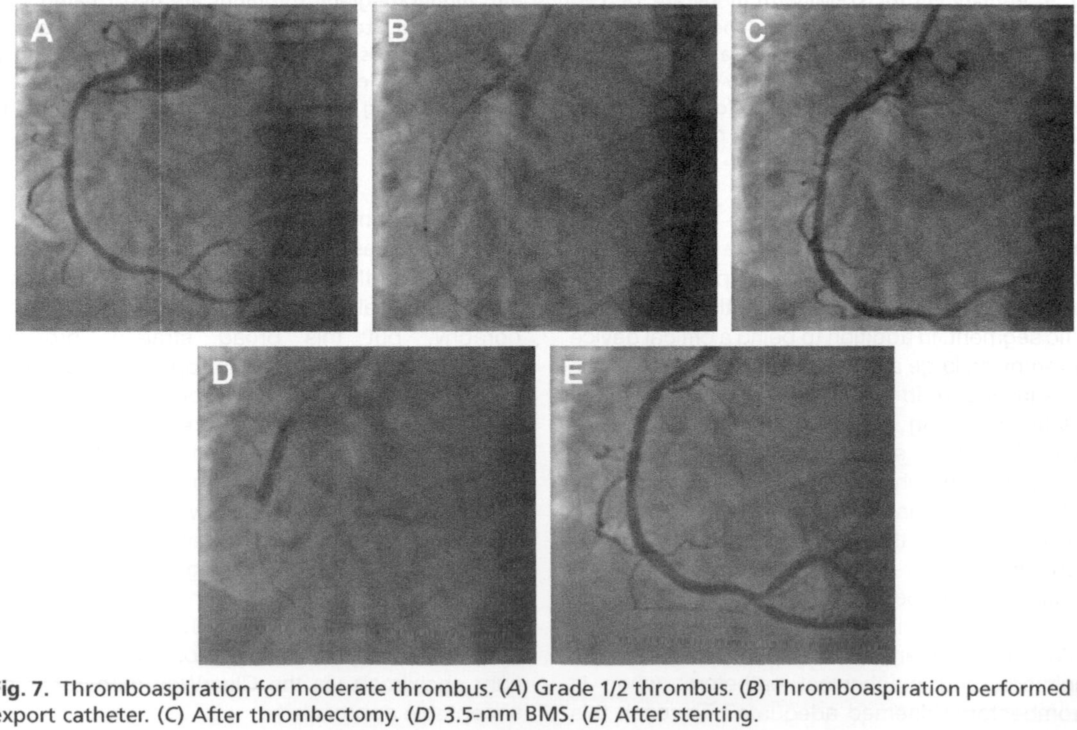

Fig. 7. Thromboaspiration for moderate thrombus. (*A*) Grade 1/2 thrombus. (*B*) Thromboaspiration performed by export catheter. (*C*) After thrombectomy. (*D*) 3.5-mm BMS. (*E*) After stenting.

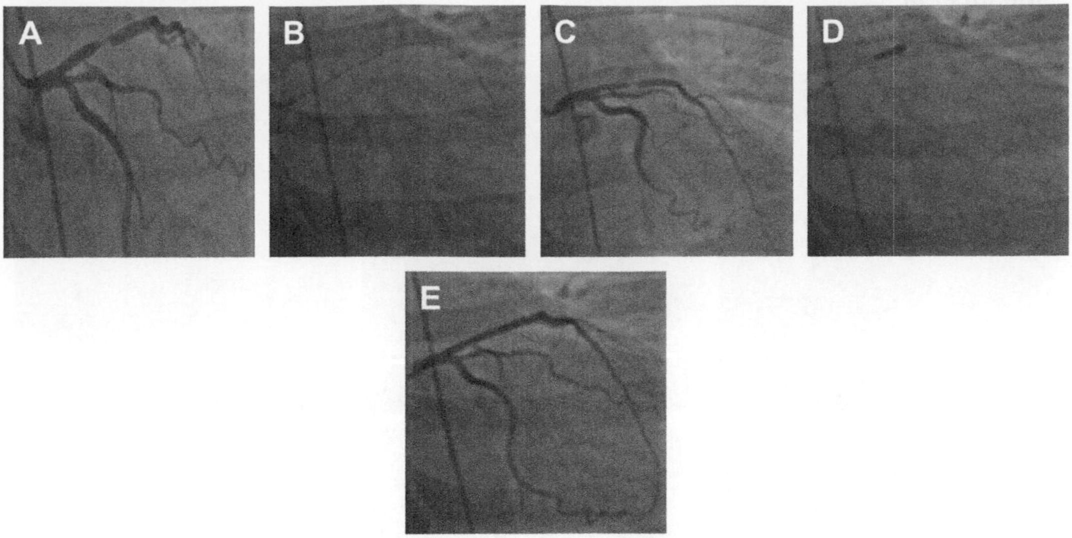

Fig. 8. Thromboaspiration for moderate thrombus. (*A*) Grade 2/3 thrombus. (*B*) Thromboaspiration performed by export catheter. (*C*) After thrombectomy. (*D*) 3.5-mm drug-eluting stent. (*E*) After stenting.

LIMITATIONS OF THE MEHTA STRATEGY

1. Several catheterization laboratories are not equipped with mechanical thrombectomy devices (AngioJet [Possis Medical Inc, Minneapolis, Minnesota], X-Sizer [eV3, White Bear Lake, Minnesota], and ThromCat [Kensey Nash Corporation, Exton, Pennsylvania]), or operators are not familiar with their use or find their use causes D2B delays. In these situations, we believe that drug delivery of abciximab via the ClearWay catheter (Atrium) provides a good alternative.
2. The same recommendation as number 1 exists with unfavorable anatomy for the AngioJet (our preferred mechanical thrombectomy device), although the newer 4F catheter has narrowed our relative contraindications for their use in STEMI interventions (<2.5-mm vessel size and severe tortuosity).
3. Although we recommend mechanical thrombectomy for large thrombus grade, we have been surprised in numerous cases in which thromboaspiration works well in large thrombus grade. We have presented numerous examples of these situations (**Figs. 13–18**); thrombus grade is high (4–5), yet excellent debulking is observed with the simple aspiration catheters. We suspect that this situation happens in patients who present very early, with fresh, red, soft thrombus that is easily and completely aspirated with these catheters. This observation is contrary to our proposed hypothesis, yet this powerful observation is shared for its tremendous practical benefit. We have observed this finding most often in thrombotic occlusions in which it made more sense to advance a small aspiration catheter than a more bulky mechanical device. This is also a rare situation in which we use a low-profile

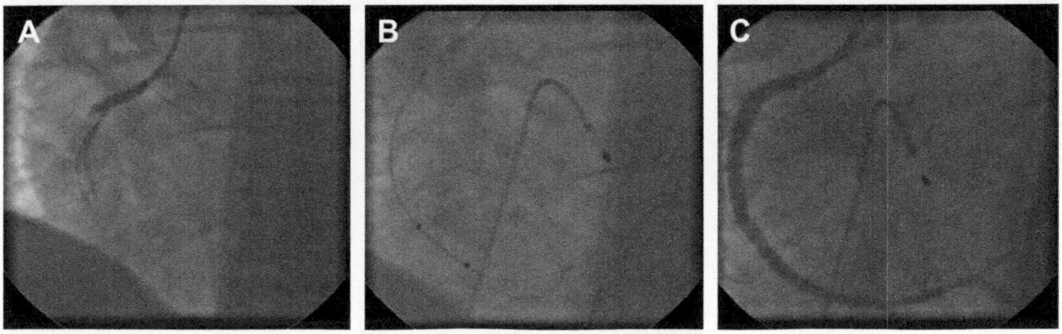

Fig. 9. Primary PCI for STEMI with large TB. Lesions with high-grade thrombus may require some thrombectomy before definitive treatment and stenting. The initial angiogram on this patient, who presented with an acute inferior wall STEMI, showed a large amount of thrombus (grade 3–4) (*A*). An AngioJet catheter (*B*) was initially used for rheolytic thrombectomy and after angioplasty and stenting, the final angiographic result was excellent (*C*).

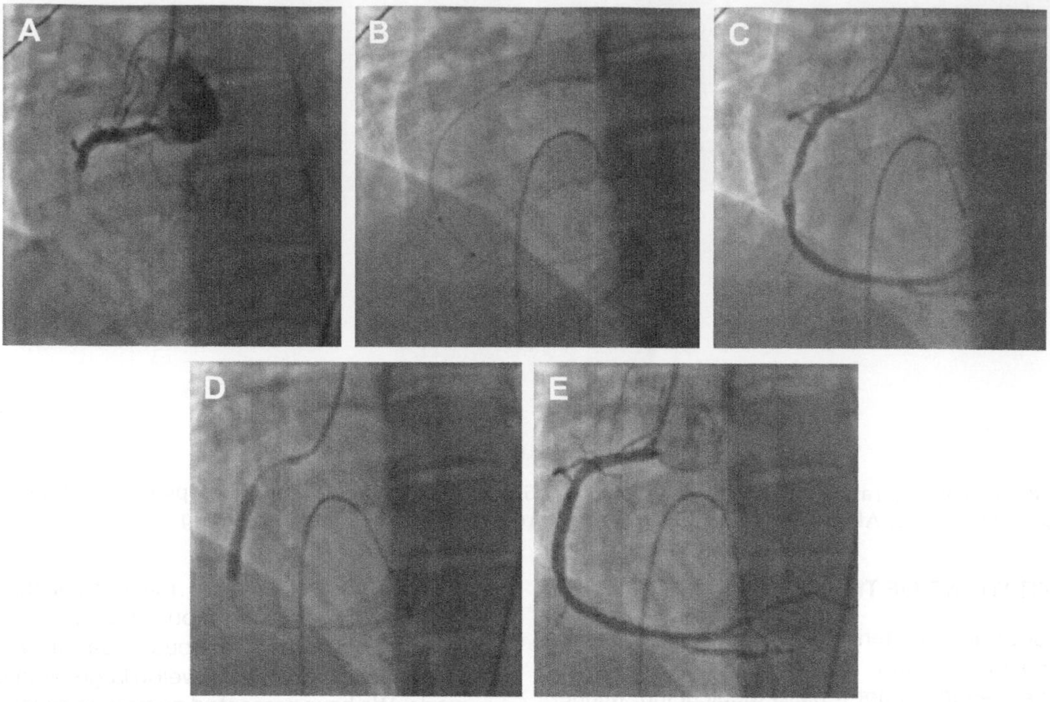

Fig. 10. Rheolytic thrombectomy for large thrombus. (*A*) Grade 5 thrombus. (*B*) Rheolytic thrombectomy performed with AngioJet. (*C*) After thrombectomy. (*D*) 4.0-mm BMS. (*E*) After stenting.

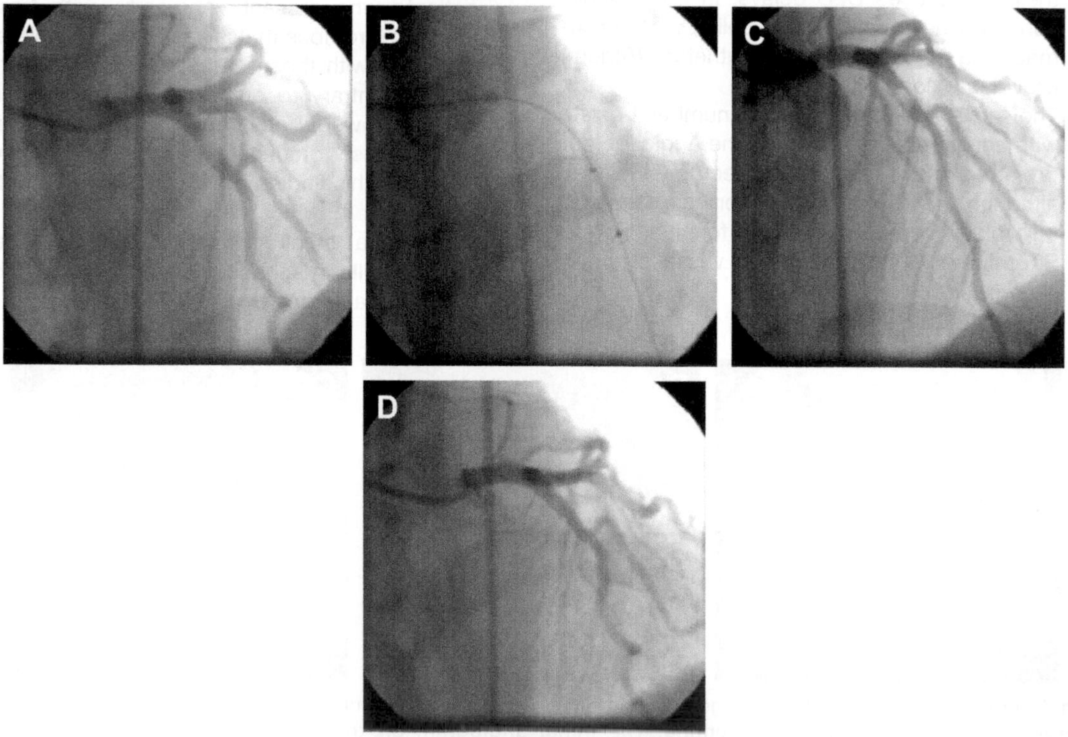

Fig. 11. Rheolytic thrombectomy for large thrombus. (*A*) Large, bulky thrombus in mid-left anterior descending artery. (*B*) Rheolytic thrombectomy performed with AngioJet. (*C*) After thrombectomy. (*D*) After stenting, final result.

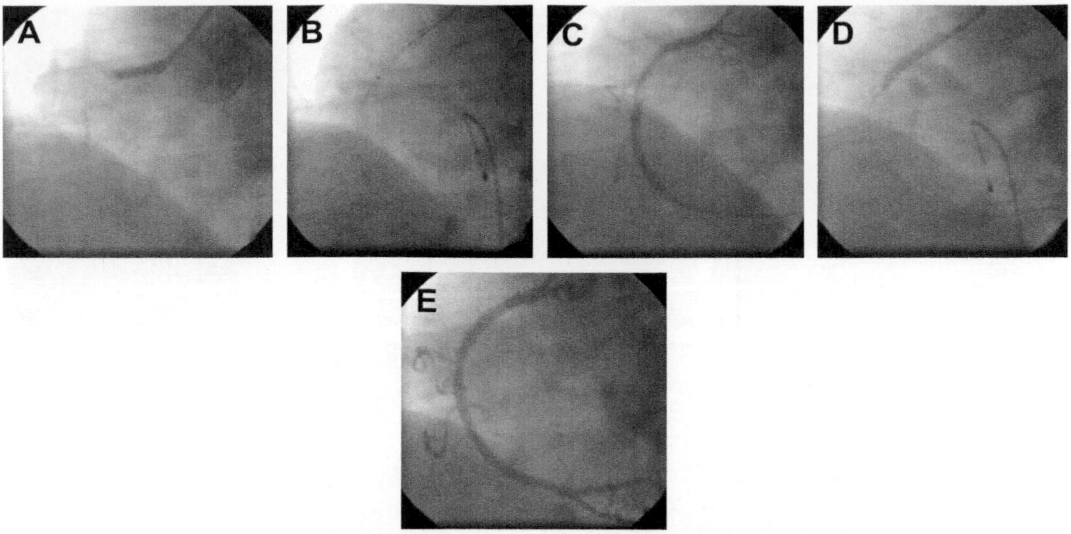

Fig. 12. Rheolytic thrombectomy for large thrombus. (*A*) Grade 5 thrombus. (*B*) Rheolytic thrombectomy performed with AngioJet. (*C*) After thrombectomy. (*D*) 4.5-mm BMS. (*E*) After stenting.

balloon to verify that the guide wire is in the true lumen. Based on an increasing number of similar cases, as shown in **Figs. 13–18**, we postulate thromboaspiration as a default strategy. The rationale for this strategy is simple: the aspiration catheters are user-friendly, relatively inexpensive, and take no more than a balloon catheter to prepare and deploy. With this methodology, we grade thrombus nevertheless, then quickly make

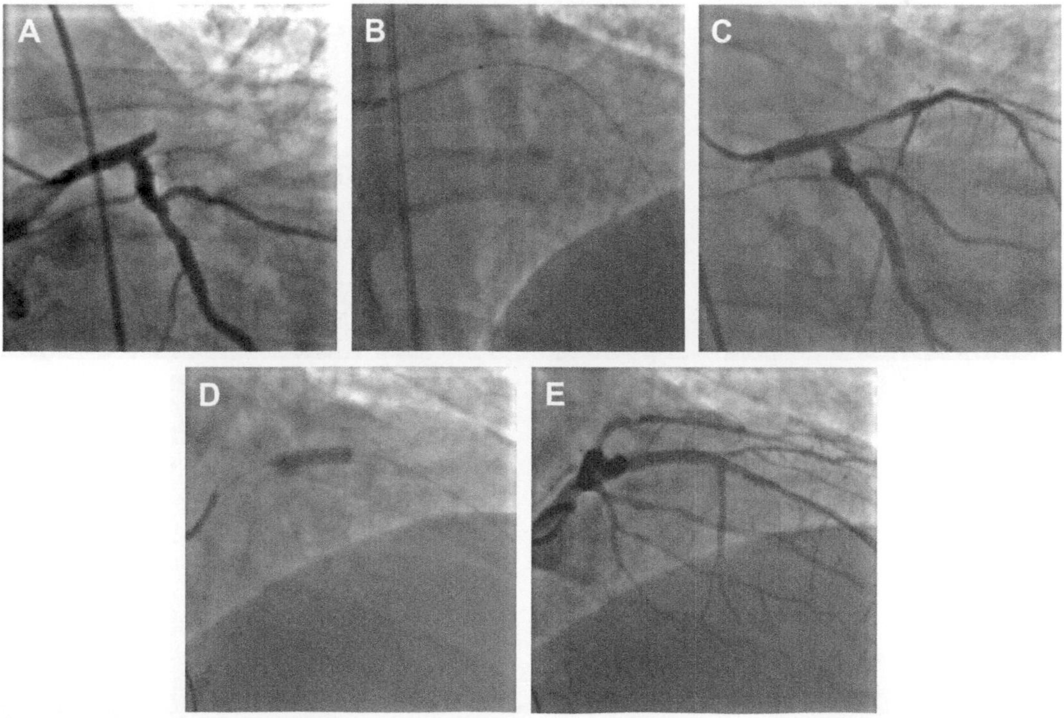

Fig. 13. Thromboaspiration as default strategy. (*A*) Grade 5 thrombus. (*B*) Thromboaspiration performed by export catheter. (*C*) After thrombectomy. (*D*) 3.5-mm Xience drug-eluting stent. (*E*) After stenting.

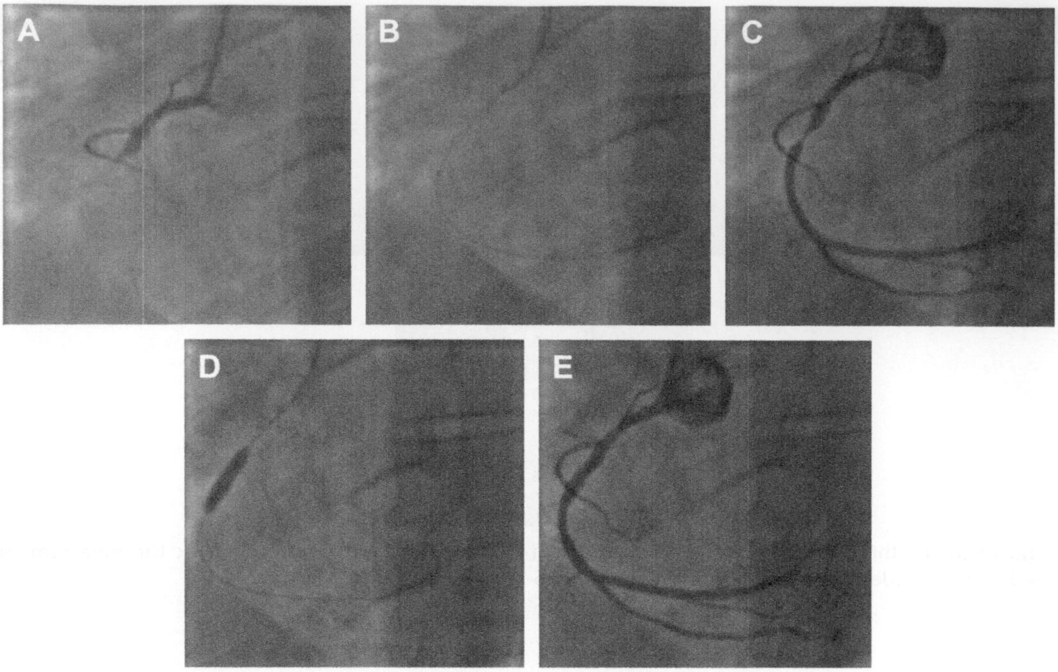

Fig. 14. Thromboaspiration as default strategy. (*A*) Grade 5 thrombus. (*B*) Thromboaspiration performed by export catheter. (*C*) After thrombectomy. (*D*) 4.0 BMS. (*E*) After stenting.

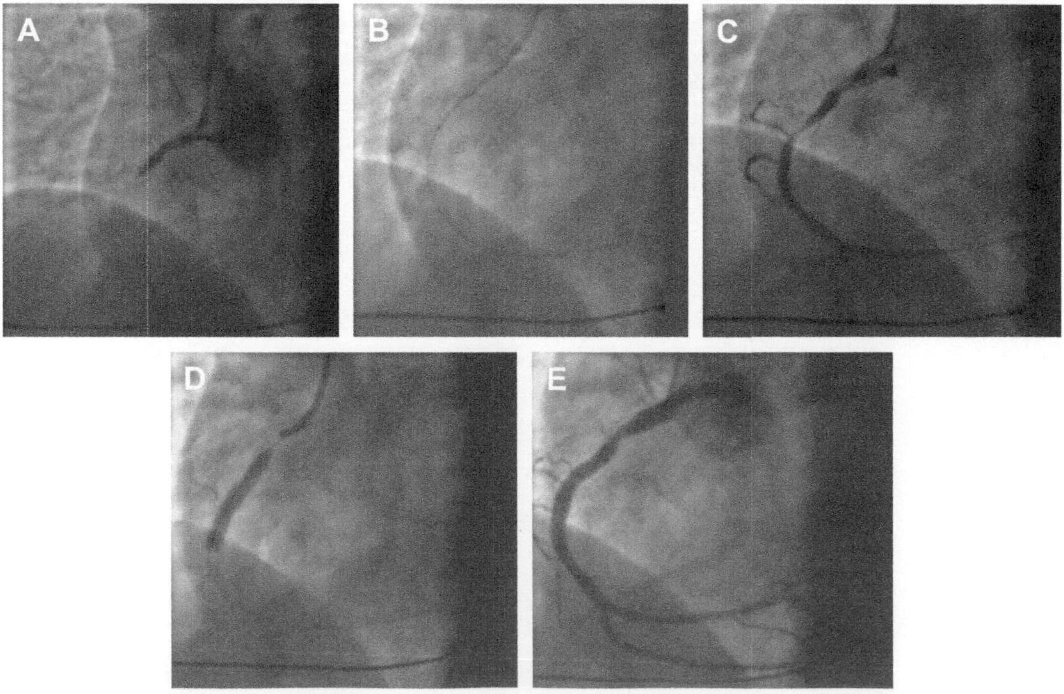

Fig. 15. Thromboaspiration as default strategy. (*A*) Grade 5 thrombus. (*B*) Thromboaspiration performed by export catheter. (*C*) After thrombectomy. (*D*) 4.0 BMS. (*E*) After stenting.

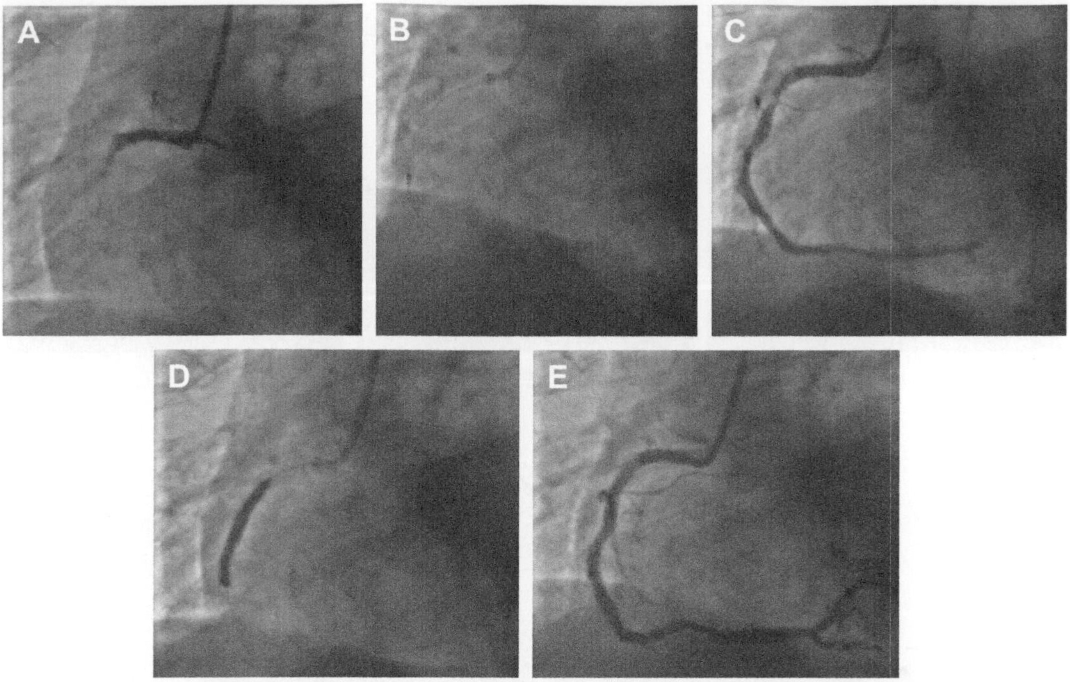

Fig. 16. Thromboaspiration as default strategy. (*A*) Grade 5 thrombus. (*B*) Thromboaspiration performed by export catheter. (*C*) After thrombectomy. (*D*) 4.0 BMS. (*E*) After stenting.

a pass with the aspiration catheter, and either persist with more thromboaspiration or advance to using mechanical thrombectomy.

4. Similarly, we have also experienced numerous cases, even with moderate TB, in which the dense, organized thrombus cannot be debulked with thromboaspiration. In these situations, the default strategy gives way to using mechanical thrombectomy, consistent with the Mehta classification.
5. Although several newer trials seem to validate our strategy with the appropriate presently available device, greater scientific validity is needed. Founded on extensive experience,

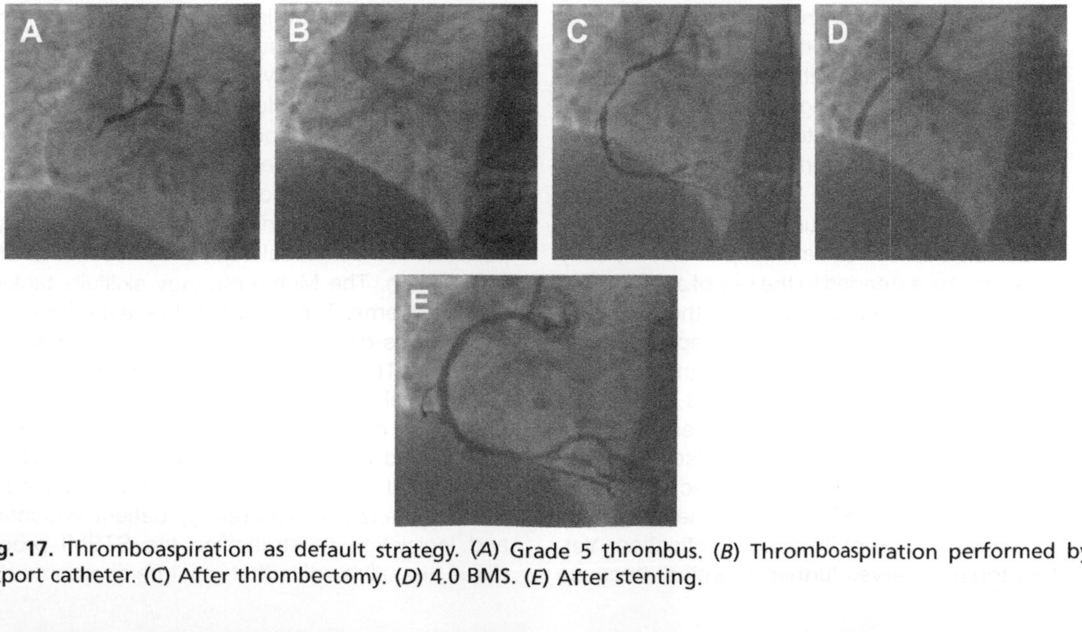

Fig. 17. Thromboaspiration as default strategy. (*A*) Grade 5 thrombus. (*B*) Thromboaspiration performed by export catheter. (*C*) After thrombectomy. (*D*) 4.0 BMS. (*E*) After stenting.

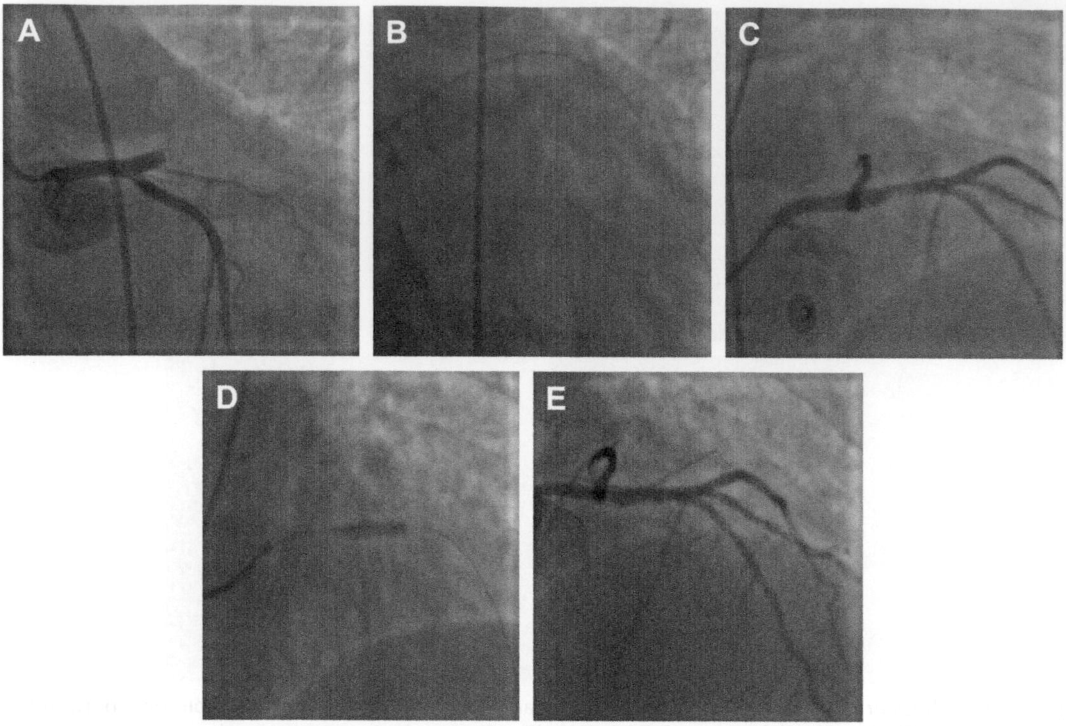

Fig. 18. Thromboaspiration as default strategy. (*A*) Grade 5 thrombus. (*B*) Thromboaspiration performed by export catheter. (*C*) After thrombectomy. (*D*) 4.0 Xience V drug-eluting stent. (*E*) After stenting.

we feel confident in our strategy for effective thrombus management for STEMI interventions; nevertheless, this strategy needs endorsement by clinical trials. A single individual experience, irrespective of its expertise, cannot substitute for data from large, randomized, clinical trials or established guidelines.

6. We have also explored the possibilities of using a time-to-presentation–based strategy for applying a thrombectomy device. This idea is akin to use of prehospital lysis, as in the CAPTIM (Comparison of Angioplasty and Prehospital Thrombolysis in Acute Myocardial Infarction) trial, in which the cohorts of patients with very early AMI benefit from very early lysis.[53] This situation probably results from effective lysis of a fresh clot. The same principles as very early lysis may be extended to the use of a thrombectomy device during STEMI, with thromboaspiration working as effective therapy for early presenters (<3 hours) and mechanical thrombectomy for late presenters (>3 hours). Of course, calculating the time to presentation is not without its challenges. We also recognize the numerous variables that affect thrombus presentation in STEMI and the heterogeneity of thrombus and of its oversimplification. Yet, this topic deserves further attention, because interventional management of soft, red, early thrombus is different than that of dense, organized thrombus.

SUMMARY

The management of thrombus in STEMI interventions is of paramount importance. To accomplish this complex task successfully, a systematic approach is necessary. Because of the dynamic nature of thrombosis formation, an interventional approach must incorporate a thrombus grading system, which also integrates mechanical adjunct devices. The limitations of equivocal clinical results from multiple trials fail to endorse the true potential of mechanical adjunct devices for STEMI intervention. The Mehta strategy skillfully tackles both problems. The algorithm has established (1) a thrombus-graded adjunct device approach to managing TB, which has already produced excellent clinical results (as shown in the SINCERE database), and (2) a scientific platform for future randomized multicenter controlled studies of the Mehta strategy. Even if perfection is obtained in the catheterization laboratory, patient education and legislation to streamline the STEMI procedures are still hurdles that must be overcome.

REFERENCES

1. Ellis SG, Roubin GS, King SB 3rd, et al. Angiographic and clinical predictors of acute closure after native vessel coronary angioplasty. Circulation 1988; 77(2):372–9.
2. Singh M, Berger PB, Ting HH, et al. Influence of coronary thrombus on outcome of percutaneous coronary angioplasty in the current era (the Mayo Clinic experience). Am J Cardiol 2001; 88(10):1091–6.
3. Mabin TA, Holmes DR Jr, Smith HC, et al. Intracoronary thrombus: role in coronary occlusion complicating percutaneous transluminal coronary angioplasty. J Am Coll Cardiol 1985;5(2 Pt 1):198–202.
4. White CJ, Ramee SR, Collins TJ, et al. Coronary thrombi increase PTCA risk. Angioscopy as a clinical tool. Circulation 1996;93(2):253–8.
5. Tamhane UU, Chetcuti S, Hameed I, et al. Safety and efficacy of thrombectomy in patients undergoing primary percutaneous coronary intervention for acute ST elevation MI: a meta-analysis of randomized controlled trials. BMC Cardiovasc Disord 2010;10:10.
6. Mongeon FP, Belisle P, Joseph L, et al. Adjunctive thrombectomy for acute myocardial infarction: a bayesian meta-analysis. Circ Cardiovasc Interv 2010;3(1):6–16.
7. Mehta S, Alfonso CE, Oliveros E, et al. Adjunct therapy in STEMI intervention. Cardiol Clin 2010; 28(1):107–25.
8. Kumar V, Abbas AK, Fausto N, et al. Robbins and Cotran pathologic basis of disease. 7th edition. Philadelphia: Elsevier Saunders; 2005.
9. Falk E, Shah PK, Fuster V. Coronary plaque disruption. Circulation 1995;92(3):657–71.
10. Furie B, Furie BC. Mechanisms of thrombus formation. N Engl J Med 2008;359(9):938–49.
11. Friedman M, Van den Bovenkamp GJ. The pathogenesis of a coronary thrombus. Am J Pathol 1966;48(1):19–44.
12. DeWood MA, Spores J, Notske R, et al. Prevalence of total coronary occlusion during the early hours of transmural myocardial infarction. N Engl J Med 1980;303(16):897–902.
13. Davies MJ, Thomas A. Thrombosis and acute coronary-artery lesions in sudden cardiac ischemic death. N Engl J Med 1984;310(18):1137–40.
14. Davies MJ, Thomas AC. Plaque fissuring–the cause of acute myocardial infarction, sudden ischaemic death, and crescendo angina. Br Heart J 1985; 53(4):363–73.
15. Horie T, Sekiguchi M, Hirosawa K. Coronary thrombosis in pathogenesis of acute myocardial infarction. Histopathological study of coronary arteries in 108 necropsied cases using serial section. Br Heart J 1978;40(2):153–61.
16. Grines CL, Browne KF, Marco J, et al. A comparison of immediate angioplasty with thrombolytic therapy for acute myocardial infarction. The Primary Angioplasty in Myocardial Infarction Study Group. N Engl J Med 1993;328(10):673–9.
17. Rezkalla SH, Kloner RA. No-reflow phenomenon. Circulation 2002;105(5):656–62.
18. Okamura A, Ito H, Iwakura K, et al. Detection of embolic particles with the Doppler guide wire during coronary intervention in patients with acute myocardial infarction: efficacy of distal protection device. J Am Coll Cardiol 2005;45(2):212–5.
19. Fukuda D, Tanaka A, Shimada K, et al. Predicting angiographic distal embolization following percutaneous coronary intervention in patients with acute myocardial infarction. Am J Cardiol 2003;91(4): 403–7.
20. Tanaka A, Kawarabayashi T, Nishibori Y, et al. No-reflow phenomenon and lesion morphology in patients with acute myocardial infarction. Circulation 2002;105(18):2148–52.
21. Barreto AD, Albright KC, Hallevi H, et al. Thrombus burden is associated with clinical outcome after intra-arterial therapy for acute ischemic stroke. Stroke 2008;39(12):3231–5.
22. Sianos G, Papafaklis MI, Daemen J, et al. Angiographic stent thrombosis after routine use of drug-eluting stents in ST-segment elevation myocardial infarction: the importance of thrombus burden. J Am Coll Cardiol 2007;50(7):573–83.
23. Ciszewski M, Pregowski J, Teresinska A, et al. Aspiration coronary thrombectomy for acute myocardial infarction increases myocardial salvage: single center randomized study. Catheter Cardiovasc Interv 2011;78(4):523–31.
24. Jolly S. Total trial: a randomized trial of routine aspiration thrombectomy with PCI versus PCI alone in patients with STEMI undergoing primary PCI. Available at: http://www.clinicaltrials.gov/ct2/show/NCT01149044. Accessed March 26, 2012.
25. The INFUSE-Anterior Myocardial Infarction (AMI) Study. ClinicalTrials.gov–a service of the U.S. National Institutes of Health. Available at: http://clinicaltrials.gov/ct2/show/NCT00976521. Accessed February 25, 2012.
26. Frobert O, Lagerqvist B, Gudnason T, et al. Thrombus Aspiration in ST-Elevation myocardial infarction in Scandinavia (TASTE trial). A multicenter, prospective, randomized, controlled clinical registry trial based on the Swedish angiography and angioplasty registry (SCAAR) platform. Study design and rationale. Am Heart J 2010;160(6):1042–8.
27. Sardella G, Mancone M, Bucciarelli-Ducci C, et al. Thrombus aspiration during primary percutaneous coronary intervention improves myocardial reperfusion and reduces infarct size: the EXPIRA (thrombectomy with export catheter in infarct-related

artery during primary percutaneous coronary intervention) prospective, randomized trial. J Am Coll Cardiol 2009;53(4):309–15.
28. Burzotta F, De Vita M, Gu YL, et al. Clinical impact of thrombectomy in acute ST-elevation myocardial infarction: an individual patient-data pooled analysis of 11 trials. Eur Heart J 2009;30(18):2193–203.
29. Liistro F, Grotti S, Angioli P, et al. Impact of thrombus aspiration on myocardial tissue reperfusion and left ventricular functional recovery and remodeling after primary angioplasty. Circ Cardiovasc Interv 2009; 2(5):376–83.
30. Lipiecki J, Monzy S, Durel N, et al. Effect of thrombus aspiration on infarct size and left ventricular function in high-risk patients with acute myocardial infarction treated by percutaneous coronary intervention. Results of a prospective controlled pilot study. Am Heart J 2009;157(3):583. e1–7.
31. Vlaar PJ, Svilaas T, van der Horst IC, et al. Cardiac death and reinfarction after 1 year in the Thrombus Aspiration during Percutaneous coronary intervention in Acute myocardial infarction Study (TAPAS): a 1-year follow-up study. Lancet 2008;371(9628):1915–20.
32. Chevalier B, Gilard M, Lang I, et al. Systematic primary aspiration in acute myocardial percutaneous intervention: a multicentre randomised controlled trial of the export aspiration catheter. EuroIntervention 2008;4(2):222–8.
33. Ikari Y, Sakurada M, Kozuma K, et al. Upfront thrombus aspiration in primary coronary intervention for patients with ST-segment elevation acute myocardial infarction: report of the VAMPIRE (VAcuuM asPIration thrombus REmoval) trial. JACC Cardiovasc Interv 2008;1(4):424–31.
34. Chao CL, Hung CS, Lin YH, et al. Time-dependent benefit of initial thrombosuction on myocardial reperfusion in primary percutaneous coronary intervention. Int J Clin Pract 2008;62(4):555–61.
35. Anzai H, Yoneyama S, Tsukagoshi M, et al. Rescue percutaneous thrombectomy system provides better angiographic coronary flow and does not increase the in-hospital cost in patients with acute myocardial infarction. Circ J 2003;67(9):768–74.
36. Andersen NH, Karlsen FM, Gerdes JC, et al. No beneficial effects of coronary thrombectomy on left ventricular systolic and diastolic function in patients with acute S-T elevation myocardial infarction: a randomized clinical trial. J Am Soc Echocardiogr 2007;20(6):724–30.
37. Kaltoft A, Bottcher M, Nielsen SS, et al. Routine thrombectomy in percutaneous coronary intervention for acute ST-segment-elevation myocardial infarction: a randomized, controlled trial. Circulation 2006;114(1):40–7.
38. Silva-Orrego P, Colombo P, Bigi R, et al. Thrombus aspiration before primary angioplasty improves myocardial reperfusion in acute myocardial infarction: the DEAR-MI (Dethrombosis to Enhance Acute Reperfusion in Myocardial Infarction) study. J Am Coll Cardiol 2006;48(8):1552–9.
39. De Luca L, Sardella G, Davidson CJ, et al. Impact of intracoronary aspiration thrombectomy during primary angioplasty on left ventricular remodelling in patients with anterior ST elevation myocardial infarction. Heart 2006;92(7):951–7.
40. Burzotta F, Trani C, Romagnoli E, et al. Manual thrombus-aspiration improves myocardial reperfusion: the randomized evaluation of the effect of mechanical reduction of distal embolization by thrombus-aspiration in primary and rescue angioplasty (REMEDIA) trial. J Am Coll Cardiol 2005; 46(2):371–6.
41. Antoniucci D. Comparison of manual aspiration with rheolytic thrombectomy in patients undergoing primary PCI. The SMART-PCI trial. Available at: http://clinicaltrials.gov/ct2/show/NCT01281033. Accessed March 26, 2012.
42. Migliorini A, Stabile A, Rodriguez AE, et al. Comparison of AngioJet rheolytic thrombectomy before direct infarct artery stenting with direct stenting alone in patients with acute myocardial infarction. The JETSTENT trial. J Am Coll Cardiol 2010;56(16):1298–306.
43. Ali A, Cox D, Dib N, et al. Rheolytic thrombectomy with percutaneous coronary intervention for infarct size reduction in acute myocardial infarction: 30-day results from a multicenter randomized study. J Am Coll Cardiol 2006;48(2):244–52.
44. Lefevre T, Garcia E, Reimers B, et al. X-sizer for thrombectomy in acute myocardial infarction improves ST-segment resolution: results of the X-sizer in AMI for negligible embolization and optimal ST resolution (X AMINE ST) trial. J Am Coll Cardiol 2005;46(2):246–52.
45. Antoniucci D, Valenti R, Migliorini A, et al. Comparison of rheolytic thrombectomy before direct infarct artery stenting versus direct stenting alone in patients undergoing percutaneous coronary intervention for acute myocardial infarction. Am J Cardiol 2004;93(8):1033–5.
46. Napodano M, Pasquetto G, Sacca S, et al. Intracoronary thrombectomy improves myocardial reperfusion in patients undergoing direct angioplasty for acute myocardial infarction. J Am Coll Cardiol 2003;42(8):1395–402.
47. Beran G, Lang I, Schreiber W, et al. Intracoronary thrombectomy with the X-sizer catheter system improves epicardial flow and accelerates ST-segment resolution in patients with acute coronary syndrome: a prospective, randomized, controlled study. Circulation 2002;105(20):2355–60.
48. Svilaas T, Vlaar PJ, van der Horst IC, et al. Thrombus aspiration during primary percutaneous

coronary intervention. N Engl J Med 2008;358(6): 557–67.
49. Mehta S, Alfonso C, Oliveros E, et al. Lesson from the single Individual Community Experience Registry for Primary PCI (SINCERE) database. In: Kappur R, editor. Textbook of STEMI interventions. 2nd edition. Malvern (PA): HMP Communications; 2010. p. 131–48.
50. Whisenant BK, Baim DS, Kuntz RE, et al. Rheolytic thrombectomy with the Possis AngioJet: technical considerations and initial clinical experience. J Invasive Cardiol 1999;11(7):421–6.
51. Margheri M, Falai M, Vittori G, et al. Safety and efficacy of the AngioJet in patients with acute myocardial infarction: results from the Florence Appraisal Study of Rheolytic Thrombectomy (FAST). J Invasive Cardiol 2006;18(10):481–6.
52. Kuntz RE, Baim DS, Cohen DJ, et al. A trial comparing rheolytic thrombectomy with intracoronary urokinase for coronary and vein graft thrombus (the Vein Graft AngioJet Study [VeGAS 2]). Am J Cardiol 2002;89(3):326–30.
53. Steg PG, Bonnefoy E, Chabaud S, et al. Impact of time to treatment on mortality after prehospital fibrinolysis or primary angioplasty: data from the CAPTIM randomized clinical trial. Circulation 2003; 108(23):2851–6.

Stenting in Acute STEMI Intervention

Ahmed Magdy, MD, FSCAI*, Hisham Selim, MD, Mona Youssef, MD

KEYWORDS

• Stenting • Acute myocardial infarction • STEMI • Intervention

KEY POINTS

- Stenting in acute myocardial infarction (AMI) has the benefits of achieving an acute optimal angiographic result and correcting any residual dissection to decrease the incidence of restenosis and reocclusion.
- Studies have shown that percutaneous transluminal coronary angioplasty for primary treatment after AMI is superior to thrombolytic therapy with regard to the restoration of normal coronary blood flow. Coronary stenting improves the initial success rate, decreases the incidence of abrupt closure, and is associated with a reduced rate of restenosis.
- In the presence of thrombus-containing lesions, coronary stenting constitutes an effective therapeutic strategy, either after failure of initial angioplasty or electively as the primary procedure.
- All data and the current guidelines recommended by the American College of Cardiology/American Heart Association and European Society of Cardiology strongly support discouraging non–infarct-related artery percutaneous coronary intervention (PCI) procedures performed at the time of primary PCI when patients are hemodynamically stable.
- Studies, such as the Trial to Assess the Use of the Cypher Stent in Acute Myocardial Infarction Treated with Balloon Angioplasty (TYPHOON) and the Paclitaxel-Eluting Stent versus Conventional Stent in Myocardial Infarction with ST-Segment Elevation (PASSION) trial, have demonstrated the safety of drug-eluting stents (DES) in patients with AMI as compared with bare-metal stents in stent thrombosis with the advantage of reducing target vessel revascularization. More recent studies, such as the Evaluation of Xience-V stent in Acute Myocardial INfArcTION (EXAMINATION) trial and subgroups of the Limus Eluted from A Durable vs ERodable Stent Coating (LEADERS) study, have shown even better results with second-generation DES in patients with AMI.

INTRODUCTION

The goals of therapy in acute myocardial infarction (AMI) are to achieve rapid and optimal restoration of flow in the infarct-related vessel and to maintain this initial result in the long term.[1] Complete (Thrombolysis in Myocardial Infarction [TIMI] grade 3) patency of the infarct-related artery is a major predictor of survival and preserved left ventricular function following reperfusion therapy.[2–4] Pharmacologic therapy with fibrinolytic agents is, for logistic reasons, the initial therapy of choice in most patients presenting with an AMI.[1] However, there are several limitations to thrombolysis. First, the main limitation is the suboptimal restoration of TIMI grade 3 flow, which is generally not reported in more than 55% to 65% of patients within 90 minutes.[2,4] Second, even within the group of patients with an open artery after fibrinolytic therapy, there is a substantial minority who has suboptimal myocardial perfusion in the territory of the infarct vessel, probably as a result of

Cardiology Department, National Heart Institute, 44 Alsharifa Dina, Maadi, Cairo 11431, Egypt
* Corresponding author.
E-mail address: amagdy2@gmail.com

Intervent Cardiol Clin 1 (2012) 507–520
http://dx.doi.org/10.1016/j.iccl.2012.06.007
2211-7458/12/$ – see front matter

a combination of distal embolization of thrombotic material and of microvascular spasm related to the release of potent thrombus-derived vasoactive substances.[5] Finally, reocclusion of the infarct-related vessel occurs in roughly one-third of the patients treated by fibrinolysis in which the artery was initially patent and this proportion is not affected by either prolonged anticoagulant or antiplatelet therapy.[6]

ADVANTAGES OF PRIMARY PERCUTANEOUS CORONARY INTERVENTION

Primary or direct angioplasty is an alternative to fibrinolytic therapy. It has the advantage that normal antegrade flow can be restored acutely in a higher proportion of patients; however, the overall benefit, as for fibrinolytic therapy, depends on the delay to reperfusion. It should, therefore, only be considered as the preferred initial therapy for patients who can be rapidly admitted to an interventional center with experienced operators. In patients who are eligible for either therapy, it is clear that an initial strategy of direct angioplasty in an experienced center is associated with a better long-term outcome than an initial strategy of fibrinolytic therapy.[1] For example, the Primary Angioplasty in Myocardial Infarction (PAMI)-1 trial evaluated a strategy of either primary angioplasty or treatment with tissue-type plasminogen activator in 395 patients. At the 2-year follow-up, patients who were randomized to primary angioplasty had significantly less recurrent ischemia (36.4% vs 48.0%) and a significantly lower rate of reintervention (27.2% vs 46.5%).[7]

Despite the evidence that primary angioplasty was superior to fibrinolytic therapy, when both options were feasible, the relatively high rate of recurrent clinical events and of restenosis after primary angioplasty was a continuing preoccupation. The demonstration that elective stent implantation was associated with a decrease in restenosis and in clinical events in selected patients led to this strategy being applied in patients with MI, both in the acute phase and in early postinfarct angioplasty. A French trial STENTing In acute Myocardial infarction (STENTIM-2) that randomized patients with AMI to a strategy of either systematic or provisional stenting showed that systematic stenting was associated with a significantly lower (25.3% vs 39.6%) restenosis rate. The trial was not powered to assess an effect on the clinical outcome. However, there was a trend toward a reduction in major cardiac events at 6 months in the patients who underwent systematic stenting (18.8% vs 23.3%, P = .14) despite the crossover rate of 36.4% to stenting in the balloon group.[8]

The introduction of stent implantation that allows mechanical stabilization of the unstable plaque made the initial result of angioplasty much more predictable and reduced acute complications.[1] Furthermore, coronary stenting was proved to be effective in reducing the rates of restenosis and acute closure and in increasing the acute gain in luminal diameter in comparison with balloon angioplasty.[9,10] In ST-segment elevation myocardial infarction (STEMI), the key performance criteria is to perform the intervention as early as possible because the sooner an occluded artery is opened and blood flow is restored, the less myocardium is lost and the lower the mortality.[11] The optimization of adjuvant pharmacologic therapy, as a result of the reevaluation of the relative importance of antiplatelet and antithrombin therapy, an advance that owes much to the experience with coronary stenting, also improved outcome, in particular, by reducing bleeding complications. These two advances set the scene for a reevaluation of the role of combined fibrinolysis and percutaneous intervention.

STENTING IN AMI

For a long time, it was thought that coronary stenting was contraindicated in the setting of AMI because the implantation of a metallic device within a thrombotic environment, such as that of plaque disruption resulting in MI, would be likely to precipitate stent thrombosis with resultant vessel reocclusion.[12] The first report of bailout stenting in AMI was published in 1991,[13] but the first studies showing the feasibility and efficacy of stenting in patients with AMI and poor or suboptimal results after conventional coronary angioplasty (percutaneous transluminal coronary angioplasty [PTCA]) appeared in 1996 in 4 small series of patients.[14,15] At that time, stent thrombosis, with a rate that could be as high as 20% in bailout procedures, had been dramatically reduced to less than 2% by improvement in stent deployment techniques and advances in antiplatelet therapy, allowing a prompt reassessment of the role of stenting in AMI. In fact, after the encouraging results of these preliminary observational studies, stent implantation in patients with AMI grew enormously, and in 1997 the results of more than 30 observational studies in more than 2000 patients appeared. At the same time, several randomized trials comparing primary infarct-artery stenting with primary PTCA started.[12]

Mechanisms of Benefit of Stenting in AMI

Although the efficacy of primary PTCA has been demonstrated, the benefits of a primary PTCA strategy are limited by the high incidence of early and late restenosis or reocclusion of the infarct vessel. As a consequence of infarct artery restenosis or reocclusion, many patients have recurrent ischemia after successful primary PTCA. Within 6 months of successful primary PTCA, restenosis or reocclusion of the infarct vessel may occur in more than 50% of patients, and the incidence of major adverse events related to recurrent ischemia, such as fatal and nonfatal reinfarction and repeat target-vessel revascularization (TVR), may be as high as 30%.[16,17] With respect to early recurrent ischemia, PAMI-1investigators have shown that a suboptimal angiographic result after successful primary PTCA is a strong predictor of early major adverse events,[18] whereas with respect to late recurrent ischemia, an acute optimal angiographic result, that is, the largest minimum luminal diameter achievable, is assumed to be inversely related to late restenosis or reocclusion.[19] Thus, the postulated mechanisms of the benefit of stenting in AMI are the achievement of an acute optimal angiographic result and correction of any residual dissection to decrease the incidence of restenosis and reocclusion and of the correlated clinical events, such as fatal reinfarction, nonfatal reinfarction, and repeat TVR for recurrent ischemia. It is important to point out that most patients with recurrent ischemia after successful primary PTCA have angina or nonfatal reinfarction, whereas death as a consequence of recurrent ischemia accounts for a minority of deaths[20,21] because most deaths of patients with AMI are caused by refractory cardiogenic shock despite a patent infarct artery. As a consequence, the expected benefit of stent in terms of the reduction of mortality rates is limited only to patients with a very large area at risk or severe left ventricular dysfunction. For patients not at high risk, the benefit of stenting may result only in a significant reduction of the incidence of nonfatal reinfarction and mainly of repeat TVR for recurrent angina. Obviously, repeat TVR is a soft end point as compared with death. Nevertheless, this soft end point has important clinical and economic implications when considering the quality of life of patients, the longer hospital stay in the acute phase, the need for readmission for late recurrence, and the adjunctive costs of a repeat revascularization procedure.[12]

Another potential benefit of stenting independent of myocardial salvage is related to the early and late open artery hypotheses.[22] By reducing the incidence of early and late reocclusion, stenting may prevent or reduce left ventricular remodeling and long-term mortality rates, as being ventricular remodeling a major determinant of survival.

APPARENT PARADOX OF PRIMARY INFARCT ARTERY STENTING AND DETERIORATION OF FLOW

After a TIMI grade 3 flow is restored by mechanical recanalization with the use of the coronary wire or, more frequently, the PTCA balloon, a deterioration of TIMI flow may occur after stent placement. The phenomenon of angiographic no-reflow (TIMI 0–1) or slow flow (TIMI 2) after primary infarct artery stenting is not frequent and is similar to that occurring in other clinical settings associated with thrombus-containing lesions or with the use of atherectomy devices that may microembolize with vessel debris and capillary plugging.[23,24] In primary infarct artery stenting, no-reflow or slow reflow respond to intracoronary calcium antagonists or adenosine in most cases and this suggests that microvascular spasm is the mechanism of microvascular dysfunction. Persistent flow impairment after calcium antagonist treatment suggests microembolization or microvascular reperfusion injury. In the Florence Randomized Elective Stenting in Acute Coronary Occlusions (FRESCO) trial, only 1 (1.3%) patient out of 75 randomly assigned to stenting had persistent slow flow despite intracoronary calcium antagonist treatment.[25] In the Stent PAMI trial, 8 (2.6%) patients out of 350 assigned to stenting with TIMI grade 3 flow after predilatation PTCA had slow flow (7 patients) or no-reflow (1 patient).[25]

High-pressure stent expansion is likely to be the mediator of microvascular dysfunction and degradation of angiographic TIMI flow. It is important to point out that microvascular dysfunction related to stent placement should not be confused with no perfusion despite removal of any coronary obstruction. The latter may also be associated with an angiographic slow flow with TIMI grade 3 flow and is likely to be the expression of reperfusion injury unrelated to stent placement.[12]

DRUG-ELUTING STENTS OR BARE-METAL STENT FOR AMI: AN ISSUE OF SAFETY?

Coronary-artery stenting is commonly performed to treat MI. Acute coronary syndromes and MI (in contrast to stable angina)[26] are the only clinical presentations in which percutaneous coronary intervention (PCI) has been shown to reduce the rate of death to a rate lower than that achieved with medical therapy alone.[27–29] Despite the important role of stenting in patients with MI and, in particular, in those who have MI with STEMI, there has been little information regarding the long-term efficacy or safety of drug-eluting stents (DES) among these patients.[30] There have been several specific concerns about using DES (thrombogenic material) in AMI (prothrombotic state), particularly after studies and case reports relating DES thrombosis occurring in patients having suffered from acute coronary syndrome.

For instance, McFadden and colleagues[31] reported that most late stent thrombosis occurred when a DES was placed in patients with acute coronary syndrome. Observational studies have shown that this risk continues at a constant rate up to at least 4 years after stenting.[32] Finn and colleagues[33] demonstrated in their laboratory that delayed healing (ie, lack of complete endothelization) is the primary pathologic substrate underlying these events and that greater than 50% of stent struts in humans are not covered by the endothelium up to 24 months after DES placement (**Fig. 1**).

Moreover, the preliminary results of the Prospective Registry Evaluating Myocardial Infarction: Events and Recovery (PREMIER) displayed a 3-fold higher mortality rate in the group treated with DES (sirolimus-eluting stent [SES]) compared with the group treated with bare-metal stent (BMS).[34] Based on these data, a cautionary approach has been promulgated to refrain from the systematic use of DES in the setting of STEMI until the publication of the two first large randomized controlled trials, the Trial to Assess the Use of the Cypher Stent in Acute Myocardial Infarction Treated with Balloon Angioplasty (TYPHOON) and Paclitaxel-Eluting Stent versus Conventional Stent in Myocardial Infarction with ST-Segment Elevation (PASSION), which are summarized next.

The TYPHOON trial[35] was a single-blind multicenter prospectively randomized trial to compare SES with BMS in primary PCI for AMI with ST-segment elevation. The trial included 712 patients at 48 medical centers. The primary end point was target-vessel failure at 1 year after the procedure, defined as target vessel–related death, recurrent MI, or TVR. A follow-up angiographic substudy was performed at 8 months among 174 patients from selected centers. In this study, the rate of the primary end point was significantly lower in the

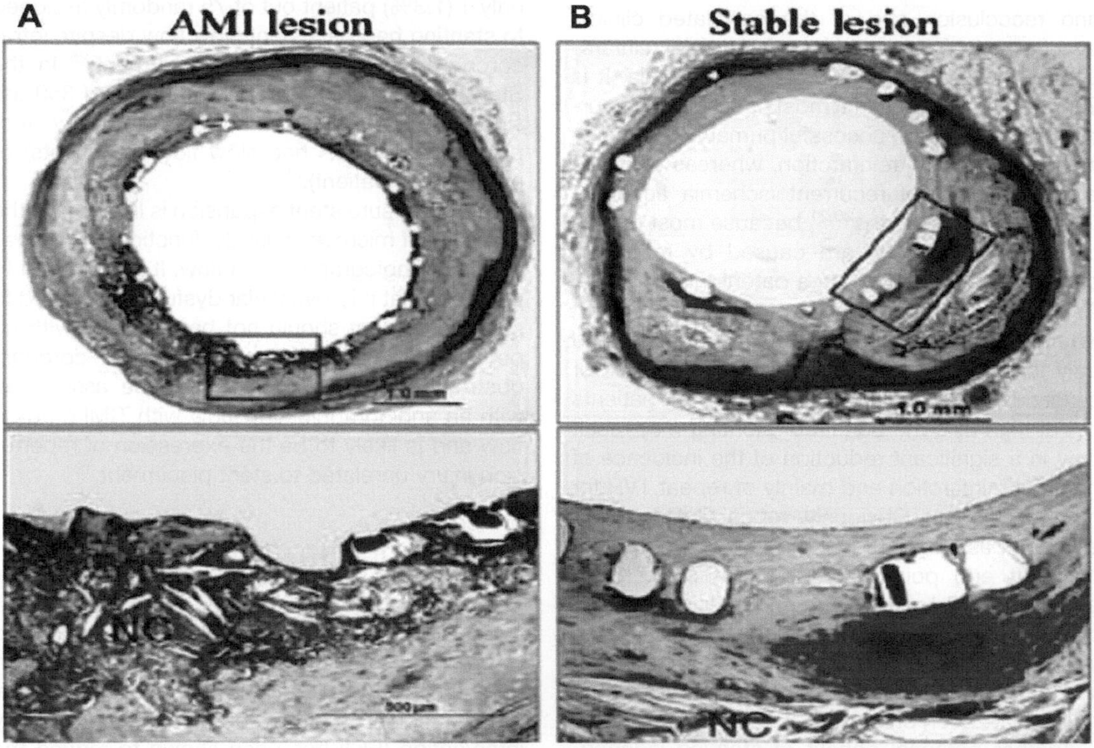

Fig. 1. (*A*) Histologic sections of the stented artery from a 64-year-old woman who died of congestive heart failure 9 months after Taxus stent implantation for AMI. Many uncovered struts are observed in the section (*upper panel*). Note that there is an underlying necrotic core with no healing above stent struts (*lower panel*). (*B*) Histologic sections of a stented artery from a 65-year-old woman with Taxus stent ([Paclitaxel-Eluting Coronary Stent] Boston Scientific) implanted 9 months earlier in the left circumflex artery (LCX) who died of stent thrombosis in another vessel. Sections from LCX demonstrate underlying stable plaque with overlying mild neointimal formation (*upper panel*) consisting of smooth muscle cells and proteoglycan matrix (*lower panel*). Note that no uncovered strut is observed.

SES group than in the BMS group (7.3% vs 14.3%, $P = .004$). This reduction was driven by a decrease in the rate of TVR (5.6% and 13.4%, respectively; $P = .001$). There was no significant difference between the two groups in the rate of death (2.3% and 2.2%, respectively; $P = 1.00$), reinfarction (1.1% and 1.4%, respectively; $P = 1.00$), or stent thrombosis (3.4% and 3.6%, respectively; $P = 1.00$).

The PASSION trial[36] randomly assigned 619 patients presenting with an AMI with ST-segment elevation to receive either a paclitaxel-eluting stent (PES) or BMS. The primary end point was a composite of death from cardiac causes, recurrent MI, or target-lesion revascularization at 1 year and did not reach the significance level. There was, however, a trend toward a lower rate of serious adverse events in the PES group than in the BMS group (8.8% vs 12.8%; adjusted relative risk, 0.63; 95% confidence interval, 0.37–1.07; $P = .09$). A nonsignificant trend was also detected in favor of the PES group, as compared with the BMS group, in the rate of death from cardiac causes or recurrent MI (5.5% vs 7.2%, $P = .40$) and in the rate of target-lesion revascularization (5.3% vs 7.8%, $P = .23$). The incidence of stent thrombosis during 1 year of follow-up was the same in both groups (1.0%). The TYPHOON and PASSION trials ultimately attest to the safety and efficacy of both SESs and PESs as compared with BMSs in the setting of STEMI. Although the studies were designed and conducted differently, the results were remarkably similar (**Table 1**).

On the other hand, Three-year results from the small, randomized Sirolimus-Eluting Stent versus Bare-Metal Stent in Acute Myocardial Infarction (SESAMI) trial suggest that three-year major adverse cardiovascular events (MACE) remain lower in acute MI patients treated with sirolimus-eluting stents than in AMI patients treated with bare-metal stents. One-year results from SESAMI had suggested that sirolimus-eluting stents were superior, driven by a lower rate of repeat procedures. In all, 320 patients were randomized to a sirolimus-eluting stent or a bare-metal stent. After three years, MACE rates (a combination of deaths, MI, CABG, and target lesion revascularization [TLR]) were almost halved in the sirolimus-stent group. Rates of Target lesion revascularization (TLR), target vessel revascularization (TVR), and target vessel failure (TVF). (TVR/recurrent MI/ target vessel-related death) were also significantly lower in the sirolimus-stent group.[37]

THE NEWER DES PERFORMANCE IN AMI

Primary angioplasty has become the standard of care for acute STEMI; however, its long-term success is limited by the occurrence of restenosis.[28,38] The introduction of DESs has greatly alleviated this problem[39] and their use in coronary intervention has markedly increased. DESs (Cypher ([Sirolimus-Eluting Stent] Cordis, Johnson & Johnson) and Taxus ([Paclitaxel-Eluting Coronary Stent] Boston Scientific)) are considered more effective and equally safe compared with BMSs for on-label use.[40–42] Despite debates over the safety of off-label use,[43–46] the Cypher and Taxus DESs seem to be superior to BMSs in improving 1-year event-free survival in patients with STEMI.[47–50] The zotarolimus-eluting stent (ZES; Endeavor (Medtronic, Minneapolis)) is a second-generation DES with an excellent safety and efficacy profile;

Table 1
Randomized trials of DES versus BMS in STEMI

		TYPHOON			PASSION		
		Active Arm (n = 355)	Control Arm (n = 357)	*P*-Value	Active Arm (n = 355)	Control Arm (n = 357)	*P*-Value
Study Design	*No. of Centers Involved Adjudication*		48 Independent			2 Authors	
Results	*TVF (Death, MI, TVR) (%)*	7.3	14.3	.04	8.8	12.8	.09
	TVR (%)	5.6	13.4	<.001	5.3	7.8	.23
	Cardiac death (%)	2.0	1.4	.58	3.9	6.2	.20
	MI (%)	1.1	1.4	1.0	1.7	2.0	.74
	Angiographically proven stent thrombosis (%)	2.0	3.4	.35	1.0	1.0	1.0

Abbreviations: TVF, target vessel failure; TVR, target vessel revascularization.

these stents contain zotarolimus, a low-profile cobalt alloy stent, and a biocompatible phosphorylcholine polymer. The Endeavor stent has been shown to decrease the need for repeat revascularization compared with BMSs, but there were no differences in the incidence of death or MI between these 2 stent types.[51–53] Although new DESs are increasingly used for the treatment of patients with STEMI, there have been few direct comparisons of outcomes among the currently approved DESs in these patients.[54] The major findings of a study conducted by Lee CW and colleagues[55] comparing the efficacy and safety of ZESs, SESs, and PESs in patients with STEMI are as follows: (1) There was no difference in the overall rate of major cardiac events at 12 months among the ZES, SES, and PES groups. (2) There was a nonsignificant trend in favor of ZESs in the rate of stent thrombosis. (3) SESs were associated with lower late loss and restenosis rates compared with ZESs or PESs. (4) The rate of ischemia-driven TVR was the same among the 3 DESs.[55] The results of this study[55] are, thus, in agreement with those of previous studies comparing different types of DESs in stable coronary artery disease, which found that late loss was significantly higher after ZES compared with SES implantation but that, below a certain threshold level, this difference did not translate to an increase in the repeat revascularization rate.[51–53]

SESs and PESs have been found to decrease the risk of restenosis compared with BMS. Although SESs and PESs are effective, SESs were found to have a somewhat greater benefit in the restenosis rate. In the setting of STEMI, SES implantation resulted in a lower angiographic restenosis rate at 6 months compared with PES implantation, although there were no differences in major adverse cardiac event rates between the 2 stents. The ZES is a second generation DES that contain Zotarolimus, a low profile cobalt alloy stent and a biocompatible phosphorylcholine polymer, may improve arterial healing with less inflammation.[56,57] Several studies have shown that ZESs provide a consistent and sustained decrease in the need for repeat procedures compared with BMSs and maintain an excellent safety profile.[51–53]

The Limus Eluted from A Durable vs ERodable Stent Coating (LEADERS)[58] trial is a prospective randomized noninferiority trial comparing the biolimus-eluting stent (BES) with the biodegradable polymer versus the SES with durable polymer. In the subgroup analysis of this trial that included patients with STEMI, there was a significant reduction of major adverse cardiac events (MACE) with BESs compared with SESs (9.6% vs 20.7%, $P = .01$). Furthermore, the very late stent thrombosis (VLST) was rare (BES 0.2% vs SES 0.9%, $P = .43$). There were no VLST events in patients with BESs between the 2- and 3-year clinical follow-up.

THE EVALUATION OF XIENCE-V STENT IN ACUTE MYOCARDIAL INFARCTION TRIAL: THE RESULTS

A lower rate of stent thrombosis was found with a second-generation DES than with the BMS.[59] The second-generation DES Xience-V (Abbott Vascular, Northern California) performs well in patients having primary PCI for STEMI and has a better safety profile than that of BMSs, according to results of the Evaluation of Xience-V Stent in Acute Myocardial INfArcTION (EXAMINATION) trial.

The study was a randomized controlled trial with an all-comers design to evaluate the Xience-V stent in the complex setting of STEMI and to provide data that may be applicable to the real-world population.

The first-generation DESs have been evaluated in randomized controlled trials in the setting of STEMI, with positive results overall. However, most of these trials lacked good generalizability to real-world circumstances because of their highly selected inclusion/exclusion criteria. Moreover, no safety and efficacy data exist for the new generation of DESs in this high-risk group of patients with STEMI. The all-comers design of the EXAMINATION trial applied wide inclusion and few exclusion criteria, "which may result in a more representative sample of the target population."[60]

The study was an investigator-initiated, multicenter, multinational trial involving 1498 patients with STEMI randomized to either a Xience-V stent (everolimus-eluting stent [EES]) or cobalt chromium BMS. The primary end point was a composite of all-cause death, any recurrent MI, and any repeat revascularization at the 1-year follow-up. Individual components of the primary end point and stent thrombosis were the main secondary end points. Patients included in the trial represented up to 70% of all the patients with STEMI present in the centers during the recruitment period, reflecting the real-world nature of the design.

Results presented during the Hot Line session in Paris at the European Society of Cardiology Congress 2011 included 98% of patients with 1-year follow-up data. In terms of the primary end point, there was a nonsignificant trend toward a benefit with the Xience-V stent by virtue of a lower rate of new revascularizations during follow-up as compared with the BMS.

In terms of safety, the rates of definite and definite/probable stent thrombosis at the 1-year follow-up were significantly lower with the Xience-V stent as compared with the BMS, accounting for 0.5% (definite) and 0.9% (definite or probable) at 1 year with the Xience-V stent and 1.9% and 2.6% with the BMS (both $P = .01$).

The use of EES in the setting of STEMI resulted in a numerically (not significantly) reduced primary end point at the expense of a trend in reduction of the repeat revascularization rate. The significant reduction observed in the definite and definite/probable stent thrombosis rates suggest an excellent safety profile of the EES in these high-risk patients presenting with STEMI. The results of this all-comer randomized trial are highly representative of the real-world population.

So in conclusion, the use of DESs in selected patients with AMI seems to be safe and, with the presence of the new generations of DESs (BES, ZESs, EES), has shown acceptable results in terms of safety and efficacy in the treatment of STEMI.

STENTS VERSUS PLAIN OLD BALLOON ANGIOPLASTY

As previously stated, PTCA for primary treatment after AMI has been demonstrated to be superior to thrombolytic therapy with regard to the restoration of normal coronary blood flow[61] and is associated with lower rates of recurrent ischemia, reinfarction, stroke, and death.[62–64] In a study comparing primary angioplasty with angioplasty accompanied by the implantation of the heparin-coated Palmaz-Schatz stent (Johnson & Johnson), Grines and colleagues[65] have demonstrated that there is a divergence between the stent group and the angioplasty group in the rate of clinical events occurring between 1 and 6 months after intervention, a finding consistent with the known time course of restenosis. As expected, they found a lower rate of restenosis in the stent group than in the angioplasty group. The rate of restenosis after emergency implantation of a stent for AMI was similar to that observed in elective cases. This finding suggests that thrombus and activated platelets already present at the time of AMI may not influence the risk of restenosis or perhaps that a reduction in platelet deposition caused by the use of the heparin-coated stent,[66] as compared with an uncoated stent, had a positive effect on the rate of restenosis. Stenting was also known to be superior to plain old balloon angioplasty (POBA) at improving coronary flow reserve (CFR).[67] Edep and colleagues[68] recently showed that coronary blood flow is increased after stenting compared with POBA in the setting of AMI as measured by the TIMI frame count method. In addition, Sasao and colleagues[69] reported that primary stenting is superior to POBA in acute anterior MI for preventing myocardial injury and restoring left ventricular function. They also speculated that primary stenting improves regional wall motion by improving the coronary vasodilator reserve. It has been shown that CFR is not commonly normalized after PTCA, although reports suggest that CFR may be normalized after stent implantation.[67] Clearly, coronary stenting improves the initial success rate, decreases the incidence of abrupt closure, and is associated with a reduced rate of restenosis. For these reasons, coronary stenting is increasingly used to treat AMI.[70]

STENTING IN THE PRESENCE OF THROMBUS

Animal studies revealed that endothelial denudation is less in direct stenting cases compared with conventional stenting, which may mean less vascular wall trauma and thrombosis risk.[71,72] In addition, Webb and colleagues[73] reported lesser atheromatous embolic debris during intervention in saphenous vein grafts with direct stenting compared with conventional stenting, which may lead to the no reflow phenomenon. They also reported that stents reduced the dislodgement of the thrombus and embolization by entrapping friable material. In their study of direct stenting in angiographically apparent thrombus-containing lesions, Timurkayanak and colleagues[74] have shown that TIMI flow grades after stenting are quite high, with the majority being TIMI 3 flow (93%). Trapping of the thrombus with the stent might also be an important factor in protecting the flow. The trauma caused by balloon predilatation might be responsible for a greater amount of distal embolization of the thrombi and debris.[74]

In the presence of thrombi, a stent may act as a jail for the thrombus and prevent distal propagation. However, the potential pitfalls of direct stenting should always be considered. Although stenosis severity was not reported to be an indicator of successful direct stenting,[75] passing a stent through a severe undilated stenosis might be more traumatic. However, direct stenting may not be an appropriate approach in all lesion subsets and requires distal opacification of the vessel for accurate assessment of lesion characteristics and stent choice.[74]

Thus, coronary stenting constitutes an effective therapeutic strategy for patients with thrombus-containing lesions, either after failure of initial angioplasty or electively as the primary procedure. Coronary stenting in this adverse anatomic setting results in a high degree of angiographic success, a low incidence of subacute thrombosis, and an acceptable restenosis rate.[76]

STENTING CULPRIT VERSUS NONCULPRIT IN AMI

Current guidelines recommend that elective PCI should not be performed in a non-infarct–related artery at the time of primary PCI of the infarct-related artery in patients without hemodynamic compromise.[77] In their study comparing culprit vessel PCI versus multivessel and staged PCI for STEMI, Hannan E and colleagues[78] found that patients with multivessel disease STEMI undergoing multivessel primary PCI at the time of the index procedure had mortality rates that were trending higher than rates for patients with culprit vessel PCI alone. Also, when outcomes for the subset of patients without hemodynamic instability, ejection fraction less than 20%, or malignant ventricular arrhythmia were examined, patients with culprit vessel PCI alone had lower in-hospital mortality rates (0.9% vs 2.4%, P = .04). Because the current guidelines of the American College of Cardiology (ACC)/American Heart Association (AHA) recommend culprit vessel PCI for patients without hemodynamic compromise, Hannan and colleagues[78] support the recommendations in their findings. Another part of this study consisted of comparing differences in mortality between patients with multivessel disease STEMI treated with culprit vessel PCI and those patients who did not undergo multivessel PCI during the index procedure but did undergo multivessel PCI within 60 days after the index procedure, either during the index admission or afterward. Conclusions from these analyses were that patients who underwent multivessel PCI within 60 days of the index procedure fared better than patients who were limited to culprit vessel PCI within 60 days. In the largest report of its kind to date, Toma and colleagues[79] have shown that nonculprit coronary interventions, when performed concurrently with primary PCI, are associated with adverse outcomes, including excess death. All data strongly support both current guideline (ACC/AHA and the European Society of Cardiology) recommendations discouraging non–infarct-related artery PCI procedures performed at the time of primary PCI when patients are hemodynamically stable.[79]

ADJUNCTIVE THERAPY: ANTITHROMBOTICS AND ANTIPLATELETS

Oral Antiplatelet Therapy

Aspirin

Aspirin reduces the frequency of ischemic complications after PCI. Although the minimum effective aspirin dosage in the setting of PCI has not been established, aspirin 325 mg given at least 2 hours, and preferably 24 hours, before PCI is recommended,[80,81] after which aspirin 81 mg daily should be continued indefinitely.

Clopidogrel

Several investigations have explored various loading doses of clopidogrel before or during PCI. Compared with a 300-mg loading dose, doses of either 600 mg or 900 mg achieve greater degrees of platelet inhibition with fewer low responders.[82] A meta-analysis of 7 studies that included 25 383 patients undergoing PCI demonstrated that intensified loading of clopidogrel with 600 mg reduces the rate of MACE without an increase in major bleeding compared with 300 mg.[83] Another study suggested that a 600-mg loading dose of clopidogrel is associated with improvements in procedural angiographic end points and 1-year clinical outcomes in patients with STEMI who undergo primary PCI compared with a 300-mg dose.[84] There is no benefit with increasing the loading dose to 900 mg compared with 600 mg.[82] Clopidogrel 75 mg daily should be given for a minimum of 4 weeks after balloon angioplasty or BMS implantation (a minimum of 2 weeks if increased bleeding risk is present)[85] and for at least 12 months after DES implantation (unless the risk of bleeding outweighs the anticipated benefit). Patients should be counseled on the need for and risks of Dual Antiplatelet Therapy (DAPT) before stent implantation, especially DES implantation, and alternative therapies pursued (BMS or balloon angioplasty) if they are unwilling or unable to comply with the recommended duration of DAPT.

Prasugrel

When prasugrel was compared with clopidogrel in patients with acute coronary syndrome (ACS) in the Trial to Assess Improvement in Therapeutic Outcomes by Optimizing Platelet Inhibition with Prasugrel–Thrombolysis In Myocardial Infarction (TRITON–TIMI 38), prasugrel was associated with a significant 2.2% reduction in absolute risk and a 19.0% reduction in relative risk in the composite end point of cardiovascular death, nonfatal MI, or nonfatal stroke, and a significant increase in the rate of TIMI major hemorrhage (1.8% vs 2.4%).[86] Prasugrel is contraindicated in patients with a history of transient ischemic attack or stroke. Patients weighing less than 60 kg have an increased risk of bleeding on the 10-mg daily maintenance dosage. The package insert suggests that consideration should be given to lowering the maintenance dosage to 5 mg daily, although the effectiveness and safety of the 5-mg dosage has not been studied. Prasugrel is not recommended for patients older than 75 years because of the increased risk of fatal and intracranial bleeding and lack of benefit, except in patients with diabetes or a history of prior MI. Prasugrel should not be started in patients likely to undergo urgent coronary artery bypass graft. Prasugrel has not been studied in elective PCI and, thus, no recommendation can be made regarding its use in this clinical setting.

Ticagrelor

Ticagrelor reversibly binds the P2Y12 receptor. Unlike clopidogrel or prasugrel, ticagrelor is not a thienopyridine. It also does not require metabolic conversion to an active metabolite. Compared with clopidogrel in patients with ACS in the Platelet Inhibition and Patient Outcomes (PLATO) trial, ticagrelor was associated with a significant 1.9% reduction in absolute risk and a 16.0% reduction in relative risk in the primary composite end point of vascular death, nonfatal MI, or nonfatal stroke.[87] Ticagrelor was associated with higher rates of transient dyspnea and bradycardia compared with clopidogrel, although only a small percentage of patients discontinued the study drug because of dyspnea. Based on post hoc analysis of the PLATO study, specifically the results in the US patient cohort, a black box warning states that maintenance doses of aspirin more than 100 mg reduce the effectiveness of ticagrelor and should be avoided. After any initial dose, ticagrelor should be used with aspirin 75 mg to100 mg per day.[88] Given the twice-daily dosing and reversible nature of the drug, patient compliance may be a particularly important issue to consider and emphasize. Ticagrelor has not been studied in elective PCI or in patients who received fibrinolytic therapy, thus, no recommendations about its use in these clinical settings can be made.

Antiplatelet Therapy

In the era before DAPT, trials of adequately dosed glycoprotein (GP) IIb/IIIa inhibitors in patients undergoing balloon angioplasty and coronary stent implantation demonstrated a reduction in the incidence of composite ischemic events with GP IIb/IIIa treatment, primarily through a reduction of enzymatically defined MI.[89–93] In some trials, the use of GP IIb/IIIa inhibitors are associated with some increased bleeding risk, and trials of these agents have generally excluded patients at high risk of bleeding (eg, coagulopathy).[89–105] Thus, recommendations about the use of GP IIb/IIIa inhibitors are best construed as applying to those patients not at a high risk of bleeding complications. Abciximab, double-bolus eptifibatide (180 mcg/kg bolus followed 10 minutes later by a second 180 mcg/kg bolus), and high-bolus dose tirofiban (25 mcg/kg) all result in a high degree of platelet inhibition,[106–110] have been demonstrated to reduce ischemic complications in patients undergoing PCI,[89–93,111–113] and seem to lead to comparable angiographic and clinical outcomes.[84,85] Trials of GP IIb/IIIa inhibitors in the setting of STEMI and primary PCI were conducted in the era before routine stenting and DAPT. The results of these and more recent trials, as well as several meta-analyses, have yielded mixed results.[102–105,114–116] Therefore, it is reasonable to administer GP IIb/IIIa inhibitors in patients with STEMI undergoing PCI, although these agents cannot be definitively recommended as routine therapy. These agents might provide more benefit in selective use, such as in patients with large anterior MI and/or large thrombus burden. Trials of precatheterization laboratory–administered (eg, ambulance or emergency department) GP IIb/IIIa inhibitors in patients with STEMI undergoing PCI, with or without fibrinolytic therapy, have generally shown no clinical benefit; GP IIb/IIIa inhibitor use in this setting may be associated with an increased risk of bleeding.[112,113,117–120] Studies of intracoronary GP IIb/IIIa inhibitor administration (predominantly using abciximab) consist of several small randomized clinical trials (RCTs), retrospective analyses, retrospective and prospective registries, cohort analyses, and case reports. Although most of these published studies have reported some benefit of intracoronary administration in terms of acute angiographic parameters, infarct size, left ventricle myocardial salvage, and composite clinical end points, several other studies have not detected any benefit with intracoronary administration.[105]

REFERENCES

1. McFadden EP. Fibrinolysis and stenting in acute MI: newlyweds destined for a "ménage a trois"? Eur Heart J 2001;22(13):1067–9.
2. The GUSTO Angiographic Investigators. The effect of tissue plasminogen activator, streptokinase, or both on coronary artery patency, ventricular function and survival after acute myocardial infarction. N Engl J Med 1993;329:1615–22.
3. Simes RJ, Topol EJ, Holmes DR, et al. GUSTO-I Investigators. Link between the angiographic substudy and mortality outcomes in a large randomized trial of myocardial reperfusion. Importance of early and complete infarct artery reperfusion. Circulation 1995;91:1923–8.
4. Granger CB, Califf RM, Topol EJ. Thrombolytic therapy for acute myocardial infarction: a review. Drugs 1992;44:293–325.

5. Ito H, Tomooka T, Sakai N, et al. Lack of myocardial perfusion immediately after successful thrombolysis. Circulation 1992;85:1699–705.
6. Meijer A, Verheugt FW, Werter CJ, et al. Aspirin versus Coumadin in the prevention of reocclusion and recurrent ischemia after successful thrombolysis: a prospective placebo-controlled study. Result of the APRICOT study. Circulation 1993;87:1524–30.
7. Nunn CM, O'Neill WW, Rothbaum D, et al. Primary Angioplasty in Myocardial Infarction I Study Group. Long term outcome after primary angioplasty: report from the Primary Angioplasty in Myocardial Infarction (PAMI-1) trial. J Am Coll Cardiol 1999; 33:1729–36.
8. Maillard L, Hamon M, Khalife K, et al. STENTIM-2 Investigators. A comparison of systematic stenting and conventional balloon angioplasty during primary percutaneous transluminal coronary angioplasty for acute myocardial infarction. J Am Coll Cardiol 2000;35:1729–36.
9. Serruys PW, de Jaegere P, Kiemeneij F, et al. A comparison of balloon-expandable stent implantation with balloon angioplasty in patients with coronary artery disease. Benstent Study Group. N Engl J Med 1994;331:489–95.
10. Fischman DL, Leon MB, Baim DS, et al. A randomized comparison of coronary stent placement and balloon angioplasty in the treatment of coronary artery disease. Stent Restenosis Study Investigators. N Engl J Med 1994;331:496–501.
11. Bradley EH, Herrin J, Wang Y, et al. Strategies for reducing the door-to-balloon time in acute myocardial infarction. N Engl J Med 2006;355:2308–20.
12. Antoniucci D, Valenti R. Current role of stenting in acute myocardial infarction. Am Heart J 1999; 138:S147–52.
13. Cannon AD, Roubin GS, Macander PJ, et al. Intracoronary stenting as an adjunct to angioplasty in acute myocardial infarction. J Invasive Cardiol 1991;3:255–8.
14. Garcia-Cantu E, Spaulding C, Corcos T, et al. Stent implantation in acute myocardial infarction. Am J Cardiol 1996;77:451–4.
15. Antoniucci D, Valenti R, Buonamici P, et al. Direct angioplasty and stenting of the infarct-related artery in acute myocardial infarction. Am J Cardiol 1996;78:568–71.
16. O'Neill WW, Brodie BR, Ivanhoe R, et al. Primary coronary angioplasty for acute myocardial infarction (the Primary Angioplasty Registry). Am J Cardiol 1994;73:627–34.
17. Nakagawa Y, Iwasaki Y, Kimura T, et al. Serial angiographic follow-up after successful direct angioplasty for acute myocardial infarction. Am J Cardiol 1996;78:980–4.
18. Stone GW, Marsalese D, Brodie BR, et al. A prospective, randomized evaluation of prophylactic intraaortic balloon counterpulsation in high risk patients with acute myocardial infarction treated with primary angioplasty: Second Primary Angioplasty in Myocardial Infarction (PAMI II) Trial Investigators. J Am Coll Cardiol 1997;29:1459–67.
19. Fooley DP, Melkert R, Serruys PW. Influence of coronary vessel size on renarrowing process and late angiographic outcome after successful balloon angioplasty. Circulation 1994;90:1239–51.
20. Brodie BR, Stuckey TD, Hansen CJ, et al. Timing and mechanism of death determined clinically after primary angioplasty for acute myocardial infarction. Am J Cardiol 1997;79:1586–91.
21. Stone GW, Grines CL, Browne KF, et al. Implications of recurrent ischemia after reperfusion therapy in acute myocardial infarction: a comparison of thrombolytic therapy and primary angioplasty. J Am Coll Cardiol 1995;26:66–72.
22. Hochman JS, Choo H. Limitation of myocardial infarct expansion by reperfusion independent of myocardial salvage. Circulation 1987;75:299–306.
23. Abbo KM, Dooris M, Glazier S, et al. No-reflow after percutaneous coronary intervention: clinical and angiographic characteristics, treatment and outcome. Am J Cardiol 1995;75:778–82.
24. Stone GW, Garcia E, Griffin J, et al. Does stent implantation in acute myocardial infarction degrade TIMI flow and result in higher early mortality than PTCA? The PAMI Stent Randomized Trial. Circulation 1998;98(Suppl I):I-151.
25. Antoniucci D, Santoro GM, Bolognese L, et al. A clinical trial comparing primary stenting of the infarct-related artery with optimal primary angioplasty for acute myocardial infarction: results from the Florence Randomized Elective Stenting in Acute Coronary Occlusions (FRESCO) Trial. J Am Coll Cardiol 1998;31:1234–9.
26. Boden WE, O'Rourke RA, Teo KK, et al. Optimal medical therapy with or without PCI for stable coronary disease. N Engl J Med 2007;356:1503–16.
27. Bavry AA, Kumbhani DJ, Quiroz R, et al. Invasive therapy along with glycoprotein IIb/IIIa inhibitors and intracoronary stents improves survival in non-ST-segment elevation acute coronary syndromes: a meta-analysis and review of the literature. Am J Cardiol 2004;93:830–5.
28. Keeley EC, Boura JA, Grines CL. Primary angioplasty versus intravenous thrombolytic therapy for acute myocardial infarction: a quantitative review of 23 randomized trials. Lancet 2003;361:13–20.
29. Mehta SR, Cannon CP, Fox KA, et al. Routine vs selective invasive strategies in patients with acute coronary syndromes: a collaborative meta-analysis of randomized trials. JAMA 2005;293:2908–17.
30. Mauri L, Silbaugh TS, Garg P, et al. Drug-eluting or bare metal stents for acute myocardial infarction. N Engl J Med 2008;359:1330–42.

31. McFadden EP, Stabile E, Regar E, et al. Late thrombosis in drug-eluting coronary stents after discontinuation of antiplatelet therapy. Lancet 2004;364: 1519–21.
32. Daemen J, Wenaweser P, Tsuchida K, et al. Early and late coronary stent thrombosis of sirolimus-eluting and paclitaxel-eluting stents in routine clinical practice: data from a large two-institutional cohort study. Lancet 2007;369:667–78.
33. Finn AV, Nakazawa G, Kolodgie F, et al. Drug eluting or bare metal stent for acute myocardial infarction: an issue of safety? Eur Heart J 2009;30:1828–30.
34. Joner M, Finn AV, Farb A, et al. Pathology of drug-eluting stents in humans: delayed healing and late thrombotic risk. J Am Coll Cardiol 2006;48: 193–202.
35. Spaulding C, Henry P, Teiger E, et al. Sirolimus-eluting versus uncoated stents in acute myocardial infarction. N Engl J Med 2006;355:1093–104.
36. Laarman GJ, Suttorp MJ, Dirksen MT, et al. Paclitaxel-eluting versus uncoated stents in primary percutaneous coronary intervention. N Engl J Med 2006;355:1105–13.
37. Violini R, Musto C, De Felice F, et al. Maintenance of long-term clinical benefit with sirolimus-eluting stents in patients with ST-segment elevation myocardial infarction: 3-year results of the SESAMI (Sirolimus-Eluting Stent versus Bare-Metal Stent in Acute Myocardial Infarction) trial. J Am Coll Cardiol 2010;55:810–4.
38. Zhu MM, Feit A, Chadow H, et al. Primary stent implantation compared with primary balloon angioplasty for acute myocardial infarction: a meta-analysis of randomized clinical trials. Am J Cardiol 2001;88:297–301.
39. Moses JW, Leon MB, Popma JJ, et al, SIRIUS Investigators. Sirolimus eluting stents versus standard stents in patients with stenosis in a native coronary artery. N Engl J Med 2003;349:1315–23.
40. Stone GW, Moses JW, Ellis SG, et al. Safety and efficacy of sirolimus- and paclitaxel-eluting coronary stents. N Engl J Med 2007;356:998–1008.
41. Kastrati A, Mehilli J, Pache J, et al. Analysis of 14 trials comparing sirolimus-eluting stents with bare-metal stents. N Engl J Med 2007;356:1030–9.
42. Tu JV, Bowen J, Chiu M, et al. Effectiveness and safety of drug-eluting stents in Ontario. N Engl J Med 2007;357:1393–402.
43. Beohar N, Davidson CJ, Kip KE, et al. Outcomes and complications associated with off-label and untested use of drug-eluting stents. JAMA 2007; 297:1992–2000.
44. Grines CL. Off-label use of drug-eluting stents putting it in perspective. J Am Coll Cardiol 2008; 51:615–7.
45. Daemen J, Tanimoto S, Kukreja N, et al. Comparison of three-year clinical outcome of sirolimus- and paclitaxel-eluting stents versus bare metal stents in patients with ST-segment elevation myocardial infarction (from the RESEARCH and T-SEARCH registries). Am J Cardiol 2007;99:1027–32.
46. Steg G. DES fall from GRACE in STEMI: patients face more than fourfold higher risk of death than bare-metal stent treated patients. Heart-wire. Available at: http://www.medscape.com. Accessed September 4, 2007.
47. Menichelli M, Parma A, Pucci E, et al. Randomized trial of sirolimus-eluting stent versus bare-metal stent in acute myocardial infarction (SESAMI). J Am Coll Cardiol 2007;49:1924–30.
48. Valgimigli M, Percoco G, Malagutti P, et al. Tirofiban and sirolimus-eluting stent vs abciximab and bare-metal stent for acute myocardial infarction: a randomized trial. JAMA 2005;293:2109–17.
49. Valgimigli M, Campo G, Percoco G, et al, Multicentre Evaluation of Single High Dose Bolus Tirofiban vs Abciximab with Sirolimus-Eluting Stent or Bare Metal Stent in Acute Myocardial Infarction Study (MULTI-STRATEGY) Investigators. Comparison of angioplasty with infusion of tirofiban or abciximab and with implantation of sirolimus-eluting or uncoated stents for acute myocardial infarction: the MULTISTRATEGY randomized trial. JAMA 2008;299:1788–99.
50. Hannan EL, Racz M, Walford G, et al. Drug-eluting versus bare-metal stents in the treatment of patients with ST-segment elevation myocardial infarction. JACC Cardiovasc Interv 2008;1:129–35.
51. Kandzari DE, Leon MB. Overview of pharmacology and clinical trials program with the zotarolimus-eluting Endeavor stent. J Interv Cardiol 2006;19: 405–13.
52. Gershlick A, Kandzari DE, Leon MB, et al, ENDEAVOR Investigators. Zotarolimus-eluting stents in patients with native coronary artery disease: clinical and angiographic outcomes in 1,317 patients. Am J Cardiol 2007;100(Suppl):S45–55.
53. Kandzari DE, Leon MB, Popma JJ, et al, ENDEAVOR III Investigators. Comparison of zotarolimus-eluting and sirolimus-eluting stents in patients with native coronary artery disease: a randomized controlled trial. J Am Coll Cardiol 2006;48:2440–7.
54. Lee JH, Kim HS, Lee SW, et al. Prospective randomized comparison of sirolimus- versus paclitaxel-eluting stents for the treatment of acute ST-elevation myocardial infarction: PROSIT trial. Catheter Cardiovasc Interv 2008;72:25–32.
55. Lee CW, Park DW, Lee SH. Comparison of the efficacy and safety of *zotarolimus*-, *sirolimus*-, and *paclitaxel*-eluting stents in patients with ST-elevation myocardial infarction. Am J Cardiol 2009; 104:1370–6.
56. Whelan DM, van der Giessen WJ, Krabbendam SC, et al. Biocompatibility of phosphorylcholine coated

stents in normal porcine coronary arteries. Heart 2000;83:338–45.
57. Nakazawa G, Finn AV, John MC, et al. The significance of preclinical evaluation of sirolimus-, paclitaxel-, and zotarolimus-eluting stents. Am J Cardiol 2007;100(Suppl):36M–44M.
58. Windecker S, Serruys PW, Wandel S, et al. Biolimus-eluting stent with biodegradable polymer versus sirolimus-eluting stent with durable polymer for coronary revascularisation (LEADERS): a randomized non-inferiority trial. Lancet 2008;372:1163–73.
59. Data presented at European Society of Cardiology Congress in Paris. 2011. Available at: http://www.escardio.org/congresses/esc-2011/congress-reports/Pages/708-3-EXAMINATION.aspx. Accessed August 30, 2011.
60. De Boer SPM. Eur Heart J May 2011; [ahead of print].
61. Grines CL. Should thrombolysis or primary angioplasty be the treatment of choice for acute myocardial infarction? Primary angioplasty — the strategy of choice. N Engl J Med 1996;335:1313–7.
62. Grines CL, Browne KF, Marco J, et al. A comparison of immediate angioplasty with thrombolytic therapy for acute myocardial infarction. N Engl J Med 1993;328:673–9.
63. Zijlstra F, de Boer MJ, Hoorntje JC, et al. A comparison of immediate coronary angioplasty with intravenous streptokinase in acute myocardial infarction. N Engl J Med 1993;328:680–4.
64. Weaver WD, Simes RJ, Betriu A, et al. Comparison of primary coronary angioplasty and intravenous thrombolytic therapy for acute myocardial infarction: a quantitative review [Erratum appears in JAMA 1998;279:1876]. JAMA 1997;278:2093–8.
65. Grines CL, Cox DA, Stone GW. Coronary angioplasty with or without stent implantation for acute myocardial infarction. N Engl J Med 1999;341:1949–56.
66. Hardhammar PA, van Beusekom HM, Emanuelsson HU, et al. Reduction in thrombotic events with heparin-coated Palmaz-Schatz stents in normal porcine coronary arteries. Circulation 1996;93:423–30.
67. Bowers TR, Safian RD, Steward RE, et al. Normalization of coronary flow reserve immediately after stenting but not after PTCA. J Am Coll Cardiol 1996;27(Suppl):19A.
68. Edep ME, Guarneri EM, Teirstein PS, et al. Differences in TIMI frame count following successful reperfusion with stenting or percutaneous transluminal coronary angioplasty for acute myocardial infarction. Am J Cardiol 1999;83:1326–9.
69. Sasao I I, Tcuchihashi K, Hase M, et al. NORTH-981 Investigators. Does primary stenting preserve cardiac function in myocardial infarction? A case-control study. Heart 2000;84:515–52.
70. Koneru S, Monsen CE, Pucillo A. Percutaneous transluminal coronary angioplasty (PTCA) combined with stenting improves clinical outcomes compared with PTCA alone in acute myocardial infarction. Heart Dis 2000;2(4):282–6.
71. Rogers C, Parikh S, Seifert P, et al. Endothelial cell seeding: remnant endothelium after stenting enhances vascular repair. Circulation 1996;94:2909–14.
72. Rogers C, Karnovsky M, Edelman E. Inhibition of experimental neointimal hyperplasia and thrombosis depends on the type of vascular injury and the site of drug administration. Circulation 1993;88:1215–21.
73. Webb J, Carere R, Virmani R, et al. Retrieval and analysis of particulate debris following saphenous vein graft intervention. J Am Coll Cardiol 1999;34:468–75.
74. Timurkayank T, Ozdemir M, Cengel A. Direct stenting in angiographically apparent thrombus—containing lesions. J Invasive Cardiol 2001;13(10):742–7.
75. Briguori C, Sheiban I, De Gregorio J, et al. Direct coronary stenting without predilation. J Am Coll Cardiol 1999;34:1910–5.
76. Alfonso F, Rodriguez P, Hernanadez R. Clinical and angiographic implications of coronary stenting in thrombus-containing lesions. J Am Coll Cardiol 1997;29:725–33.
77. Smith SC Jr, Feldman TE, Hirshfield JW Jr, et al. ACC/AHA/SCAI 2005 guideline update for percutaneous coronary intervention: a report of the American College of Cardiology/American Heart Association Task Force on Practice Guidelines (ACC/AHA/SCAI Writing Committee to Update the 2001 Guidelines for Percutaneous Coronary Intervention). J Am Coll Cardiol 2006;47:e1–121.
78. Hannan EL, Walford G, Holmes DR. Culprit vessel percutaneous coronary intervention versus multivessel and staged percutaneous coronary intervention for ST-segment elevation myocardial infarction patients with multivessel disease. JACC Cardiovasc Interv 2010;3:22–31.
79. Toma M, Buller CE, Cynthia M, et al. Non-culprit coronary artery percutaneous coronary intervention during acute ST-segment elevation myocardial infarction: insights from the APEX—AMI trial. Eur Heart J 2010;31:1701–7.
80. Jolly SS, Pogue J, Haladyn K, et al. Effects of aspirin dose on ischaemic events and bleeding after percutaneous coronary intervention: insights from the PCI-CURE study. Eur Heart J 2009;30:900–7.
81. Popma JJ, Berger P, Ohman EM, et al. Antithrombotic therapy during percutaneous coronary intervention: tho Seventh ACCP Conference on Antithrombotic and Thrombolytic Therapy. Chest 2004;126:576S–99S.

82. von Beckerath N, Taubert D, Pogatsa-Murray G, et al. Absorption, metabolization, and antiplatelet effects of 300-, 600-, and 900-mg loading doses of clopidogrel: results of the ISAR-CHOICE (Intracoronary Stenting and Antithrombotic Regimen: Choose Between 3High Oral Doses for Immediate Clopidogrel Effect) trial. Circulation 2005;112: 2946–50.
83. Siller-Matula JM, Huber K, Christ G, et al. Impact of clopidogrel loading dose on clinical outcome in patients undergoing percutaneous coronary intervention: a systematic review and meta-analysis. Heart 2011;97:98–105.
84. Mangiacapra F, Muller O, Ntalianis A, et al. Comparison of 600 versus 300-mg clopidogrel loading dose in patients with ST-segment elevation myocardial infarction undergoing primary coronary angioplasty. Am J Cardiol 2010;106:1208–11.
85. Berger PB, Mahaffey KW, Meier SJ, et al. Safety and efficacy of only 2 weeks of ticlopidine therapy in patients at increased risk of coronary stent thrombosis: results from the Antiplatelet Therapy alone versus Lovenox plus Antiplatelet therapy in patients at increased risk of Stent Thrombosis (ATLAST) trial. Am Heart J 2002;143:841–6.
86. Wiviott SD, Braunwald E, McCabe CH, et al. Prasugrel versus clopidogrel in patients with acute coronary syndromes. N Engl J Med 2007;357:2001–15.
87. Wallentin L, Becker RC, Budaj A, et al. Ticagrelor versus clopidogrel in patients with acute coronary syndromes. N Engl J Med 2009;361:1045–57.
88. AstraZeneca. Brilinta REMS document [package insert]. NDA 22–433. Reference ID: 2976456. a. Available at: http://www1.astrazeneca-us.com/pi/brilinta.pdf. Accessed September 9, 2011.
89. The EPILOG Investigators Platelet glycoprotein IIb/IIIa receptor blockade and low-dose heparin during percutaneous coronary revascularization. N Engl J Med 1997;336:1689–96.
90. Hamm CW, Heeschen C, Goldmann B, et al. Benefit of abciximab in patients with refractory unstable angina in relation to serum troponin T levels. c7E3 Fab Antiplatelet Therapy in Unstable Refractory Angina (CAPTURE) Study Investigators. N Engl J Med 1999;340:1623–9.
91. The EPIC Investigators. Use of a monoclonal antibody directed against the platelet glycoprotein IIb/IIIa receptor in high-risk coronary angioplasty. The EPIC Investigation. N Engl J Med 1994;330: 956–61.
92. EPISTENT Investigators. Randomised placebo-controlled and balloon-angioplasty-controlled trial to assess safety of coronary stenting with use of platelet glycoprotein-IIb/IIIa blockade. Lancet 1998;352:87–92.
93. ESPIRIT Investigators. Novel dosing regimen of eptifibatide in planned coronary stent implantation (ESPRIT): a randomised, placebo-controlled trial [published correction appears in Lancet 2001;357:1370]. Lancet 2000;356:2037–44.
94. Boersma E, Akkerhuis KM, Theroux P, et al. Platelet glycoprotein IIb/IIIa receptor inhibition in non-ST-elevation acute coronary syndromes: early benefit during medical treatment only, with additional protection during percutaneous coronary intervention. Circulation 1999;100:2045–8.
95. Kastrati A, Mehilli J, Neumann FJ, et al. Abciximab in patients with acute coronary syndromes undergoing percutaneous coronary intervention after clopidogrel pretreatment: the ISAR-REACT 2 randomized trial. JAMA 2006;295:1531–8.
96. Roffi M, Chew DP, Mukherjee D, et al. Platelet glycoprotein IIb/IIIa inhibitors reduce mortality in diabetic patients with non-ST-segment-elevation acute coronary syndromes. Circulation 2001;104:2767–71.
97. Kastrati A, Mehilli J, Schuhlen H, et al. A clinical trial of abciximab in elective percutaneous coronary intervention after pretreatment with clopidogrel. N Engl J Med 2004;350:232–8.
98. Mehilli J, Kastrati A, Schuhlen H, et al. Randomized clinical trial of abciximab in diabetic patients undergoing elective percutaneous coronary interventions after treatment with a high loading dose of clopidogrel. Circulation 2004;110:3627–35.
99. Hausleiter J, Kastrati A, Mehilli J, et al. A randomized trial comparing phosphorylcholine-coated stenting with balloon angioplasty as well as abciximab with placebo for restenosis reduction in small coronary arteries. J Intern Med 2004;256: 388–97.
100. De Luca G, Cassetti E, Verdoia M, et al. Bivalirudin as compared to unfractionated heparin among patients undergoing coronary angioplasty: a meta-analysis of randomised trials. Thromb Haemost 2009;102:428–36.
101. Stone GW, Moliterno DJ, Bertrand M, et al. Impact of clinical syndrome acuity on the differential response to 2 glycoprotein IIb/IIIa inhibitors in patients undergoing coronary stenting: the TARGET Trial. Circulation 2002;105:2347–54.
102. Antoniucci D, Migliorini A, Parodi G, et al. Abciximab-supported infarct artery stent implantation for acute myocardial infarction and long-term survival: a prospective, multicenter, randomized trial comparing infarct artery stenting plus abciximab with stenting alone. Circulation 2004;109: 1704–6.
103. Montalescot G, Barragan P, Wittenberg O, et al. Platelet glycoprotein IIb/IIIa inhibition with coronary stenting for acute myocardial infarction. N Engl J Med 2001;344:1895–903.
104. De Luca G, Suryapranata H, Stone GW, et al. Abciximab as adjunctive therapy to reperfusion in acute ST-segment elevation myocardial infarction:

a meta-analysis of randomized trials. JAMA 2005; 293:1759–65.
105. Mehilli J, Kastrati A, Schulz S, et al. Abciximab in patients with acute ST-segment-elevation myocardial infarction undergoing primary percutaneous coronary intervention after clopidogrel loading: a randomized double-blind trial. Circulation 2009; 119:1933–40.
106. Danzi GB, Capuano C, Sesana M, et al. Variability in extent of platelet function inhibition after administration of optimal dose of glycoprotein IIb/IIIa receptor blockers in patients undergoing a high-risk percutaneous coronary intervention. Am J Cardiol 2006;97:489–93.
107. Steinhubl SR, Kottke-Marchant K, Moliterno DJ, et al. Attainment and maintenance of platelet inhibition through standard dosing of abciximab in diabetic and nondiabetic patients undergoing percutaneous coronary intervention. Circulation 1999;100:1977–82.
108. Gilchrist IC, O'Shea JC, Kosoglou T, et al. Pharmacodynamics and pharmacokinetics of higher-dose, double-bolus eptifibatide in percutaneous coronary intervention. Circulation 2001;104:406–11.
109. Gurm HS, Tamhane U, Meier P, et al. A comparison of abciximab and small-molecule glycoprotein IIb/IIIa inhibitors in patients undergoing primary percutaneous coronary intervention: a meta-analysis of contemporary randomized controlled trials. Circ Cardiovasc Interv 2009;2:230–6.
110. De Luca G, Ucci G, Cassetti E, et al. Benefits from small molecule administration as compared with abciximab among patients with ST-segment elevation myocardial infarction treated with primary angioplasty: a meta-analysis. J Am Coll Cardiol 2009;53:1668–73.
111. Valgimigli M, Percoco G, Barbieri D, et al. The additive value of tirofiban administered with the high-dose bolus in the prevention of ischemic complications during high-risk coronary angioplasty: the ADVANCE Trial. J Am Coll Cardiol 2004;44:14–9.
112. Van't Hof AW, ten Berg JM, Heestermans T, et al. Prehospital initiation of tirofiban in patients with ST-elevation myocardial infarction undergoing primary angioplasty (On-TIME 2): a multicentre, double-blind, randomised controlled trial. Lancet 2008;372:537–46.
113. ten Berg JM, van 't Hof AW, Dill T, et al. Effect of early, pre-hospital initiation of high bolus dose tirofiban in patients with ST-segment elevation myocardial infarction on short- and long-term clinical outcome. J Am Coll Cardiol 2010;55:2446–55.
114. Neumann FJ, Kastrati A, Schmitt C, et al. Effect of glycoprotein IIb/IIIa receptor blockade with abciximab on clinical and angiographic restenosis rate after the placement of coronary stents following acute myocardial infarction. J Am Coll Cardiol 2000;35:915–21.
115. Stone GW, Grines CL, Cox DA, et al. Comparison of angioplasty with stenting, with or without abciximab, in acute myocardial infarction. N Engl J Med 2002;346:957–66.
116. De Luca G, Navarese E, Marino P. Risk profile and benefits from Gp IIb-IIIa inhibitors among patients with ST-segment elevation myocardial infarction treated with primary angioplasty: a meta-regression analysis of randomized trials. Eur Heart J 2009;30: 2705–13.
117. El Khoury C, Dubien PY, Mercier C, et al. Prehospital high-dose tirofiban in patients undergoing primary percutaneous intervention. The AGIR-2 study. Arch Cardiovasc Dis 2010;103:285–92.
118. Montalescot G, Borentain M, Payot L, et al. Early vs late administration of glycoprotein IIb/IIIa inhibitors in primary percutaneous coronary intervention of acute ST-segment elevation myocardial infarction: a meta-analysis. JAMA 2004;292:362–6.
119. Maioli M, Bellandi F, Leoncini M, et al. Randomized early versus late abciximab in acute myocardial infarction treated with primary coronary intervention (RELAx-AMI Trial). J Am Coll Cardiol 2007;49: 1517–24.
120. Keeley EC, Boura JA, Grines CL. Comparison of primary and facilitated percutaneous coronary interventions for ST-elevation myocardial infarction: quantitative review of randomised trials. Lancet 2006;367:579–88.

Door-to-Balloon ST-Elevation Myocardial Infarction Interventions: Illustrated Cases

Sameer Mehta, MD, MBA[a,b,d,*], Rebecca Rowen, BS[c], Estefania Oliveros, MD[d], Camilo Pena, MD[d], Jennifer C. Kostela, MS, MD[c,e], Kevin Treto, BS[f], Ana Isabel Flores, MD[d], Salomon Cohen, MD[g]

KEYWORDS

- ST-elevation myocardial infarction • Primary percutaneous coronary intervention
- Acute myocardial infarction • Thrombus • Thrombectomy

KEY POINTS

- STEMI intervention is constituted by STEMI: "procedure" and "process". We focus on absolute and unequivocal strategies utilized in SINCERE database to improve the procedure.
- Essential tools for STEMI interventions are: illustrated cases with teaching highlights, "Ten Commandments for Short D2B-Time STEMI Interventions" and "Mehta Strategy for Thrombus Management."
- The Mehta Strategy for Thrombus Management is based upon thrombus grade, with direct stenting recommended for low-grade, thrombo-aspiration for moderate-grade, and thrombectomy for high-grade.
- Thrombectomy catheters (manual or mechanical) should comprise the first device, applied to treat thrombus. Thrombo-aspiration maybe used as a default strategy for thrombus management.
- Achievement of a successful STEMI intervention should include relief of chest pain, ST segment resolution, TIMI 3 flow and MPG 3.

INTRODUCTION

No amount of didactics can substitute for real case studies as far as the practical lessons are concerned. With this paramount belief, this article presents 15 illustrative cases. The methodology used for performing ST-elevation myocardial infarction (STEMI) interventions remains almost unchanged in the last 600 of the 1034 procedures recorded in the Single INdividual Community Experience Registry (SINCERE) database.[1]

Three important observations are important to share at this stage. First, to reiterate, all procedures, from administering local anesthesia to achieving successful results, were performed by a single experienced operator, without assistance from fellows, colleagues, or nurse practitioners. This approach made possible the use of standardized

Disclosure: Sameer Mehta is Chief Medical Officer, Asia-Pacific region, for the Medicines Company. The other authors report no conflict of interest regarding the content herein.

[a] Miller School of Medicine, University of Miami, 1400 Northwest 12th Avenue, Miami, FL 33136, USA; [b] Mercy Medical Center, 3663 South Miami Avenue, Miami, FL 33133, USA; [c] Ross University School of Medicine 630 US Highway 1, North Brunswick, NJ 08902, USA; [d] Lumen Foundation, 55 Pinta Road Miami, FL 33133, USA; [e] Internal Medicine New York Hospital Queens, 56-45 Main Street, Flushing, NY 11355, USA; [f] Ross University School of Medicine, 786 Seneca Meadows Road, Winter Springs, FL 32708, USA; [g] Departamento de Neurocirugia, Instituto Mexicano del Seguro Social, Avenida Club de Golf#3 Torre A Dep. 1501, Lomas Country, Huixquilucan Edo de Mexico 52779

* Corresponding author. 185 Shore Drive South, Miami, FL 33133.
E-mail address: mehtas@bellsouth.net

Intervent Cardiol Clin 1 (2012) 521–557
http://dx.doi.org/10.1016/j.iccl.2012.07.002

techniques and constant improvement in efficiency. Second, the procedures were performed at 5 community hospitals, which presented huge strategic challenges as well as maintaining utmost familiarity with different imaging and percutaneous coronary intervention (PCI) equipment and with different staff. The greatest difference among the institutions was in their imaging equipment (GE Medical, Phillips, and Siemens); the availability of the Angiojet (Medrad Interventional/Possis, Minneapolis, MN) device (initially at 2 of the institutions, now at all 5, but the new Spiro Flex [Medrad Inc, Warrendale, PA] equipment is present at only 2 institutions); Clearway catheter, the Impella device, and the different repertoire of coronary stents. Several institutions have vendor contracts mandating use of restricted drug-eluting stents (DES) at the institution.

Although many operators perform interventions at several institutions, the primary operator found it extremely challenging to factor in these unique nuances in the earlier part of the SINCERE experience, particularly in the rushed environment of an STEMI intervention. The logistics of driving and parking posed additional process challenges, sometimes being more exigent than performing the STEMI procedure. Third, and most importantly, the SINCERE database remains completely without any conflict of interest. These presented cases are therefore presented without bias, with the sole aim of educating the reader about unique STEMI skills.

All procedures had one unique common denominator: the door-to-balloon (D2B) clock was ticking, and every procedure was constrained with enormous pressure to achieve successful recanalization in record times! In addition, numerous procedures were performed off hours, and they have been collected from 5 institutions with different imaging equipment. This factor has affected the quality of some digital images. The authors of this article (henceforth we) apologize, as some left ventriculograms are not sharp, and some were obtained by hand injections of contrast agent to limit dye load. Nevertheless, the images emphasize only one single fact: the prompt and superior restoration of left ventricular function with primary percutaneous intervention. Overall, the techniques remain the same and standardization is emphasized. Mean procedure time (needle stick to reperfusion) was 13 minutes. The absolute and unequivocal strategy was to abort the infarct with rapid restoration of Thrombolysis in Myocardial Infarction (TIMI) flow and myocardial perfusion.

Based on our experience with the SINCERE database, now spanning over a period of 10 years, we suggest the following standardized, stepwise technique for performing short D2B STEMI interventions:

1. Maintain the discipline of deciphering the culprit lesion before beginning the procedure. This cannot be always achieved, but its quick and methodical search begins the STEMI procedure in an optimal fashion.
2. With both the radial or femoral route, an excellent arterial stick is mandatory, a clean mid-anterior wall stick that will facilitate a smooth procedure and reduce bleeding. We suggest the best-trained team member to perform this critical task. Clearly radial access reduces bleeding and outcomes, but it should be guided by experience in this approach. It is not recommended to do otherwise, as this will institute a needless complex variable in a procedure that is routinely challenged by severe time constraints.
3. Endeavor to perform a complete coronary evaluation, beginning with angiography of the nonculprit lesion with a diagnostic catheter.
4. 6-French (6F) access and 6F guiding catheters suffice in the majority, the exceptions being severe tortuosity or dense organized thrombus that may require a 7F thrombectomy device.
5. Bivalirudin serves as default anticoagulation, on account of very robust data for superior outcomes in STEMI interventions. Prasugrel (avoid in age >75 years, low body weight, and previous transient ischemic attack/cerebrovascular accidents) and ticagrelor are the superior antiplatelets, and they should be initiated early in the course of an STEMI intervention.
6. Thrombectomy catheters, either manual or mechanical, should philosophically comprise the first STEMI device, applied to treat the lesion. Our recommendations are the Export thrombectomy catheter for manual thrombectomy and the Angiojet device for the mechanical thrombectomy group.
7. DES should be preferred for treating long lesions, small vessels, in diabetics, and for proximal left anterior descending (LAD) artery. Bare-metal stents (BMS) should suffice for large lesions in the right coronary artery (RCA) or left circumflex (LCX) lesions, in patients who cannot take or afford long-term antiplatelets (difficult to discern in an STEMI intervention).
8. Liberal use of intracoronary vasodilators, either through the guiding catheter or through infusion catheters. Our preferred agent is nitroprusside.
9. Left ventriculography is critical for early risk stratification; we also use it to triage patients for intensive care and for early discharge.
10. Most access sheaths can be removed early with closure devices, and early ambulation is possible.

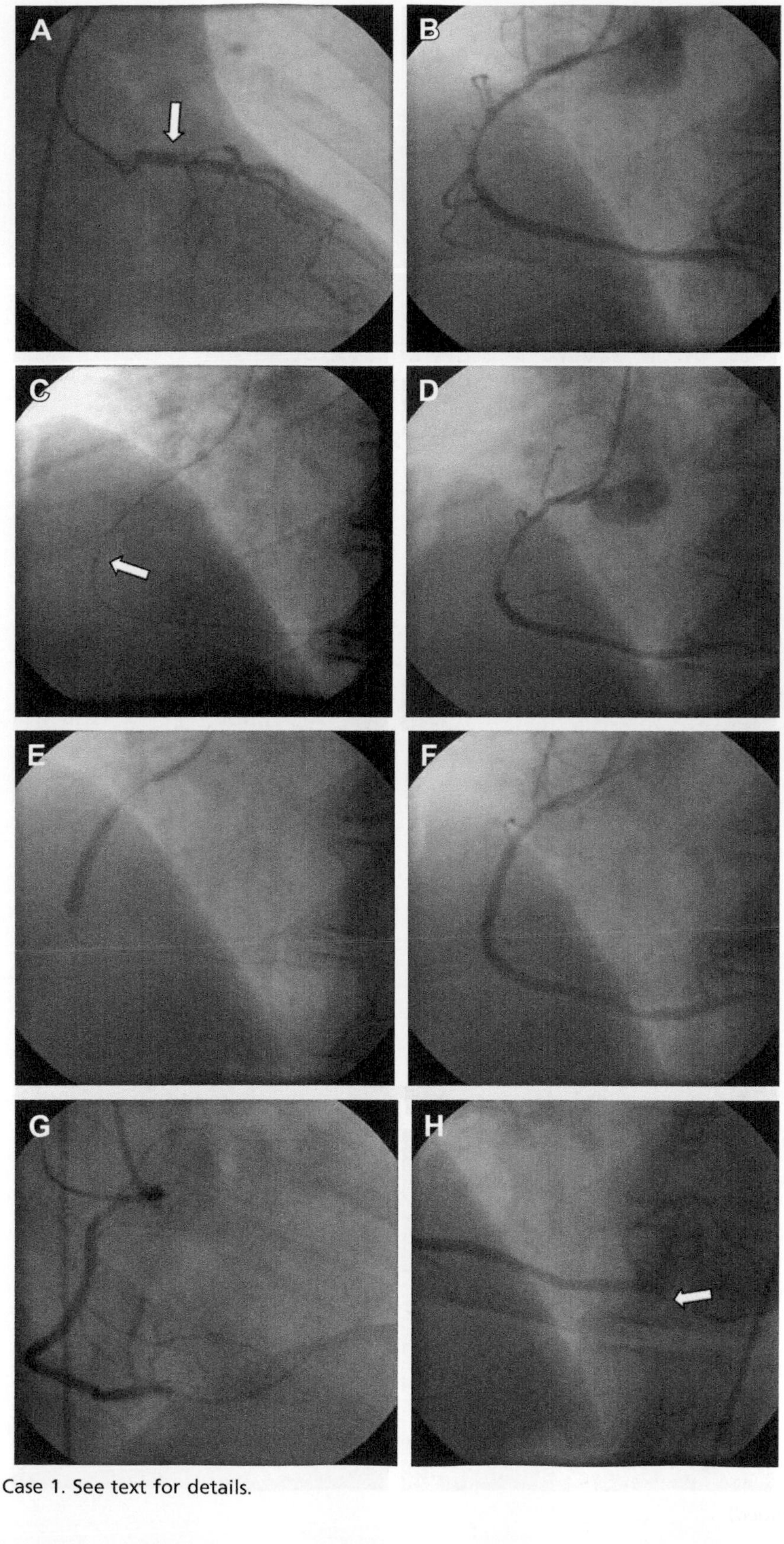

Fig. 1. (*A–P*) Case 1. See text for details.

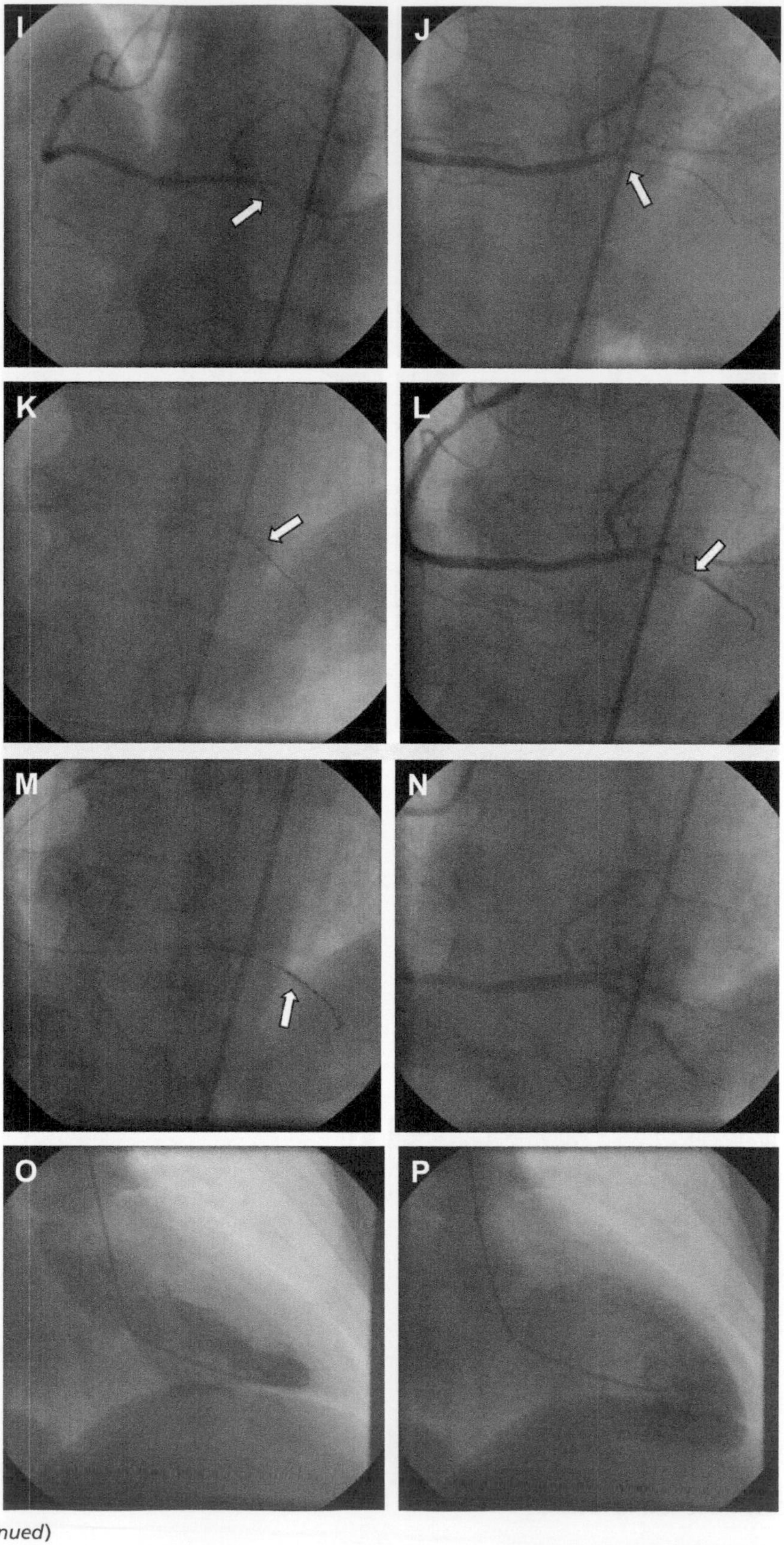

Fig. 1. (*continued*)

ILLUSTRATED CASES

Case 1

Tips and tricks

Several important lessons are embedded in this first illustrated procedure (**Fig. 1**). By electrocardiographic analysis, the culprit vessel is the RCA. In addition, moderate left main coronary artery (LMCA) disease is present. Herein lies the value of obtaining complete angiography beyond the culprit lesion. During the index STEMI procedure, however, there is no need to interrogate the LMCA. The RCA is the straightforward culprit and this vessel is rapidly recanalized with thrombectomy, stenting, and by use of intracoronary nitroprusside. Using these standardized strategies, a good angiographic result is obtained.

However, at this time, despite the apparent successful procedure, the ST segments did not resolve and the patient continued to have chest pain.

This critical information should be sought in every STEMI intervention. We believe a successful STEMI intervention should include relief of chest pain, ST-segment resolution, TIMI 3 flow, and myocardial perfusion grade (MPG) 3. In this case, the first 2 parameters have not been achieved. Although all 4 parameters will not be 100% met in every STEMI intervention, they must be sought. In this particular case, careful attention to these parameters was paramount. It was troubling why the chest pain had not been relieved and why there was persistent, and almost unchanged, ST-segment elevation.

This dilemma is quite simple to solve, and all it needed was a mere careful review of the angiograms and another anteroposterior cranial view. This view clearly demonstrates occlusion with thrombus (distal embolization) of the posterior descending branch. First, additional intracoronary nitroprusside was used, with slight improvement. Dilatation was next performed with a 2.0-mm balloon catheter and a further, final bolus of intracoronary nitroprusside was administered. This action restored of patency of the occluded vessel and there was now concomitant relief of chest pain and ST-segment resolution.

On day 3, the patient was brought back. The RCA was widely patent; intravascular ultrasonography (IVUS) of the LMCA revealed nonsevere disease. Medical management and stress testing were recommended after an early hospital discharge.

Teaching highlights from case 1 are shown in **Box 1**.

> **Box 1**
> **Case 1 teaching highlights**
>
> Culprit lesion intervention only, except in cardiogenic shock or for strict financial reasons (no insurance, inability to return for staged procedure)
>
> Achieve 4 parameters of successful STEMI interventions
>
> - Relief of chest pain
> - ST-segment resolution
> - TIMI 3 flow
> - MPG 3
>
> Pay particular attention to achieving MPG 3: often this is neglected in the rush to achieve D2B times

Case 2

Tips and tricks

This STEMI thrombotic occlusion was successfully crossed with 2 hydrophilic wires using a parallel wire technique (**Fig. 2**). For occluded STEMI lesions at bifurcations, we have sometimes found a parallel wire technique particularly useful.

We wish to emphasize the use of the parallel wire technique and its excellent application in this demonstration, rather than dwell on the advantages of hydrophilic wires, in navigating STEMI lesions. We do believe that as well as the hydrophilic wires, various other guide wires exist today that will do a superb job too. Preference is probably more about what guide wire an operator feels more comfortable with. Our preference for hydrophilic wires relates to their ability of tracking through thrombus particularly well.

Before advancing the second guide wire, several unsuccessful attempts were made to first cross the occluded lesion with a single, hydrophilic guide wire. This guide wire was reshaped, but this was not helpful either. It was clear, however, that the first guide wire had not penetrated subintimally and that it was in a small side branch. At this stage, a second hydrophilic wire was introduced along the first guide wire, which crossed the lesion and advanced distally in the true lumen with surprising ease. Once the major vessel was canalized with the second guide wire, the first wire was removed, as it was in a very small side branch that did not require any treatment.

The remaining procedure was performed in our customary manner. The circumflex lesion (see **Fig. 2**B) was deliberately left alone. Good myocardial blush resulted after liberal use of intracoronary nitroprusside. Left ventricular function was well preserved. D2B time was 61 minutes.

Teaching highlights from case 2 are shown in **Box 2**.

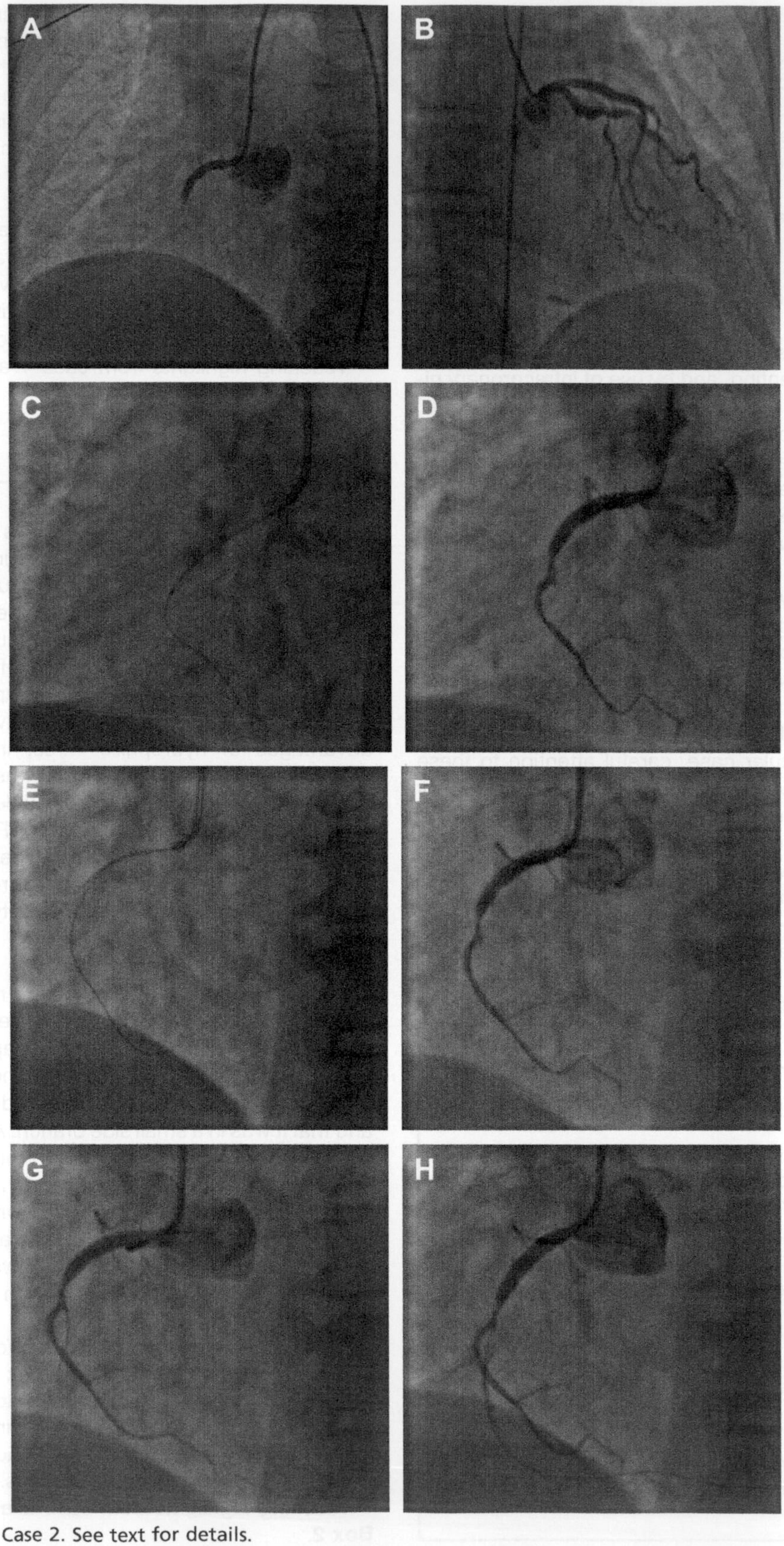

Fig. 2. (*A–P*) Case 2. See text for details.

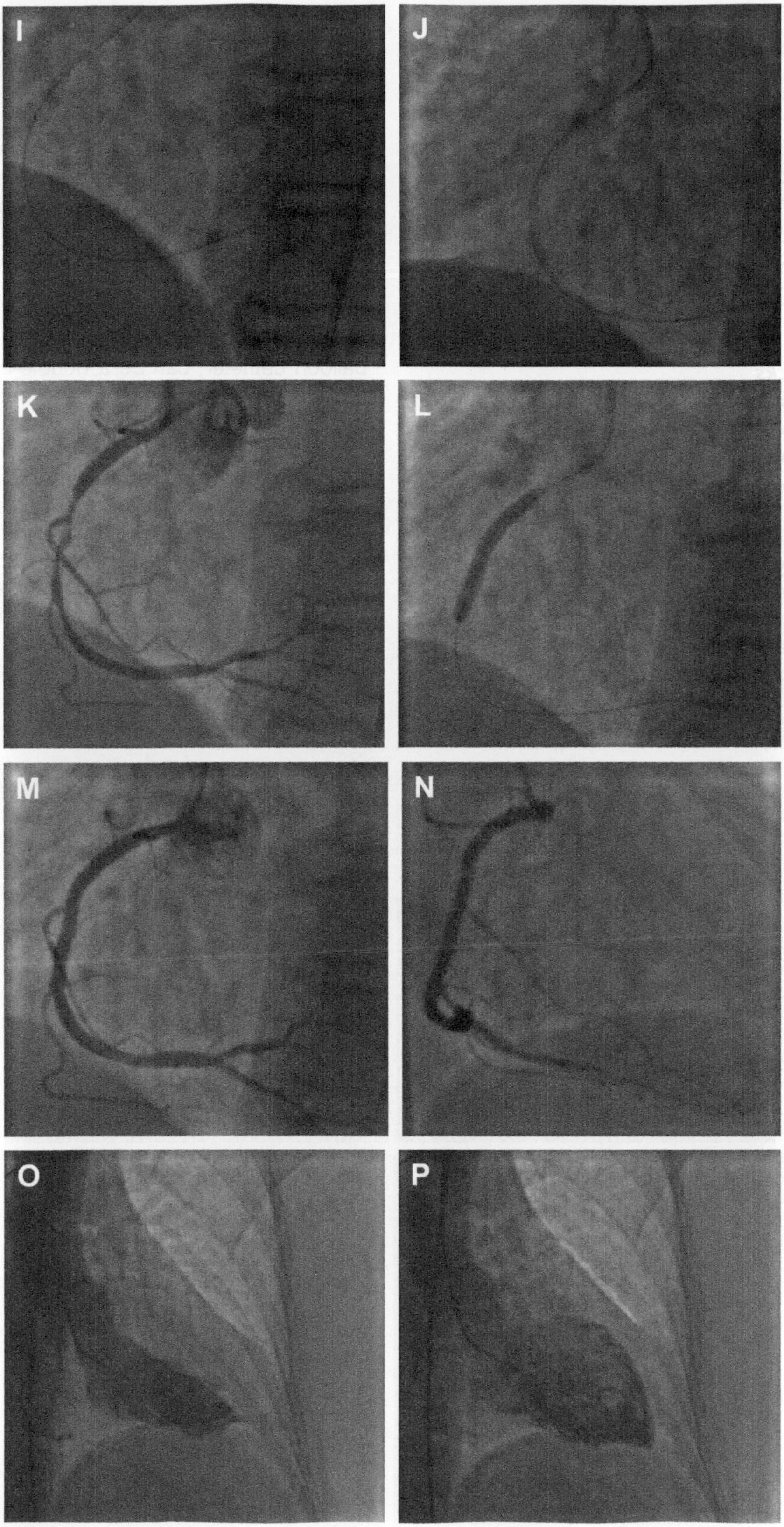

Fig. 2. (*continued*)

Box 2
Case 2 teaching highlights

Consider using a parallel wire technique in bifurcating STEMI lesions if the first guide wire stubbornly seeks the side branch

Hydrophilic guide wires are particularly useful in navigating thrombotic lesions

Leave nonculprit lesions alone

Case 3

Tips and tricks

This case subjected us with all the challenges of an STEMI intervention; it was done at 4 AM on a weekend when the entire staff was exhausted. The patient presented with crushing chest pain and severe anxiety that were incompletely controlled with narcotics; their maximal use was interrupted because of hypotension. Intravenous fluids were rapidly infused, in addition to the usual maneuvers.

Two adverse markers for crossing with the guide wire were present: severe tortuosity and organized thrombus. Panels D to F in **Figs. 3** and **4** demonstrate these angiographic challenges.

In such situations, resist the temptation to use stronger guiding catheters (AL1) and stiffer wires. Of course, you may need to move to a stronger guiding catheter, but that should not be your first choice. Stiffer wires probably have no role in STEMI interventions. In more than 1000 consecutive D2B interventions, we have never needed to use a stiff wire for crossing occluded STEMI lesions.

A support catheter (Transit, Transfer, Mini, Trail Blazer, Skyway Rx support) can be very useful to direct the distal tip of the wire. When using these catheters, be sure that the distal wire tip is moving freely. These catheters, as well as a low-profile balloon catheter, can be a double-edged sword, as careless advancement or overzealous force will likely cause subintimal passage.

In our procedure, after making some progress, we injected through the balloon catheter to confirm that the guide wire was in the true lumen (see **Fig. 3**J). Once this was confirmed, we slowly advanced the guide wire into the distal lumen.

Management thereafter was simple with thromboaspiration, DES deployment, and intracoronary nitroprusside.

Teaching highlights from case 3 are shown in **Box 3**.

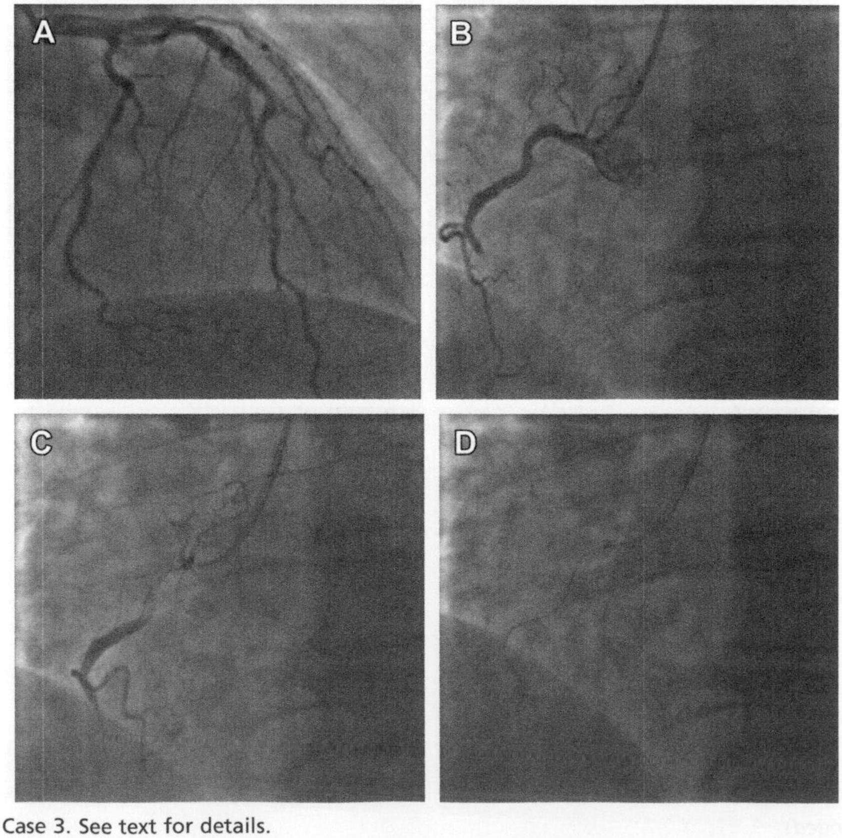

Fig. 3. (*A–S*) Case 3. See text for details.

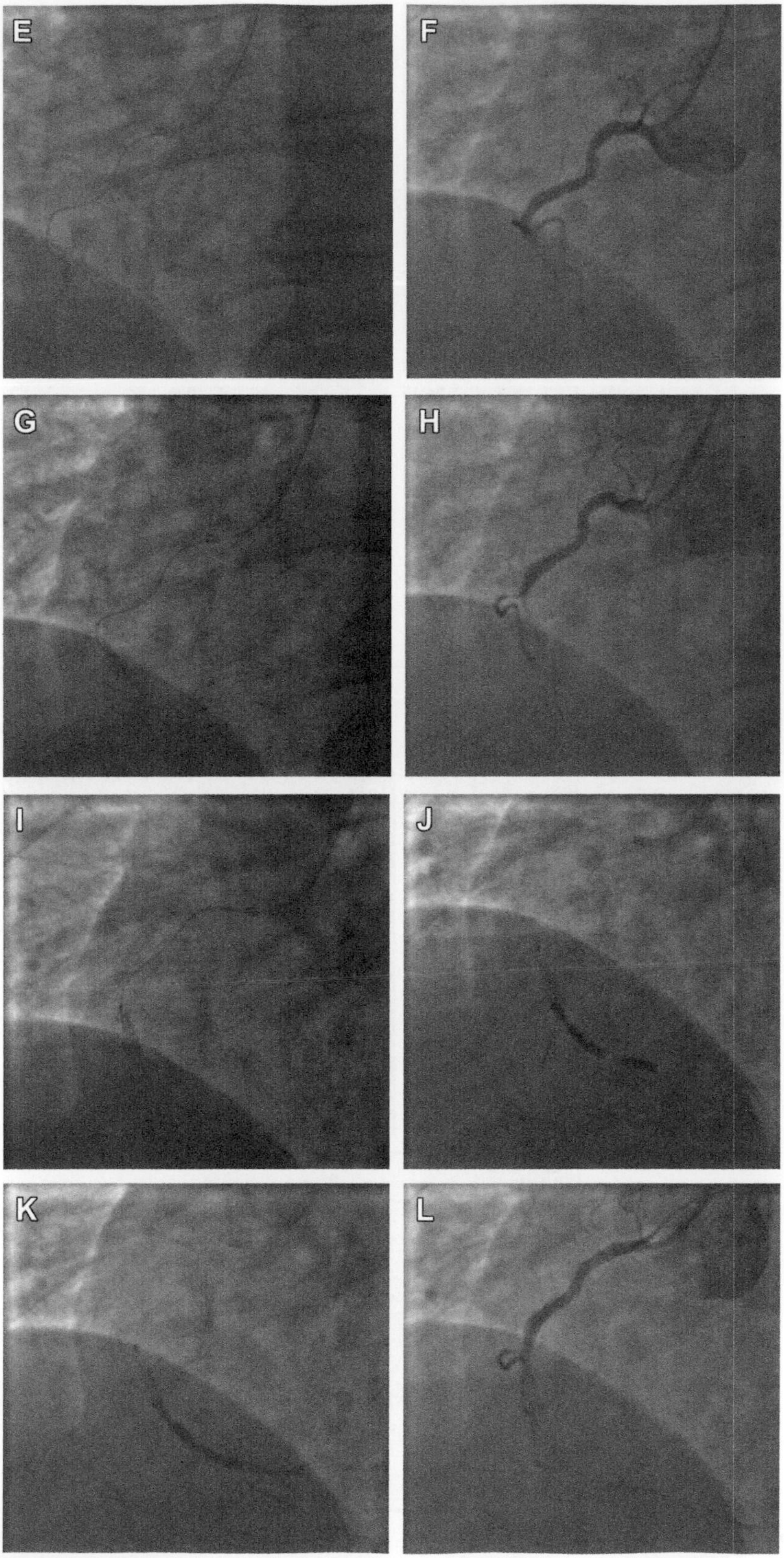

Fig. 3. (*continued*)

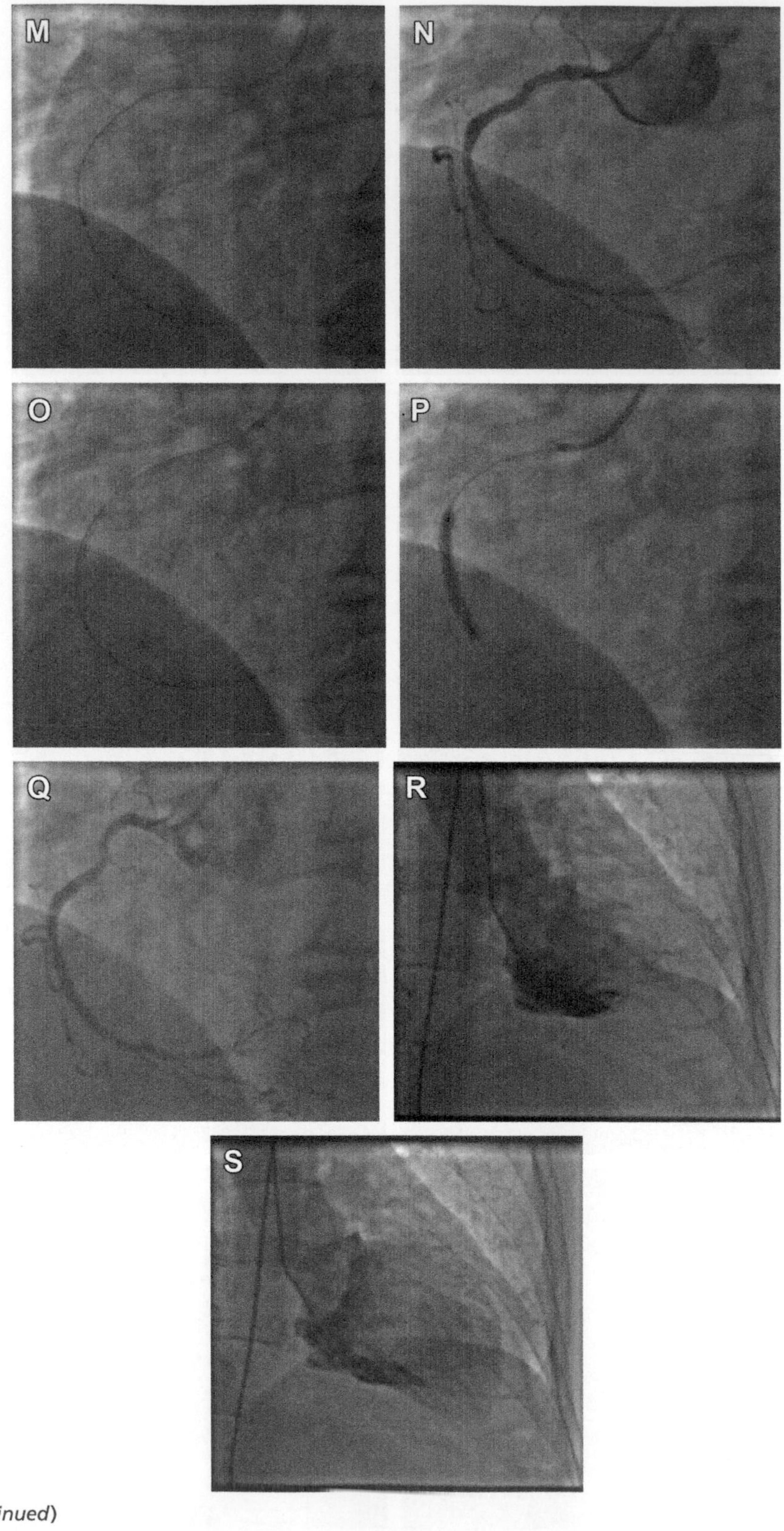

Fig. 3. (*continued*)

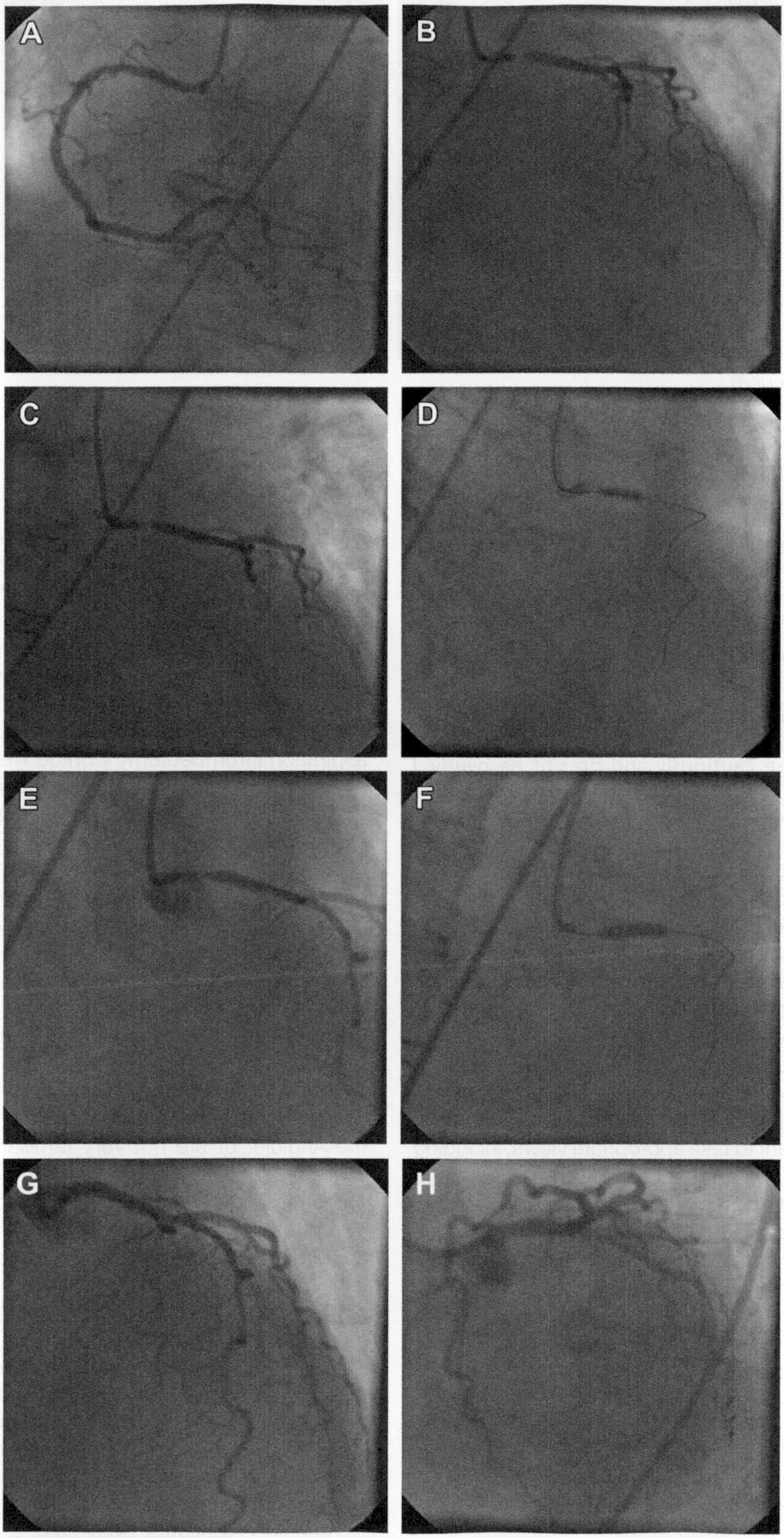

Fig. 4. (*A–J*) Case 4. See text for details.

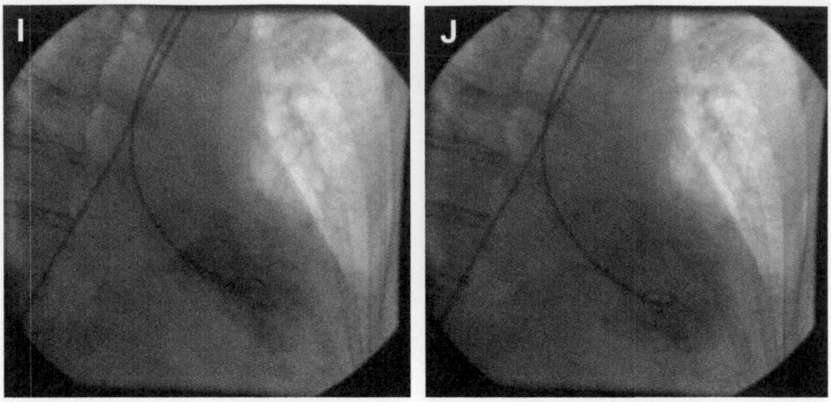

Fig. 4. (*continued*)

> **Box 3**
> **Case 3 teaching highlights**
>
> Tortuosity and organized thrombus present challenging situations in STEMI lesions: when both are simultaneously present, approach the occluded segment with great caution, as guide wire control is lost
>
> Resist use of strong guiding catheters and stiff wires
>
> Support catheter and over-the-wire balloon catheters are useful in these situations; however, use cautiously and do not be overly aggressive, as subintimal passage can occur

Case 4

Tips and tricks

Do not be intimidated by LMCA lesions presenting as STEMI. Often they are extremely easy to treat, in particular if they involve the ostia or the body. The real challenging ones are occluded, bifurcating LMCA lesions.

In this procedure, a simple, 10-minute ostial LMCA procedure was performed for an 87-year-old woman who presented with an extensive infarct.

It is important to take appropriate views, including a left anterior oblique (LAO) caudal; to use DES; and to bring back the patient for a follow-up angiography.

If there is any doubt, interrogate with IVUS.

Teaching highlights from case 4 are shown in **Box 4**.

> **Box 4**
> **Case 4 teaching highlights**
>
> It is critical to obtain optimal views for LMCA interventions, including LAO caudal
>
> Always use DES and surveillance angiography
>
> Use IVUS to interrogate, if result appears suboptimal

Case 5

Tips and tricks

We have selected this procedure to emphasize our strategy of using thromboaspiration as default strategy for thrombus management for STEMI lesions (**Fig. 5**). The rationale for this is simple: the aspiration catheters are user-friendly, effective, and relatively inexpensive. Burgeoning data from clinical trials and guidelines also supports their use in STEMI lesions.

This procedure illustrates a situation whereby aspiration thrombectomy worked well in situations where we would traditionally use mechanical thrombectomy (high thrombus grade in large vessels).

We have extensively used this default thromboaspiration strategy, and have found it to be a very simple and expedient solution to managing thrombus in STEMI lesions.

Of the 5 institutions where the SINCERE work was performed, one hospital did not, until recently, have the capability to perform mechanical thrombectomy with the Angiojet.

Similarly, across the nation and internationally, several institutions do not have the availability of the Angiojet or are not very familiar with its use. We advocate the use of the simpler aspiration catheters as default, first-line management for thrombus, even for high-grade thrombus. Should these catheters fail to aspirate thrombus (delayed presentation, organized thrombus), and if the anatomy is suitable, proceed with mechanical thrombectomy with the Angiojet or X-Sizer (EV3, Plymouth, MN); we prefer the former. For unsuitable anatomy or with the unavailability of the Angiojet, the use of a Clearway catheter (Machet Inc, Santa Barbara, CA) to administer abciximab is another suitable option for managing these difficult lesions.

Teaching highlights from case 5 are shown in **Box 5**.

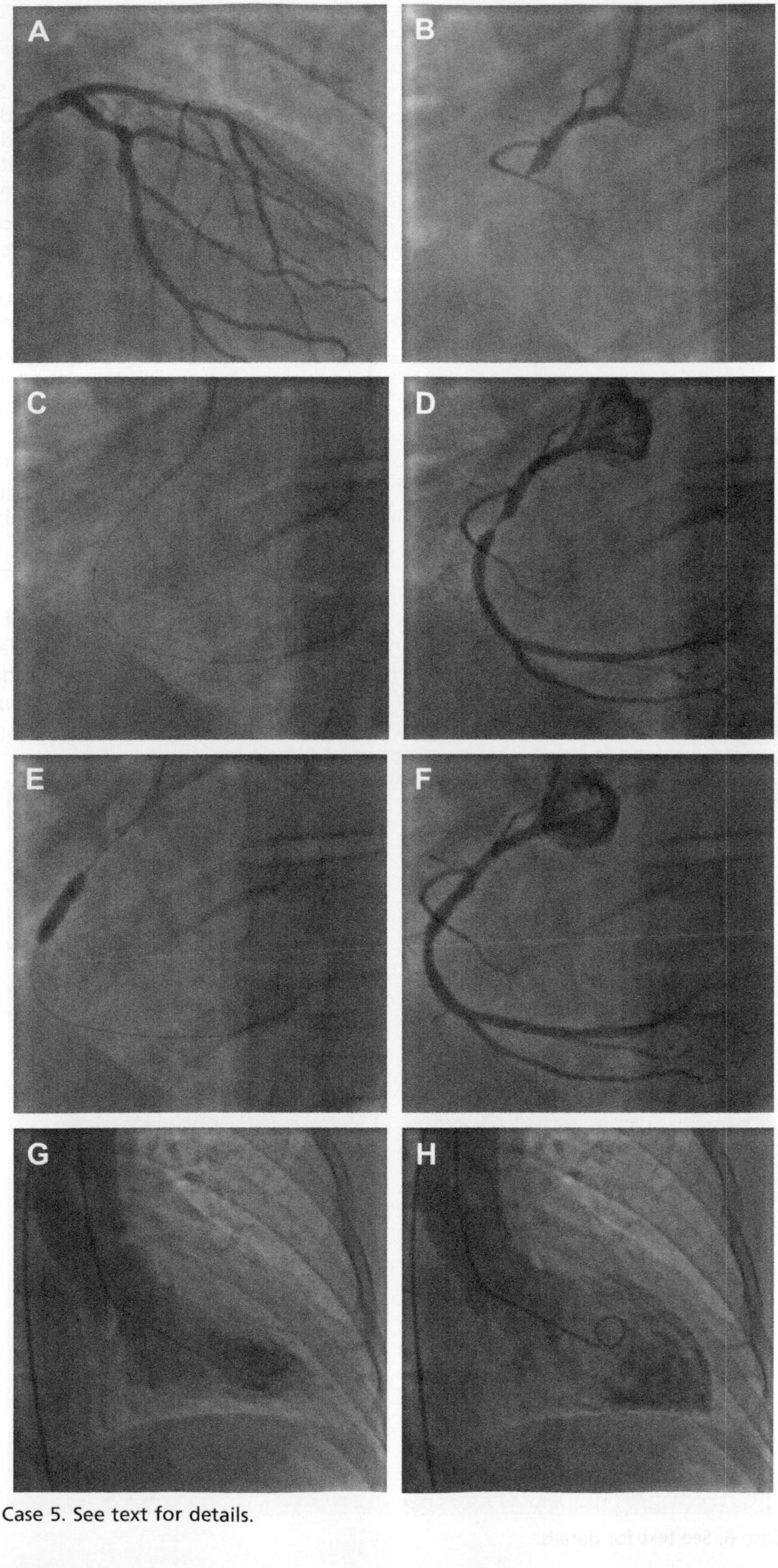

Fig. 5. (*A–H*) Case 5. See text for details.

Box 5
Case 5 teaching highlights

Aspiration catheters should be used as default, first-line management for aspirating thrombus in STEMI lesions

Mechanical thrombectomy should be considered if the aspiration strategy does not work. Avoid severe tortuosity and vessels smaller than 2.5 mm for the Angiojet

The Atrium Clearway catheter can also be used in these situations to inject abciximab into the thrombus

Case 6

Tips and tricks

Three important lessons can be gained from this extraordinary case (**Box 6**):

1. Mechanical thrombectomy, primarily the Angiojet, must be an essential arsenal in every STEMI program. We have undertaken numerous procedures (several in this illustrated article) whereby thromboaspiration will be insufficient in debulking voluminous or organized thrombus; this provides a strong, practical rationale for our making this recommendation which, we state again, is without any conflict of interest. As a follow-up to this recommendation, STEMI institutions should be proficient in quickly setting up the Angiojet and the various operators well versed with the techniques of using the device.

Box 6
Case 6 teaching highlights

The Angiojet is an invaluable tool in STEMI interventions, in particular for treating dense, organized thrombus in large vessels and for lesions with large thrombus burden and suitable anatomy that do not yield to aspiration thrombectomy

The ability of the team to quickly set up a mechanical thrombectomy device, such as an Angiojet, and the operator's capability with this equipment, are both imperative for the success of mechanical thrombectomy

For optimal use, the thrombectomy catheter must traverse through the entire length of the thrombus distally to achieve maximal thrombus removal

The catheter should be passed through the lesion numerous times until no additional gains are demonstrated by angiography and by retrieval of thrombus

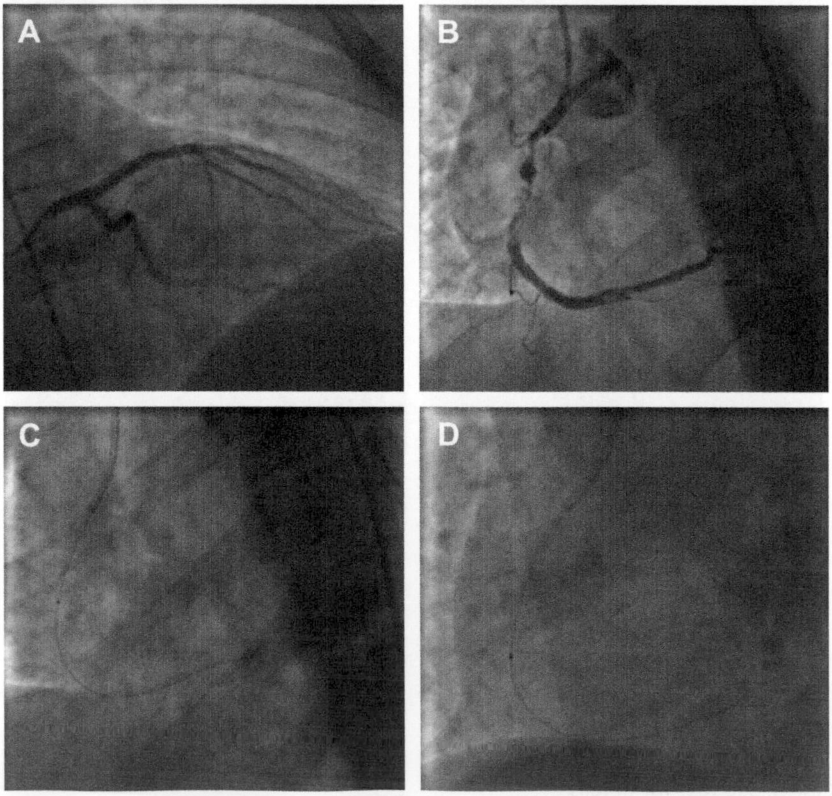

Fig. 6. (*A–N*) Case 6. See text for details.

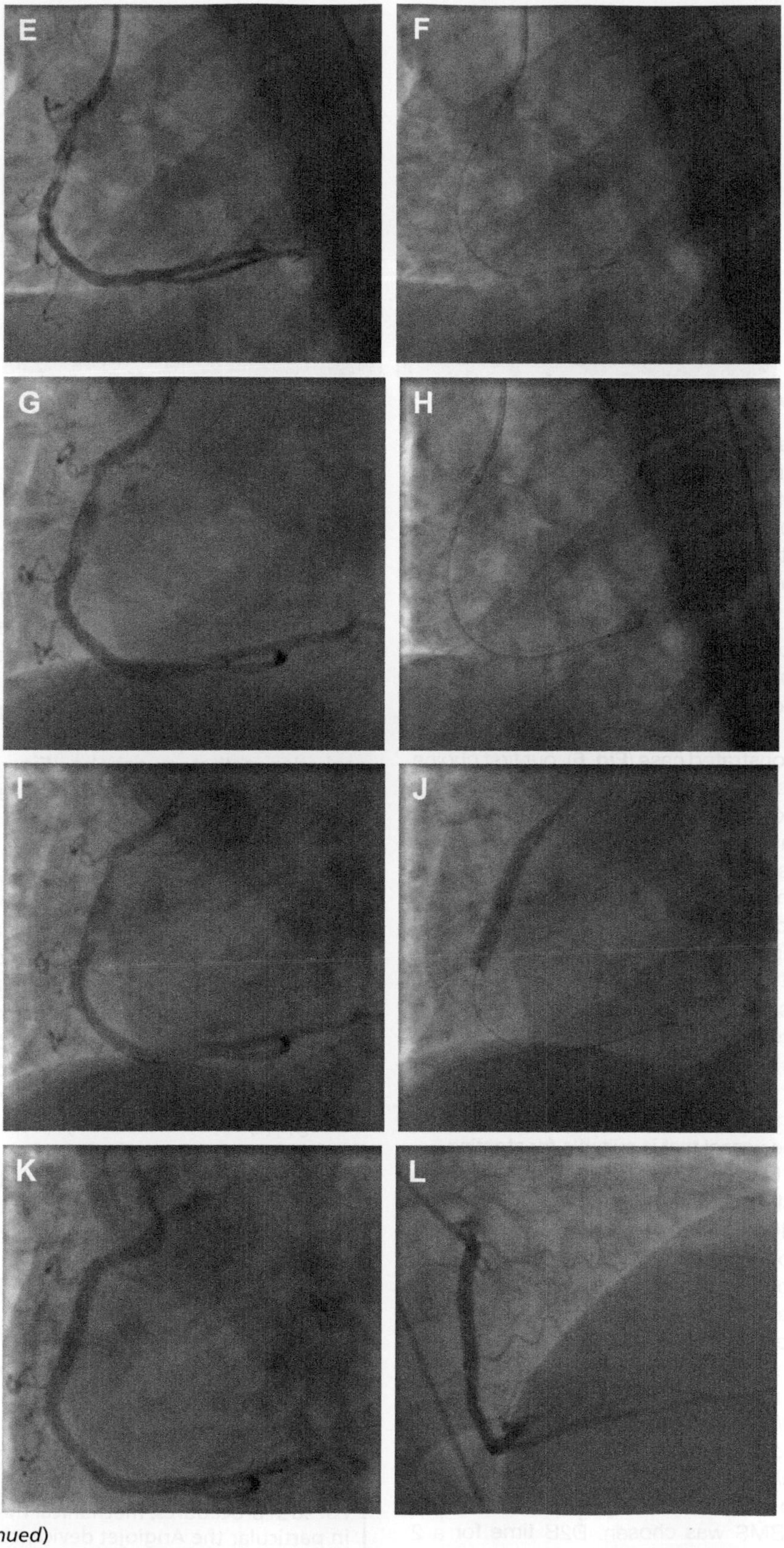

Fig. 6. (*continued*)

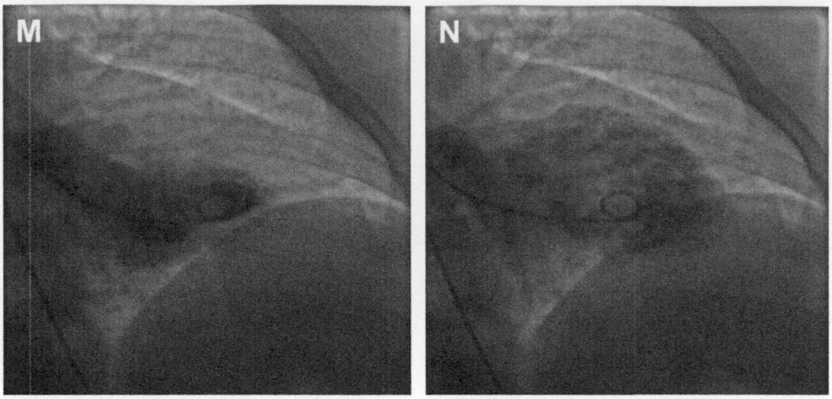

Fig. 6. (*continued*)

2. Thromboaspiration, for the reasons stated earlier in this article, is a viable default strategy, as is amply demonstrated in this case.
3. It is important to perform optimal thrombectomy, both with the mechanical devices and with thromboaspiration.

To do so, *the thrombectomy catheters should traverse through the entire length of thrombus and additional passes made until no gains are demonstrated by angiography and by retrieval of thrombus by the catheter.*

In the demonstrated case (**Fig. 6**), our first choice of device was the Angiojet. The lesion was complex and ulcerated, with a large thrombus burden, and the RCA was a large vessel. All these features were ideally suited for the use of mechanical thrombectomy with the Angiojet. However, the laboratory where this particular procedure was performed was not equipped with the Angiojet.

The Export Aspiration catheter was used instead; multiple passes were made and a large amount of debris retrieved. Each catheter passage, as shown in the various panels, removes thrombus, and modifies the lesion from a complex, large thrombus–containing, ulcerated lesion to a very large, relatively thrombus-free vessel that is suitable for stenting.

The major learning tip of this case is the need to make several passes (see **Fig. 6**C, D, F, and H) and to advance distally enough (see **Fig. 6**H) to achieve maximal thrombus removal.

As our experience in performing thrombectomy has increased, these are the 2 biggest lessons that we have learned: to make additional passes and to advance more distally.

We remain firm in our belief that before stent placement, meticulous thrombus retrieval is critical; stenting in the midst of residual thrombus will probably result in distal embolization and slow or no reflow.

Abciximab was used during the procedure and a 4.50 mm BMS was chosen. D2B time for a 2 AM presentation was 81 minutes, with a procedure time (administering local anesthesia to achieving recanalization) of 16 minutes.

Case 7

Tips and tricks

One of the 5 community hospitals where the SINCERE procedures have been performed does not possess the Angiojet. This procedure was performed at this institution.

The results with aspiration were gratifying, and also demonstrate how simple and effective the aspiration catheters can be (**Fig. 7**). However, there can be no excuse for a catheterization laboratory performing round-the-clock STEMI interventions to not have the Angiojet, and for the staff to be not well trained in its use.

Our experience with D2B times is equally replete with cases whereby simple manual, aspiration thrombectomy failed. Often it failed additionally with the more effective 7F catheters too. *We firmly believe that such a patient's occluded vessels contain dense, organized, erythrocyte-rich thrombus that is often seen with delayed presentations.* In such cases, we suggest the following escalated strategy: (1) 6F thrombectomy, preferably with the Export catheter; (2) moving to either the 7F device or administering abciximab with the Clearway catheter; (3) if both these measures fail, as will often happen with voluminous organized thrombus, the

Box 7
Case 7 teaching highlights

Manual aspiration catheters work well as default devices

However, they may be ineffective in the presence of dense, organized thrombus in patients presenting late with their STEMI

For such procedures, mechanical thrombectomy, in particular the Angiojet device, can be vital

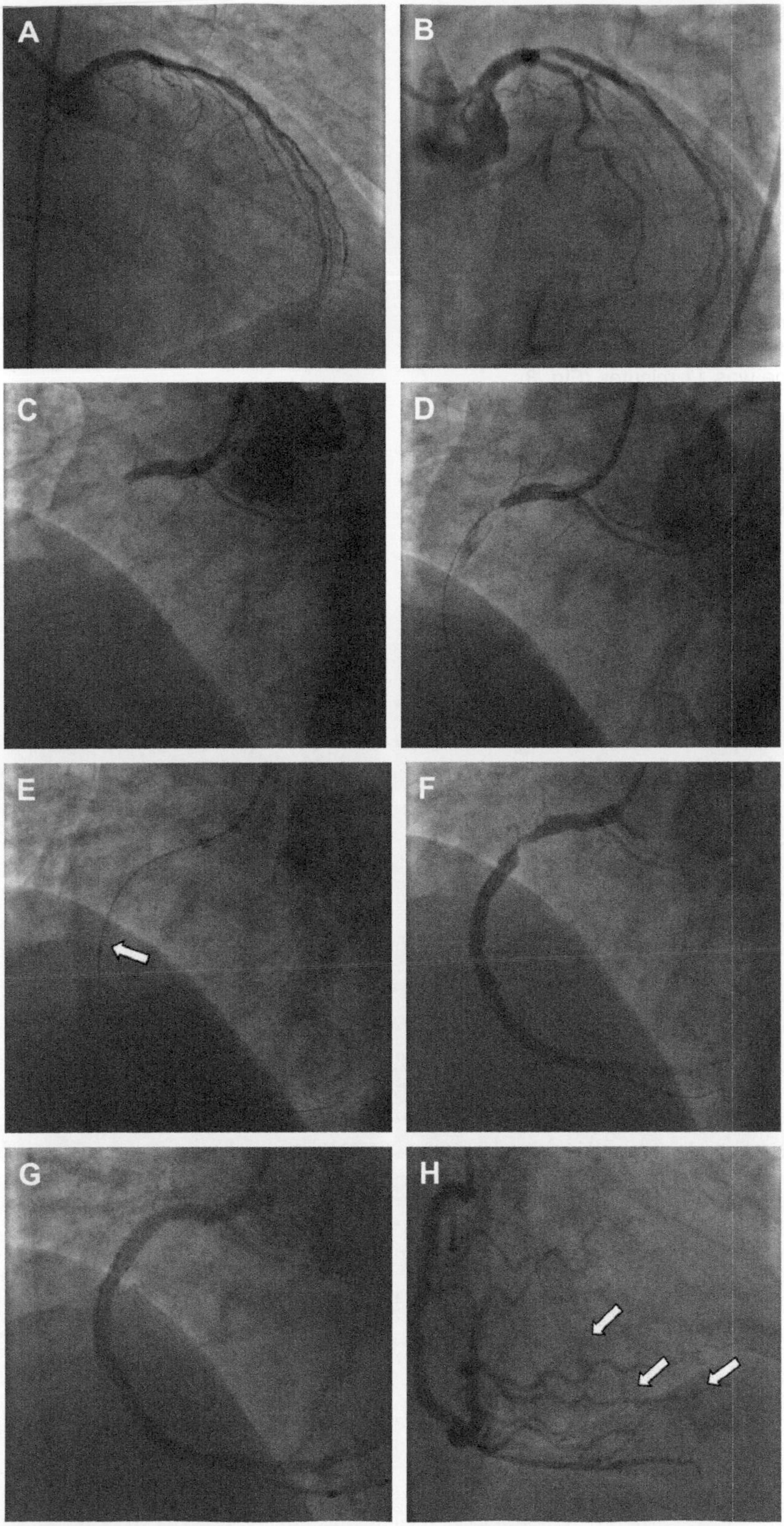

Fig. 7. (*A–H*) Case 7. See text for details.

Angiojet is the best device and often the only one that will salvage these difficult procedures.

We would have done this case with the Angiojet in view of bulky thrombus in a very large RCA. A 4.0 BMS was used. Note the excellent blush in the right anterior oblique view in **Fig. 7**H.

Teaching highlights from case 7 are shown in **Box 7**.

Case 8

Tips and tricks

This is a typical short D2B STEMI intervention: D2B time (off hours) was 76 minutes and the procedure time was 11 minutes (**Fig. 8**).

Box 8
Case 8 teaching highlights

Hydrophilic wires are particularly effective for traversing thrombotic STEMI lesions

Hydrophilic wires seek the lumen and they virtually trace the course of the vessel as the guide wire advances

A rapid, spinning, to-and-fro motion of the hydrophilic guide wire can be particularly useful to grind through thrombus

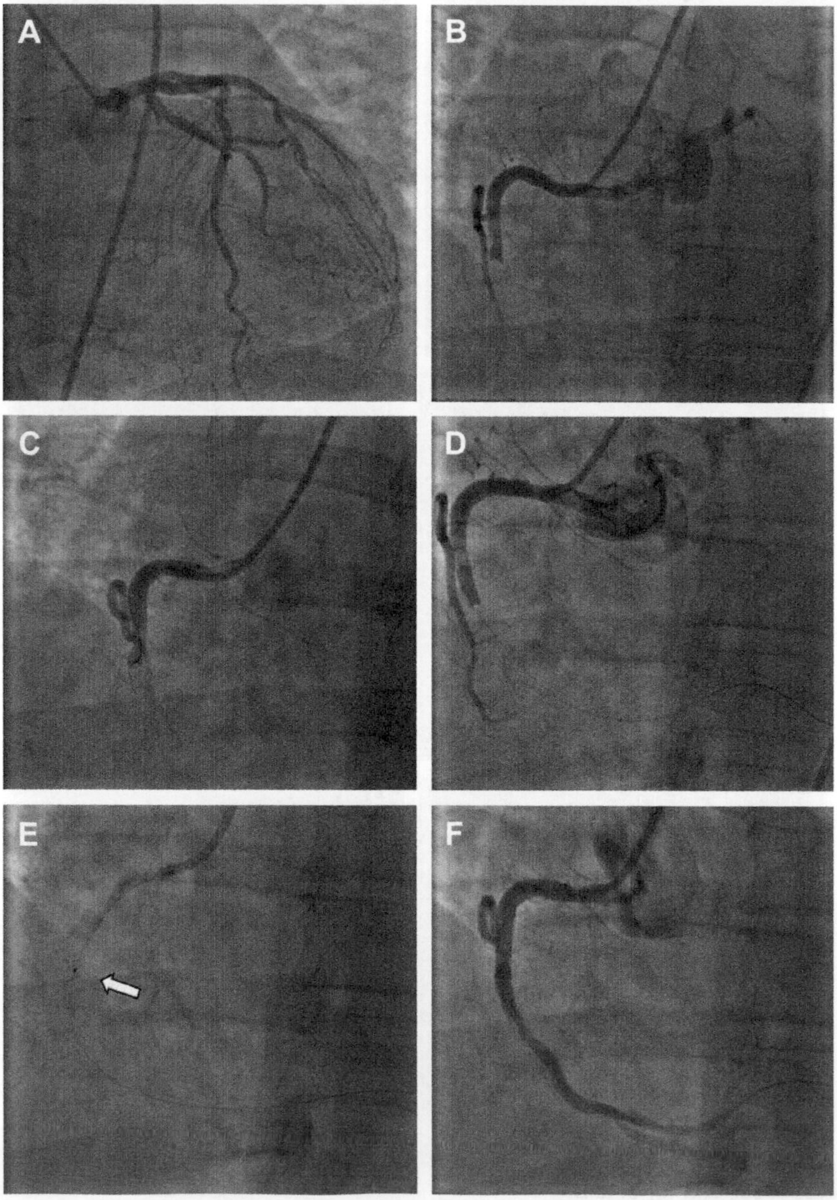

Fig. 8. (*A–H*) Case 8. See text for details.

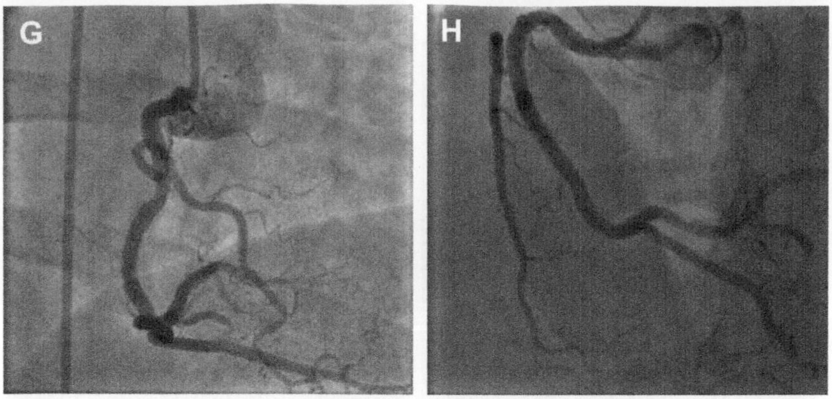

Fig. 8. (*continued*)

While navigating dense thrombus, sometimes the guide wire will buckle and not advance easily. We find the hydrophilic wires to be extremely useful in these situations; our technique is a rapidly spinning, back-and-forth movement that gently grinds its way through the thrombus. Hydrophilic wires have a propensity to seek the lumen, and the operator is virtually tracing the course of the vessel as the hydrophilic wire advances.

This procedure could also be done with the Angiojet, but the results with the simple Pronto Aspiration catheter were excellent. Again, this demonstrates the utility of manual aspiration thrombectomy as front-line management for debulking thrombus in STEMI lesions.

The ST segments were fully restored, and TIMI 3 flow and MPG 3 were established.

Teaching highlights from case 8 are shown in **Box 8**.

Case 9

Tips and tricks

Voluminous thrombus is present in this large, dominant RCA (**Fig. 9**). Thrombus grade is 5 and

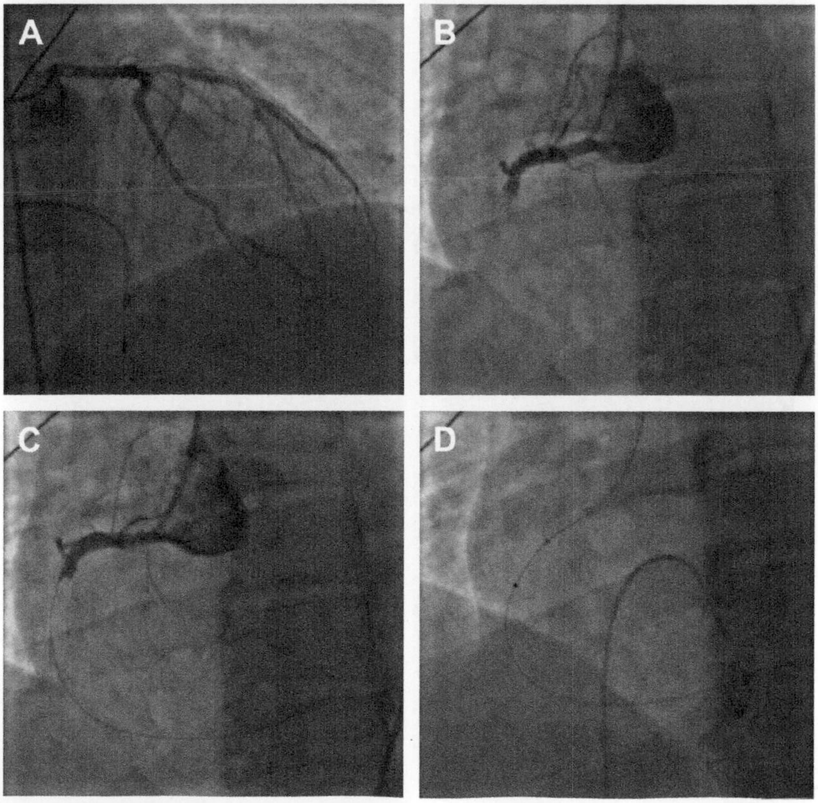

Fig. 9. (*A–N*) Case 9. See text for details.

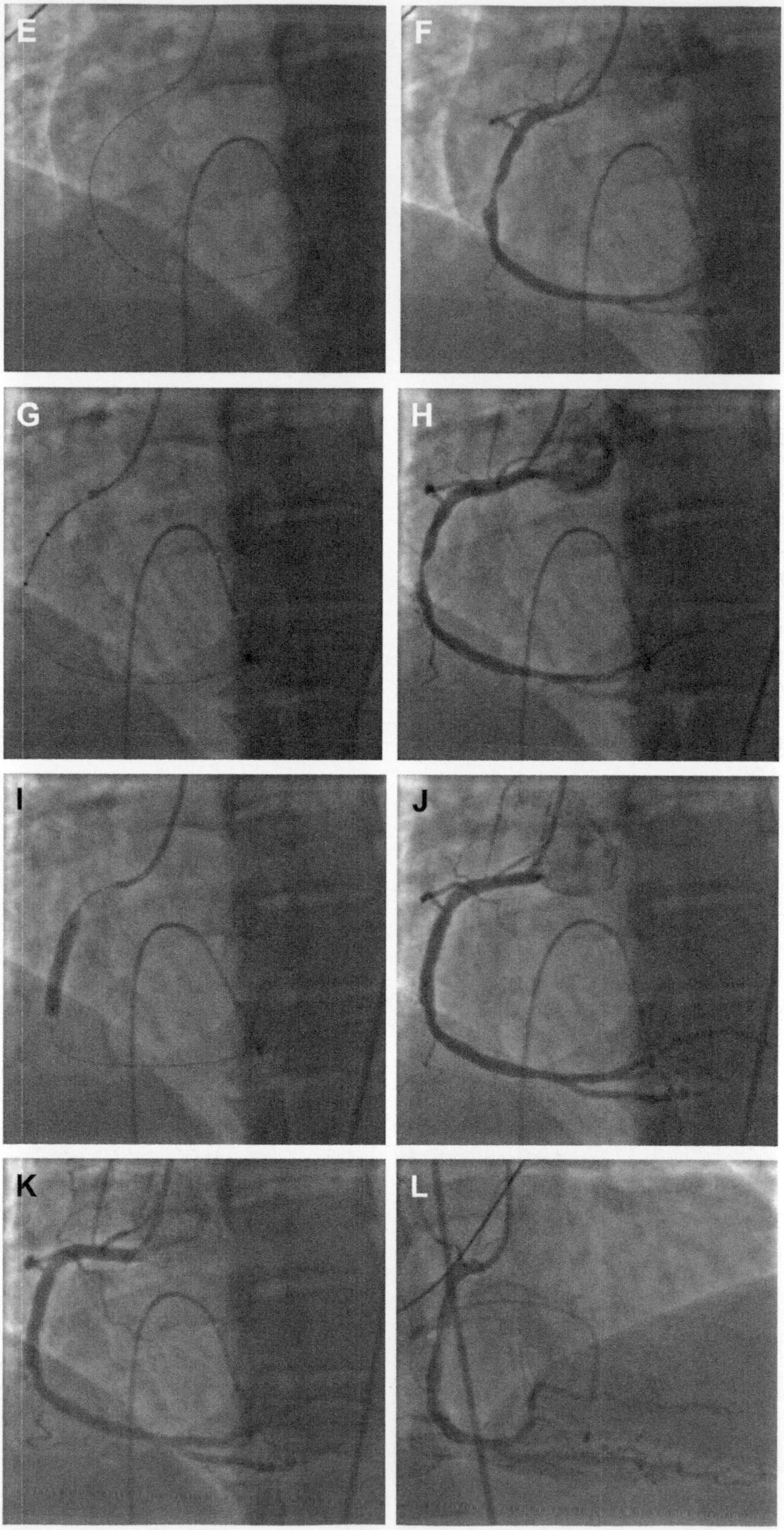

Fig. 9. (*continued*)

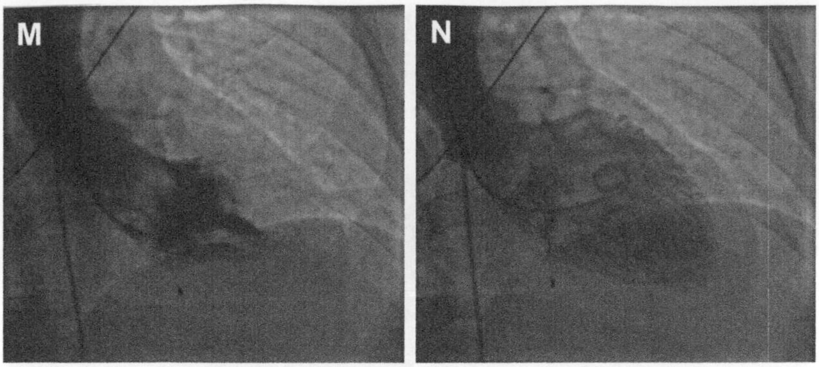

Fig. 9. *(continued)*

unchanged after wiring the lesion. A temporary pacemaker is placed, the Angiojet is rapidly set up, and 3 passes are made with the mechanical thrombectomy device. A large BMS stent is deployed, 400 μg of intracoronary nitroprusside provide MPG 3, and left ventriculography is performed.

We use a temporary pacer for all Angiojet cases, but suspect that this universal use will be significantly reduced based on experience from other institutions. Several operators place the pacer only when treating RCA and dominant LCX, and have abolished the routine use of pacemakers.

The essential understanding of using the Angiojet relies on the principle that thrombectomy occurs when the Angiojet is turned on, and that advancing the system in the off position will simply Dotter the lesion and result in distal embolization. Therefore, we fastidiously turn the system on as the catheter approaches the lesion. In our early experience, when we were less certain of the precise location of the thrombotic lesion, we would turn the system on as the thrombectomy device emerged out of the guiding catheter. This technique is good for treating proximal lesions in particular. The Angiojet is a forward debulking device; therefore, it needs to be activated as the lesion is confronted and maintained entirely in the on position during advancement through the lesion. We are also very particular about advancing the Angiojet through the entire length of the thrombus (several cases will highlight this special point). Often, we will advance and withdraw the device through the voluminous thrombus and keep the Angiojet on during this entire maneuver. This technique will minimize distal embolization.

Teaching highlights from case 9 are shown in **Box 9**.

Box 9
Case 9 teaching highlights

The essential principle of using the Angiojet relies on understanding that thrombectomy occurs when the Angiojet is activated and that advancing the device in the off position will cause Dottering and result in distal embolization

The Angiojet is a forward debulking device; therefore, it needs to be on as the lesion is confronted and maintained in the on position during advancement through the entire length of thrombus

Be sure that the catheter has traversed through the entire length of thrombus

Case 10

Tips and tricks

We consider this the best case in our SINCERE database, so we may indulge in a detailed description of this remarkable procedure.

A 52-year-old man presented with massive inferior wall ST elevation (**Fig. 10**). On presentation to the emergency room, the patient suffered a cardiac arrest. Cardiopulmonary resuscitation (CPR) was immediately initiated and runs of VT/VF were observed along with periods of asystole. With ongoing CPR, the patient was immediately transferred to the catheter laboratory—the entire STEMI intervention was performed with ongoing CPR.

An occluded RCA was identified with a 6F JR4 guiding catheter and easily crossed with a hydrophilic guide wire. A 2.5-mm balloon catheter was rapidly inflated. It did exactly what we expect balloon catheters to do: nothing! CPR was continued and an Export catheter was quickly advanced through the lesion (see **Fig. 10**F). This

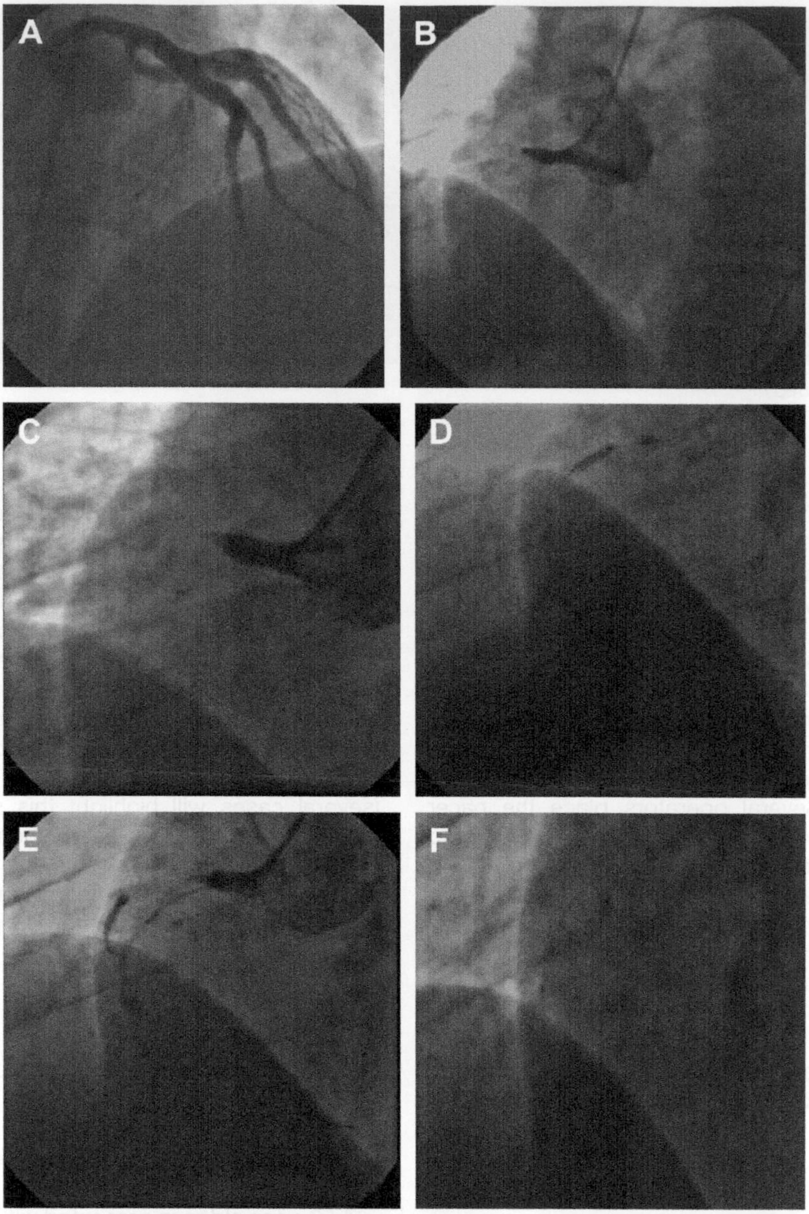

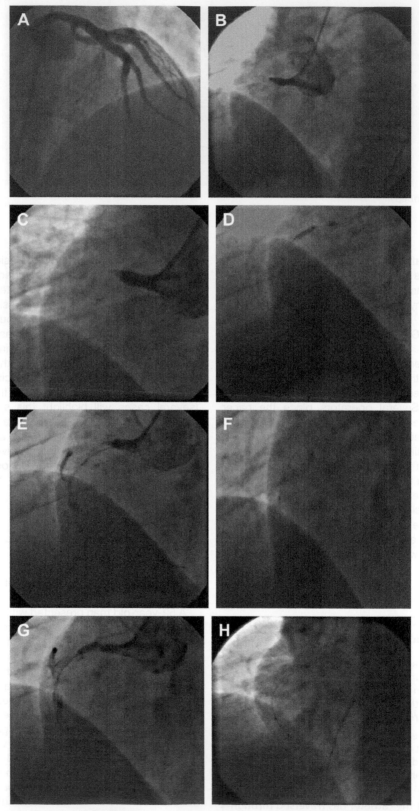

Fig. 10. (*A–T*) Case 10. See text for details.

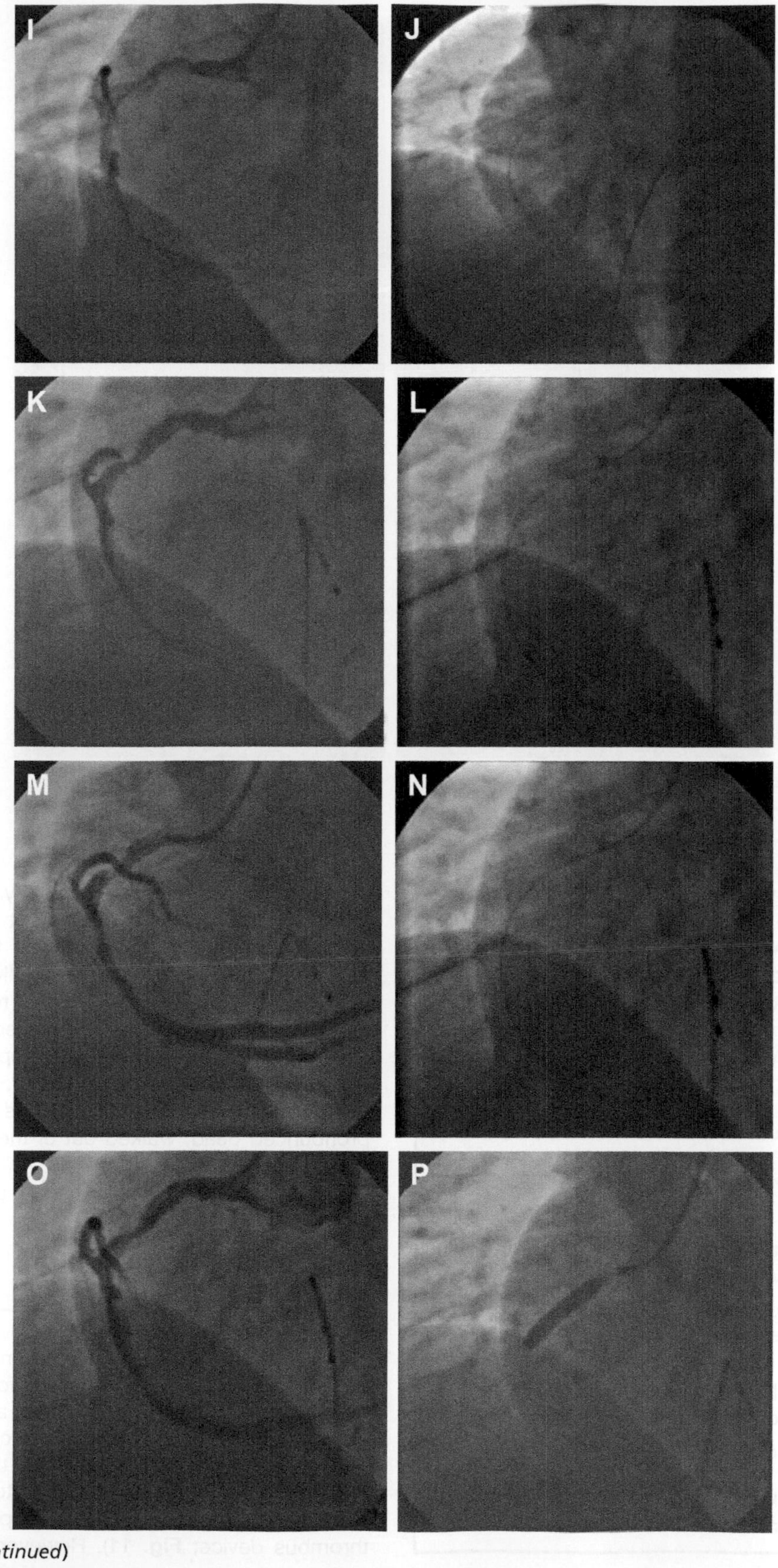

Fig. 10. (*continued*)

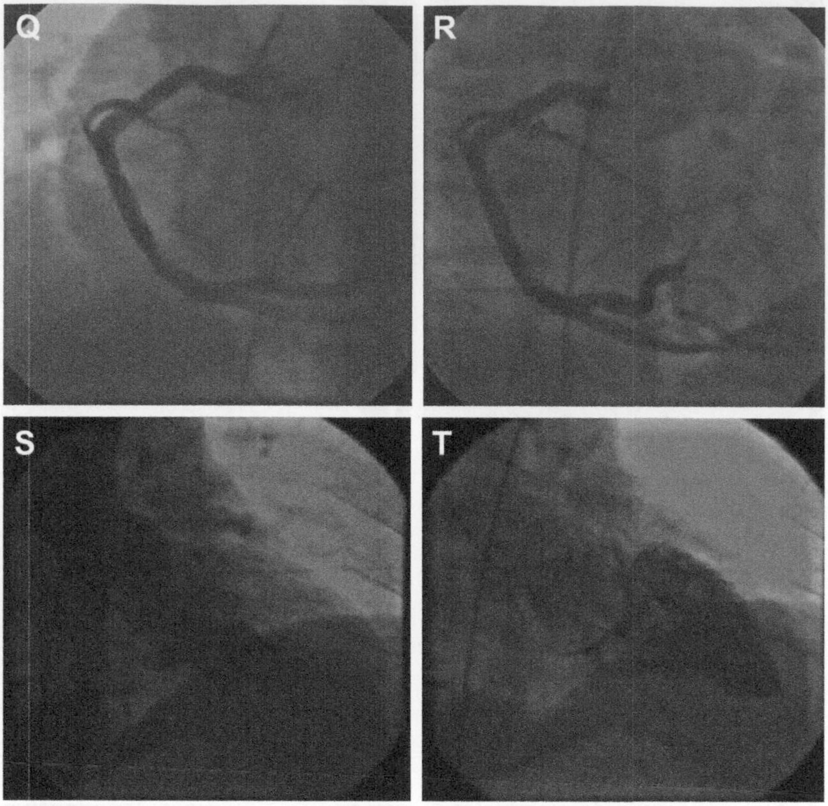

Fig. 10. (*continued*)

catheter too was ineffective; 2 quick passes were made, which made no difference at all. CPR was continued. At this stage we speedily prepared the Angiojet and used the Spiroflex catheter to debulk the voluminous and dense, organized thrombus. The first 2 passes were ineffective, but the subsequent ones restored flow. The patient dramatically regained his hemodynamics and CPR was discontinued. The most outstanding result is achieved after advancing the Angiojet catheter distally (see **Fig. 10**N). TIMI 3 flow is restored with this maneuver. The remainder of the case is simple: a large BMS is used, and excellent TIMI flow, MPG grade, and complete restoration of left ventricular function occur.

This 52-year-old patient, who was about to be pronounced dead, walked out of the hospital on day 4.

Teaching highlights from case 10 are shown in **Box 10**.

Box 10
Case 10 teaching highlights

For large vessels with dense, organized thrombus, the use of Angiojet is mandatory in debulking voluminous thrombus

The staff must be proficient in rapidly setting up the Angiojet and the operator well versed in techniques of using it

It is critical to advance the Angiojet distally enough to debulk the entire occluded segment

Thromboaspiration could be ineffective for such cases; consequently, it must not be the sole debulking therapy available for STEMI interventions

Case 11

Tips and tricks

This is another depiction of why thromboaspiration will not work as sole therapy for thrombus management in STEMI lesions. It also demonstrates the role of mechanical devices that may be needed to debulk voluminous thrombus. In this illustrated procedure, thrombectomy with the aspiration catheter is first attempted (default thrombus device; **Fig. 11**). However, despite its

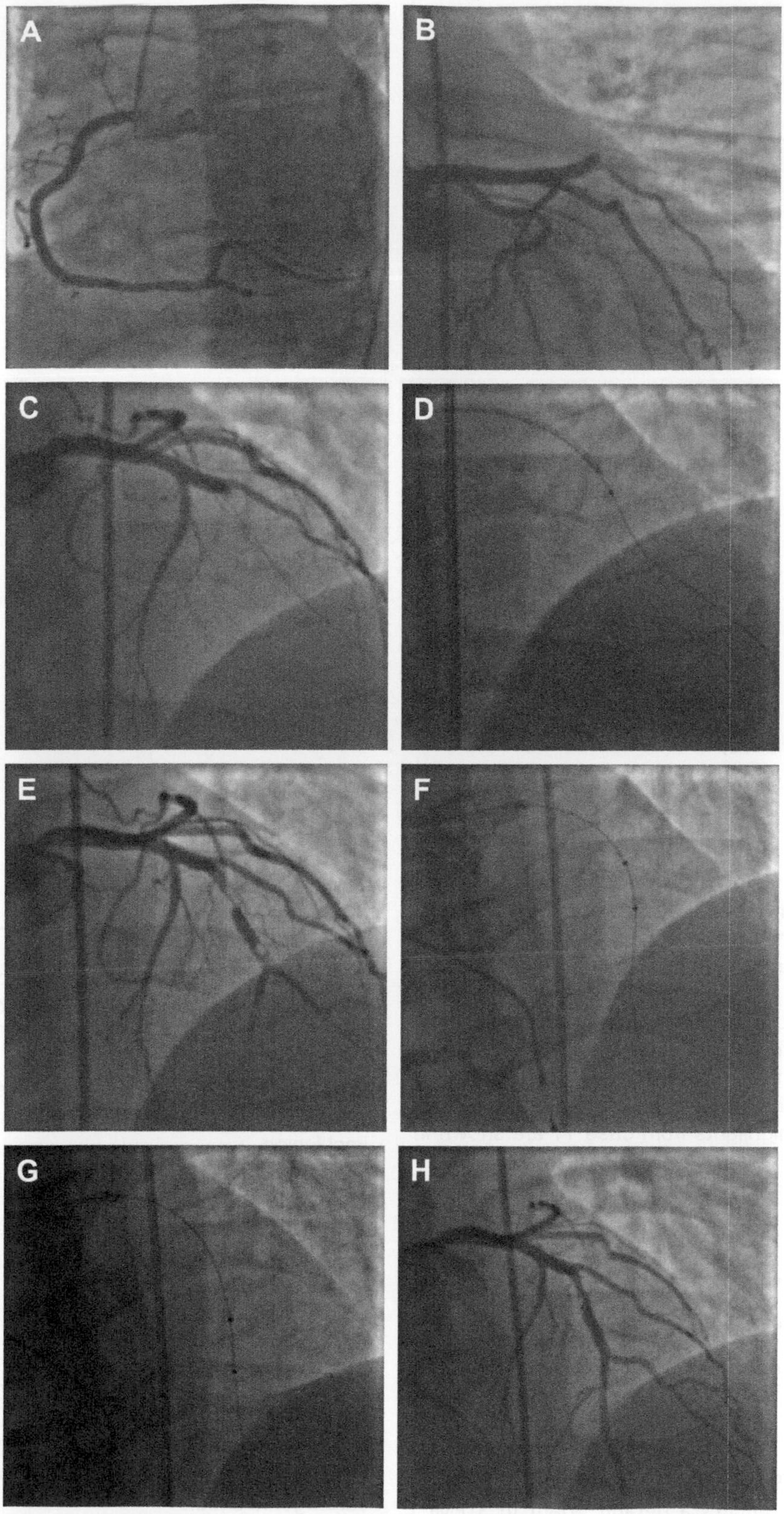

Fig. 11. (*A–L*) Case 11. See text for details.

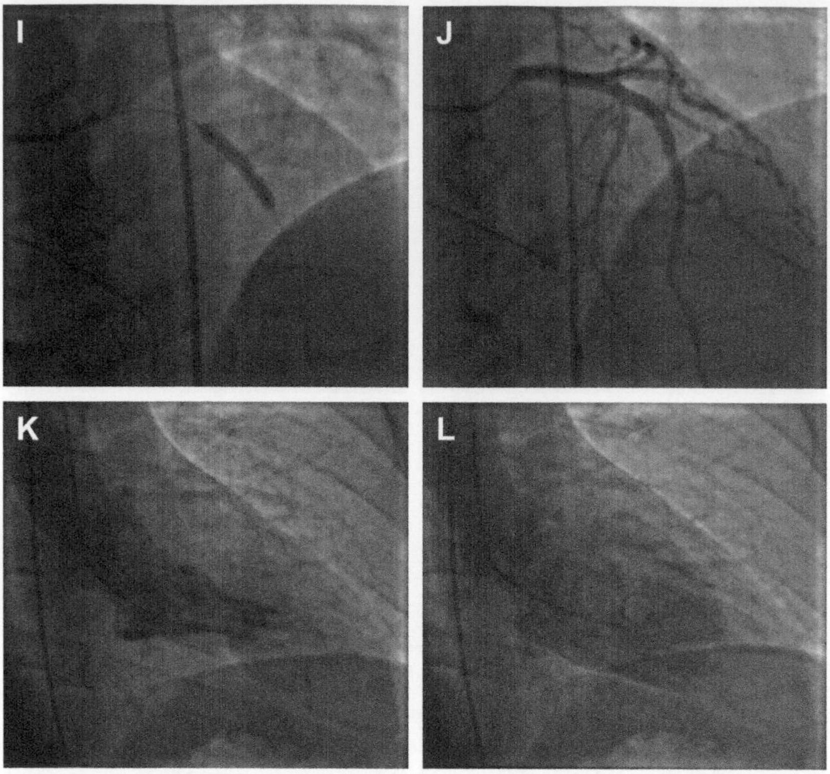

Fig. 11. (*continued*)

careful use and repeat passes, there is significant residual thrombus. It was decided to use the Angiojet at this stage; a single pass cleared most of the residual thrombus. A DES was used with a good result and intracoronary nitroprusside was administered to improve distal, microvasculature flow. As in all previous cases, Bivalirudin was used as an anticoagulant.

Teaching highlights from case 11 are shown in **Box 11**.

Box 11
Case 11 teaching highlights

In addition to organized thrombus, voluminous thrombus in large vessels is incompletely removed by aspiration thrombectomy

Mechanical devices may be useful to manage residual thrombus in such cases

Bivalirudin remains a default agent in STEMI interventions

Case 12

Tips and tricks

This case was more dramatic, the patient having STEMI, profound cardiogenic shock, and very complex coronary lesions (**Fig. 12**). The LAD was tortuous, thrombotically occluded, and poorly visible; the LCX was a very severely angulated lesion, and the RCA demonstrated a severe proximal lesion.

An Impella catheter first placed from the right groin, without difficulty, and it promptly reduced the filling pressures and dramatically improved the hemodynamics.

The RCA was superdominant and contained an eccentric, very proximal, and severe lesion. It was decided to treat this as the first target: it was thought that this large vessel would improve perfusion that in turn would assist in the PCI of the technically challenging LAD and the LCX. *This strategy is a departure from our "culprit only" dictum, and we have used it for managing coronary lesions in cardiogenic shock.*

Stenting the RCA was very simple, and was easily and rapidly performed.

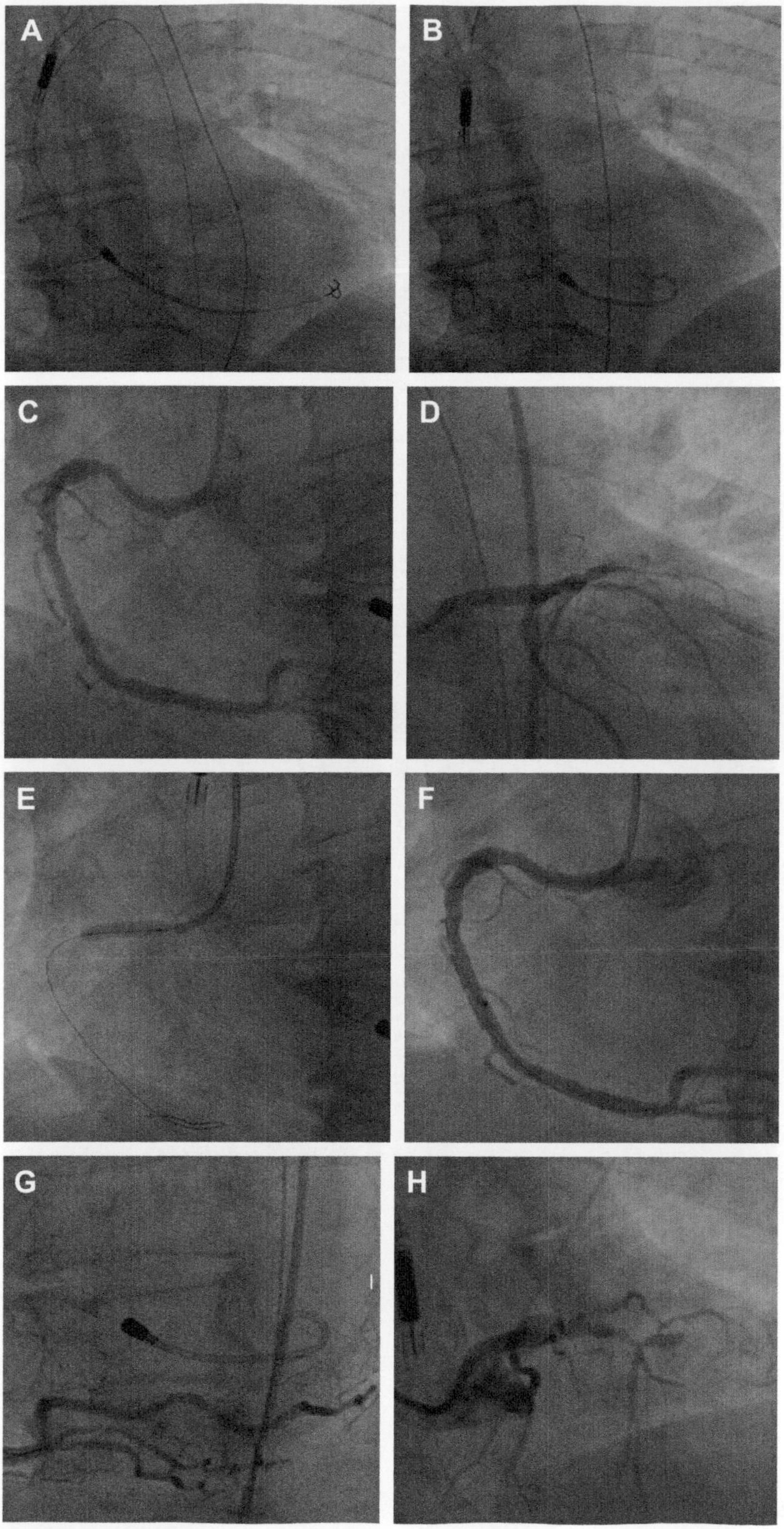

Fig. 12. (*A–R*) Case 12. See text for details.

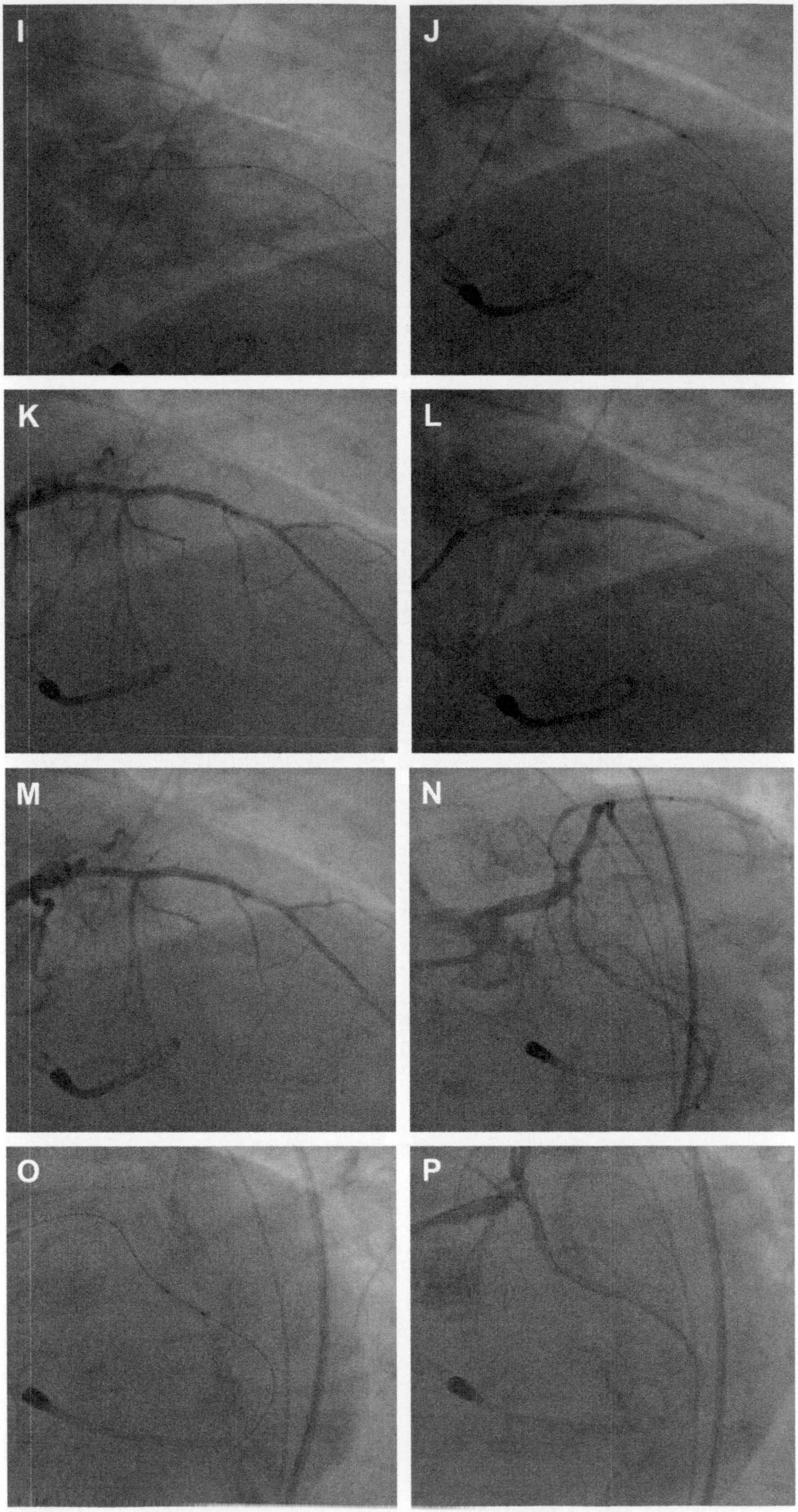

Fig. 12. (*continued*)

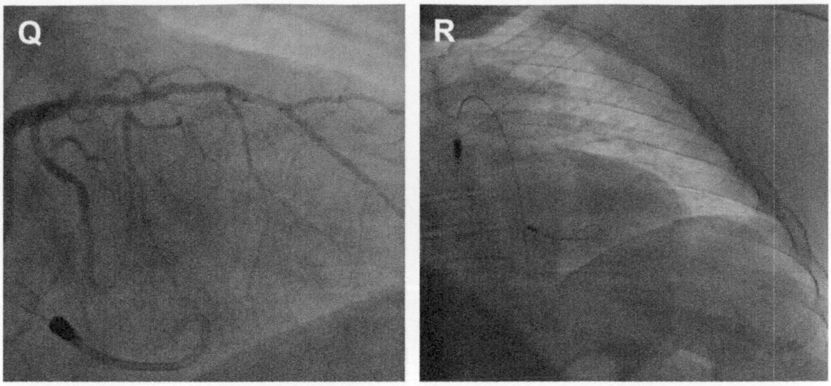

Fig. 12. *(continued)*

Box 12
Case 12 teaching highlights

For true cardiogenic shock, a strategy of treating beyond the culprit lesion may be useful

Treat lesions beyond the culprit lesion in vessels distributing large territories based on the patient's hemodynamic status

The Impella left ventricular support device appears very useful for managing cardiogenic shock

Wiring the LAD, as expected, was difficult, and multiple views and multiple wires were required. Thromboaspiration was performed before stenting.

The decision to further treat the LCX was more difficult. Because the patient was better tolerating the procedure with the Impella catheter, we proceeded with treating the mid-LCX lesion, and did not encounter much difficulty.

Abciximab was administered in addition to bivalirudin (our default agent for STEMI interventions) and 3 DES were used, 1 for each vessel.

The Impella device was removed the following morning; the patient ambulated early and was discharged home on day 6.

D2B time was not chased, being 114 minutes; left ventricular ejection fraction was estimated at 40% with mild, diffuse hypokinesis.

Teaching highlights from case 12 are shown in **Box 12**.

Case 13

To further engage the reader in the management of the very difficult STEMI procedures in the midst of cardiogenic shock, we provide a series of 4 patients with cardiogenic shock. The critical questions that can arise in the midst of management of these very difficult procedures are highlighted.

Tips and tricks

These 4 examples (**Fig. 13**) have been selected to help in some difficult decisions regarding hemodynamic support for STEMI patients in cardiogenic shock.

We hope they will assist in resolving some critical questions that arise in managing such critically ill patients, in particular about the appropriate use of left ventricular support devices.

One such dilemma is whether the hemodynamic support should be provided before or after the STEMI intervention. The operator will never be wrong to first place the support device. However, we believe that this must not be a universal mandate, as some patients will dramatically improve with recanalization of their infarct-related vessel. In these situations the operator is able to avoid cannulating the second groin and thus does not have to deal with the additional morbidity and mortality that accompanies the use of support devices.

Another critical matter pertains to the D2B times. In regard of this, we recommend not being overzealous with D2B times. Cardiogenic shock accompanying acute myocardial infarction presents a cohort of patients with the highest morbidity and mortality, and these patients require very meticulous care of their hemodynamic management and vascular access. Numerous other medications such as inotropes will be required as well, as may be intubation, placing Swan-Ganz and Foley catheters.

The strategy we propose with illustrating these 4 procedures attempts to answer the biggest dilemma: is a support device always needed and should it always be placed before PCI?

A

a

51 yr old Hispanic male, smoker, diabetic, hypertensive with 1 hour of crushing chest pain; 8 mm ST elevation in anterior leads; BP 86/50; HR 112/min; Diaphoretic

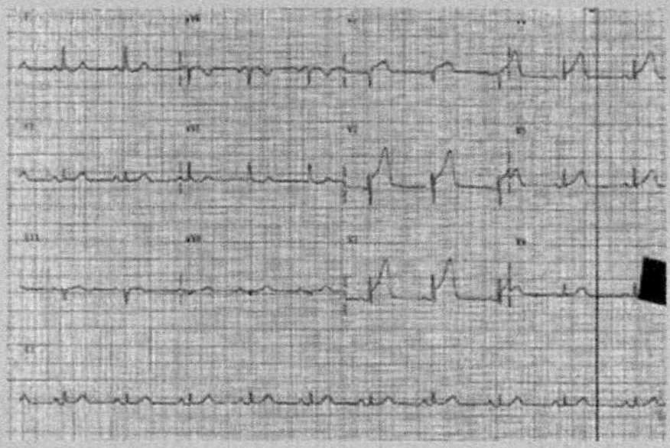

Presented at 4:35 am; Aspiration Thrombectomy available; Mechanical Thrombectomy not available

b

66 yr old Hispanic female, NIDDM with severe chest pain of several hour duration; 5-6 mm ST elevation in inferior leads; BP systolic 80; Feeble pulses

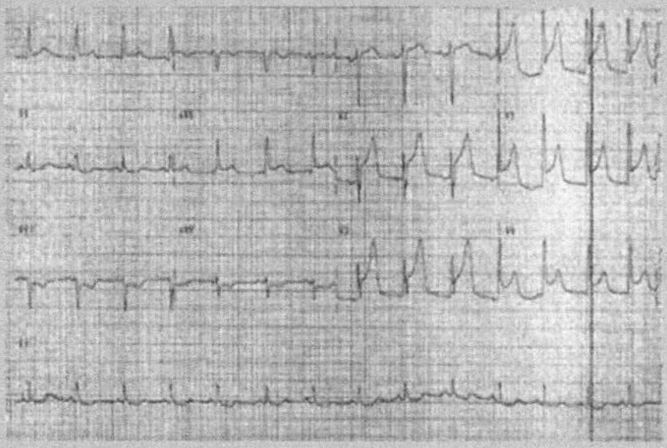

Presented at 10:10 am; Aspiration Thrombectomy available; Mechanical Thrombectomy available

Question: Should you place an IABP or LVAD?
Answer: Need coronary information, fast!

c

84 yr old Afro American Male , with previous PCI, smoker, diabetic, hypertensive, with history of COPD, with 2 hours of crushing chest pain; 8 mm ST elevation in inferior leads; BP 78/40; HR 112/min

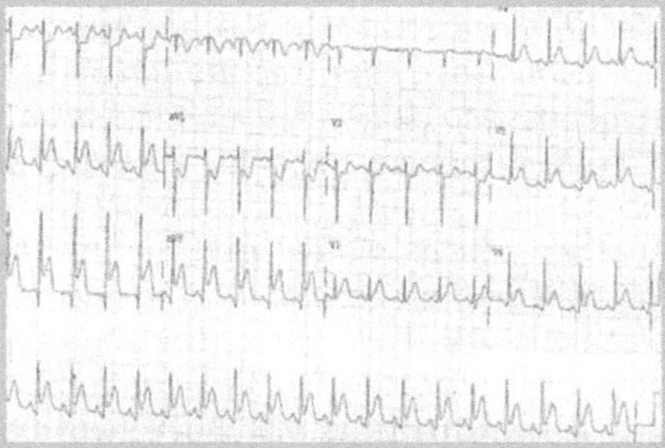

Presented at 3:26 am; Aspiration Thrombectomy available; Mechanical Thrombectomy available

d

71 yr old Hispanic female with acute onset of severe chest pain; no other history available, 8 mm ST elevation in inferior leads; BP 80/46; HR 114/min

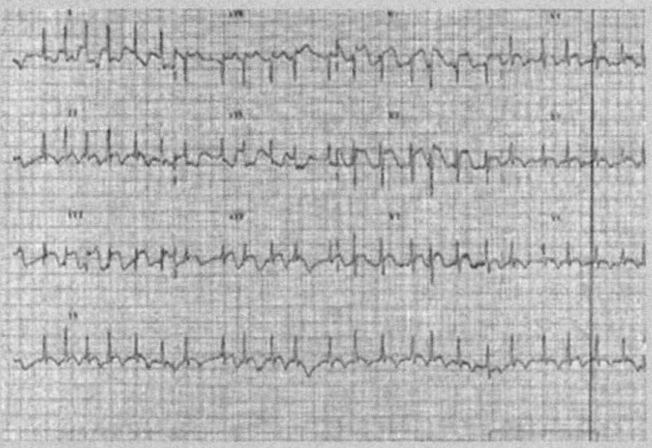

Presented at 1:58 am; Aspiration Thrombectomy available; Mechanical Thrombectomy not available

Fig. 13. (*A*) (*a–d*), (*B*) (*a–d*), (*C*) (*a d*). Case 13. See text for details.

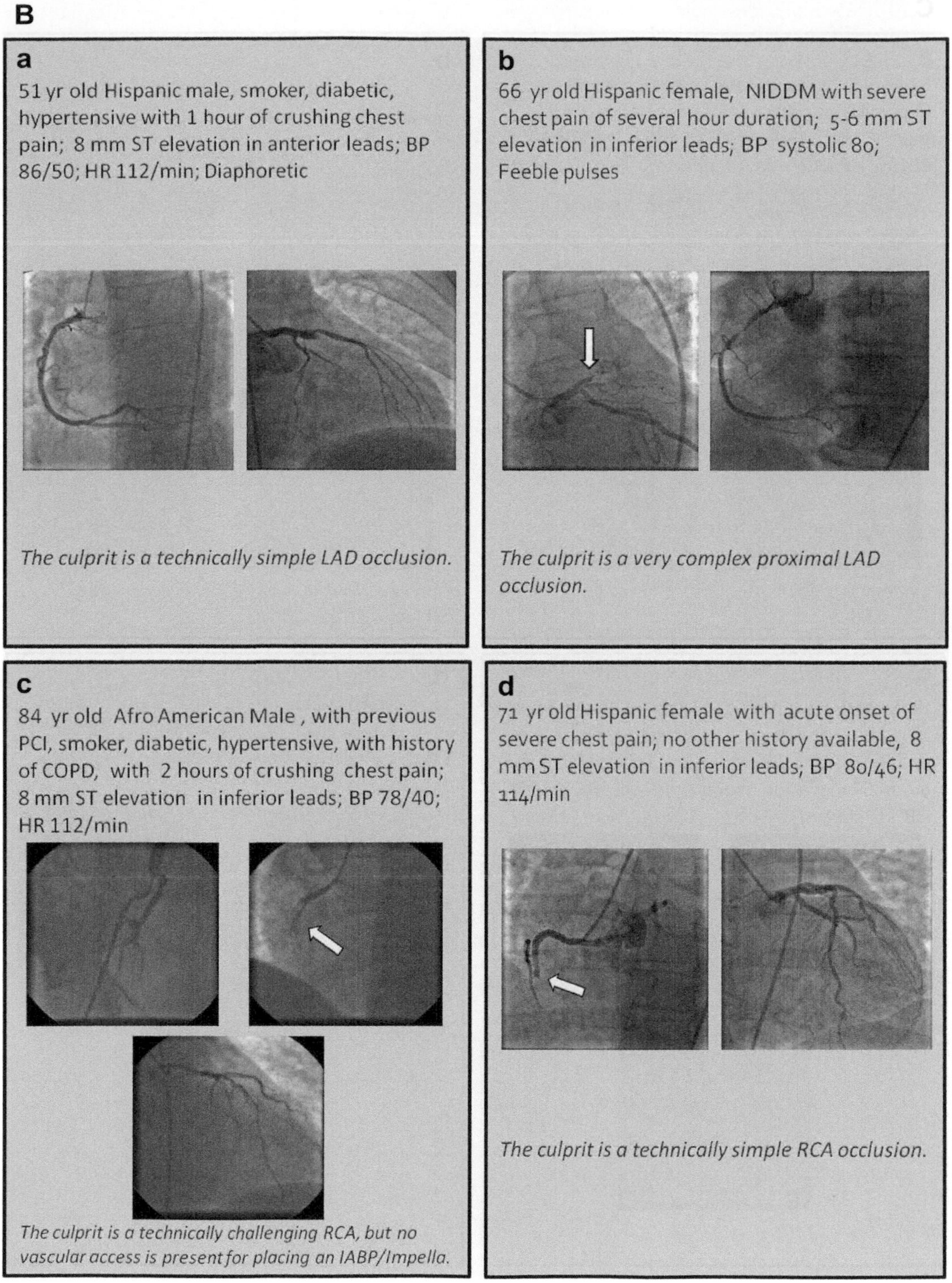
B
a
51 yr old Hispanic male, smoker, diabetic, hypertensive with 1 hour of crushing chest pain; 8 mm ST elevation in anterior leads; BP 86/50; HR 112/min; Diaphoretic
The culprit is a technically simple LAD occlusion.
b
66 yr old Hispanic female, NIDDM with severe chest pain of several hour duration; 5-6 mm ST elevation in inferior leads; BP systolic 80; Feeble pulses
The culprit is a very complex proximal LAD occlusion.
c
84 yr old Afro American Male , with previous PCI, smoker, diabetic, hypertensive, with history of COPD, with 2 hours of crushing chest pain; 8 mm ST elevation in inferior leads; BP 78/40; HR 112/min
The culprit is a technically challenging RCA, but no vascular access is present for placing an IABP/Impella.
d
71 yr old Hispanic female with acute onset of severe chest pain; no other history available, 8 mm ST elevation in inferior leads; BP 80/46; HR 114/min
The culprit is a technically simple RCA occlusion.

Fig. 13. (*continued*)

Based on our extensive work with such patients we are leaning toward the following strategy, which is based on first obtaining coronary angiography. If the lesion appears technically simple, then the operator can proceed with the STEMI intervention first. If hemodynamics dramatically improve, as may occur with relieving ischemia of large territories, one may

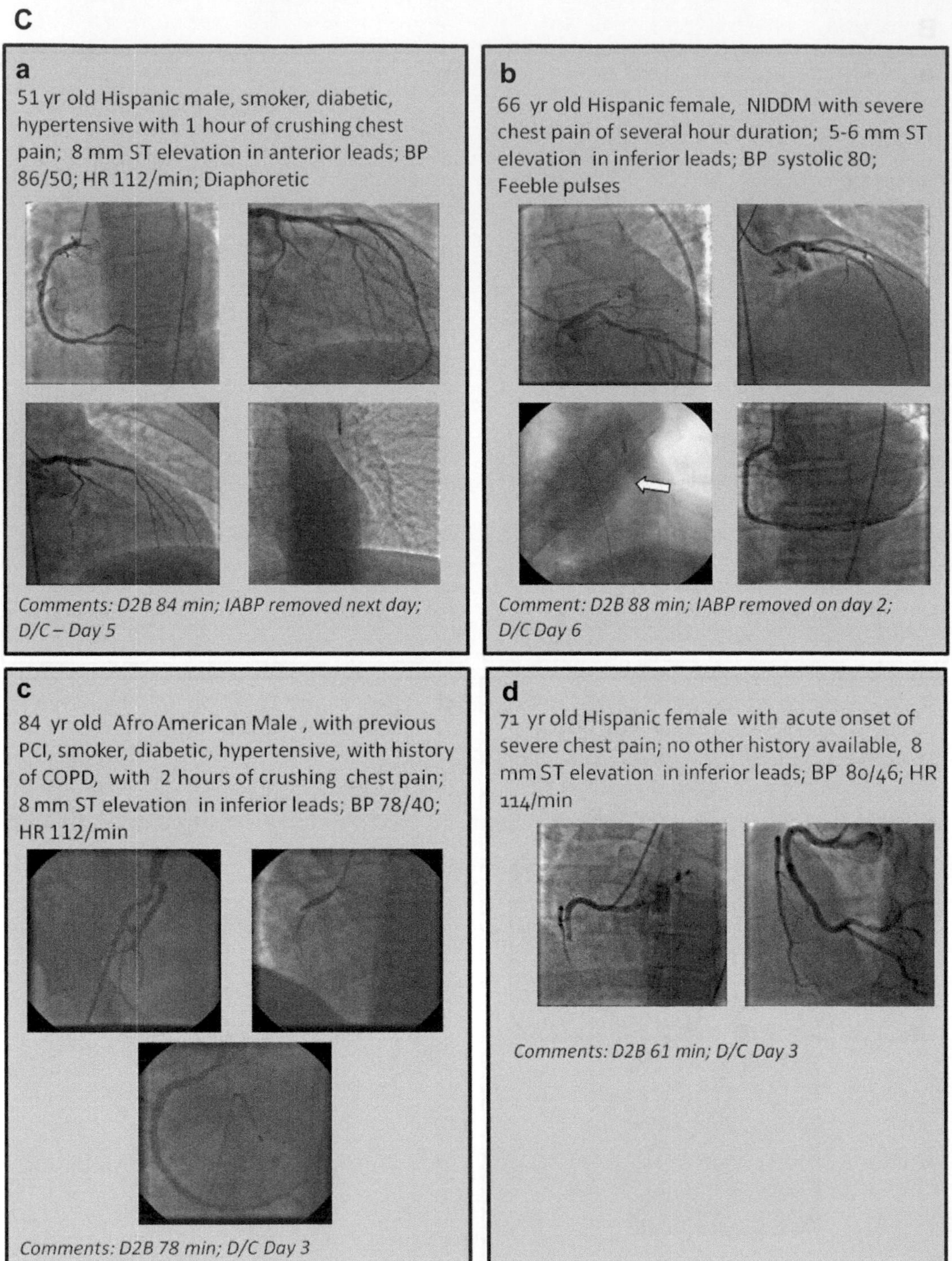
C
a
51 yr old Hispanic male, smoker, diabetic, hypertensive with 1 hour of crushing chest pain; 8 mm ST elevation in anterior leads; BP 86/50; HR 112/min; Diaphoretic
Comments: D2B 84 min; IABP removed next day; D/C – Day 5
b
66 yr old Hispanic female, NIDDM with severe chest pain of several hour duration; 5-6 mm ST elevation in inferior leads; BP systolic 80; Feeble pulses
Comment: D2B 88 min; IABP removed on day 2; D/C Day 6
c
84 yr old Afro American Male , with previous PCI, smoker, diabetic, hypertensive, with history of COPD, with 2 hours of crushing chest pain; 8 mm ST elevation in inferior leads; BP 78/40; HR 112/min
Comments: D2B 78 min; D/C Day 3
d
71 yr old Hispanic female with acute onset of severe chest pain; no other history available, 8 mm ST elevation in inferior leads; BP 80/46; HR 114/min
Comments: D2B 61 min; D/C Day 3

Fig. 13. (*continued*)

not even need a support device (case 13d). In other situations, if the patient remains unstable after the STEMI intervention, the support device can be placed via the same access site, preventing the cannulation of the second groin (case 13a). In other situations where the PCI appears technically challenging (case 13b), the support device is placed first.

Almost always, while taking care of such patients and despite the availability of support devices that can be rapidly set up, we turn our backs to the D2B clock.

Case 14

Tips and tricks

With cases 14 (**Fig. 14**) and 15, we present 2 procedures where mistakes were made and lessons learned. Both are exceptional teaching cases that teach invaluable lessons on how to avoid stent thrombosis in STEMI interventions.

Often, in the midst of rushing for a STEMI and in the middle of all the prevailing chaos, one may momentarily lose concentration, as the operator did in this case.

There were inexplicable delays in the emergency department and with transportation, and

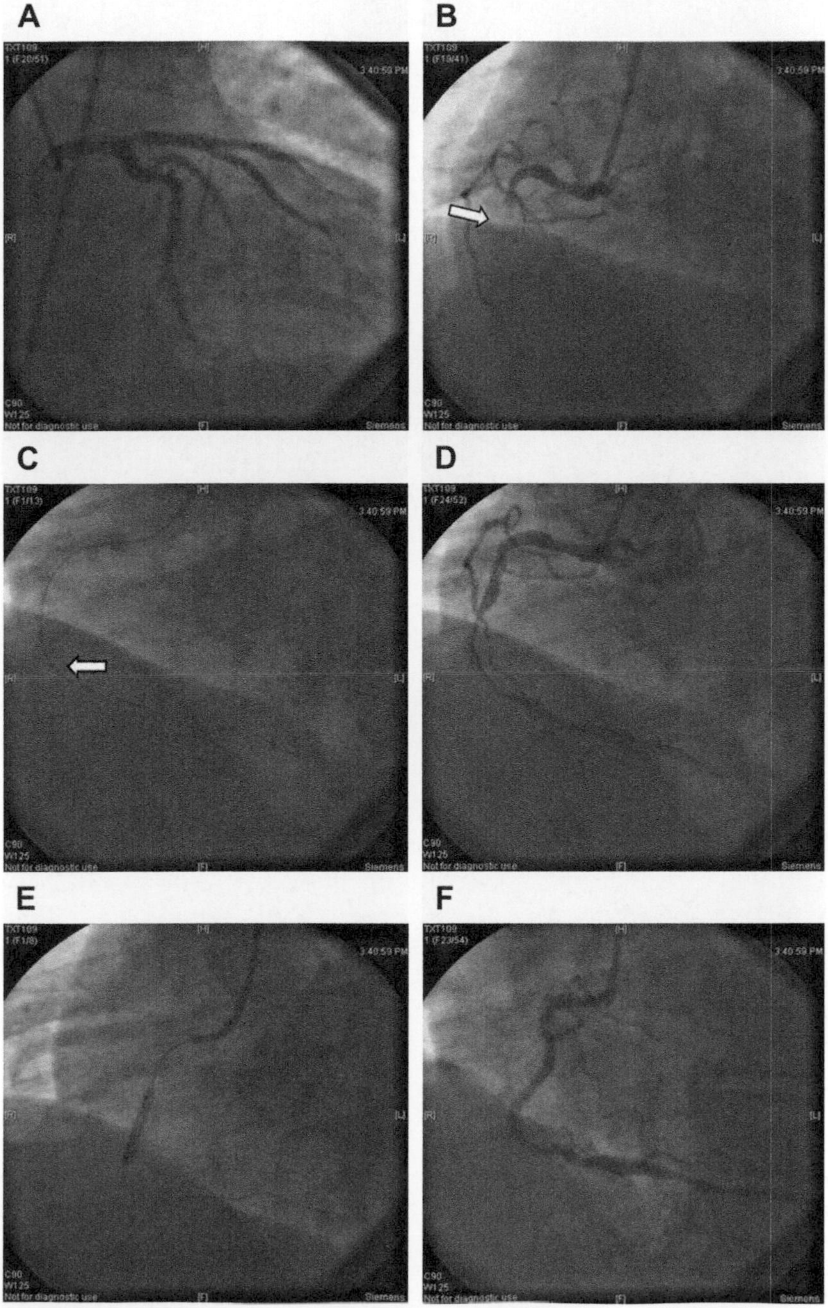

Fig. 14. (*A–L*) Case 14. See text for details.

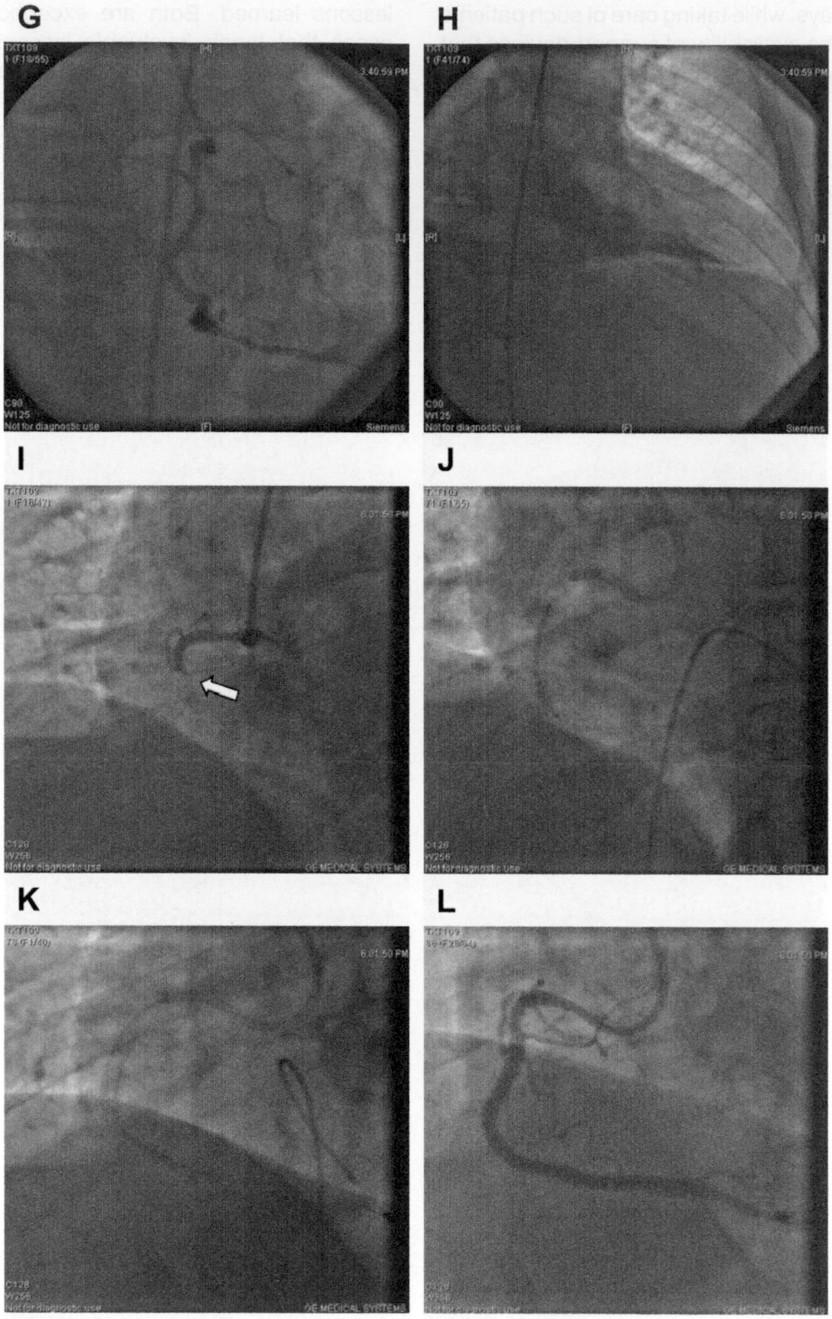

Fig. 14. (*continued*)

the procedure was at 4 AM. Nevertheless, the procedure was completed with a D2B time of 88 minutes and a procedure time of 8 minutes. The final result appeared acceptable (see **Fig. 14**F and G). Even left ventricular function was restored, as was the ST-segment elevation. Direct stenting was used and a 2.5-mm BMS was expanded at 16 atm, yielding a final diameter of 2.81 mm.

Two hours later, the patient complained of severe chest pain and accompanying ST elevation in inferior leads. The stent was occluded, compulsive

Box 13
Case 14 teaching highlights

A vessel can be underfilled as a result of spasm and diffuse disease, therefore the operator must take care not to undersize the stent

This situation occurs primarily with occluded STEMI lesions where reference diameters may be difficult to ascertain

additional thrombectomy was meticulously performed with the Angiojet, and a 4.0-mm stent was deployed. Abciximab was additionally used. The patient had an uncomplicated stay in intensive care and an uneventful discharge occurred on day 5.

Clearly the error was in undersizing the stent. *Often an occluded vessel in a STEMI intervention will be underfilled as a result of spasm and diffuse disease,* as was observed in this case. We remain highly mindful of the possibility of undersizing STEMI lesions.

Teaching highlights from case 14 are shown in **Box 13**.

Case 15

Tips and tricks

We present another stent thrombosis that was related to a common error encountered with STEMI interventions: inadequate debulking of thrombus.

The procedure involves a 56-year-old man who presents with an inferior wall myocardial infarction, and a culprit lesion is identified in the distal RCA (**Fig. 15**). The patient has been treated with antiplatelets orally, and bivalirudin has been administered. For some reason, the surgeon decides to stent directly, clearly underappreciating the presence and extent of thrombus. An adequate result is achieved, chest pain is improved, ST segment resolved, and flow and perfusion seem adequate.

Two hours later, there is stent thrombosis (see **Fig. 15**F).

The cineangiograms were carefully reviewed from the index procedure. Stent sizing appeared appropriate (a 3.5-mm Vision had been expanded at 16 atm), making malapposition less likely (it cannot be definitely ruled out without IVUS).

Would thrombectomy have prevented this complication or would the additional use of abciximab have made a difference in the outcome?

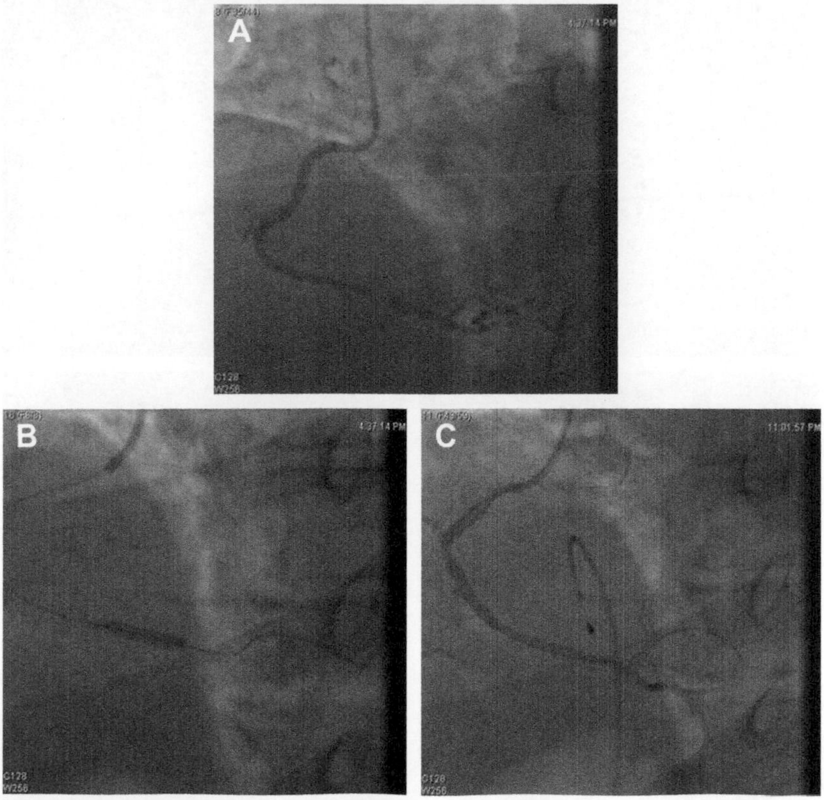

Fig. 15. (*A–K*) Case 15. See text for details.

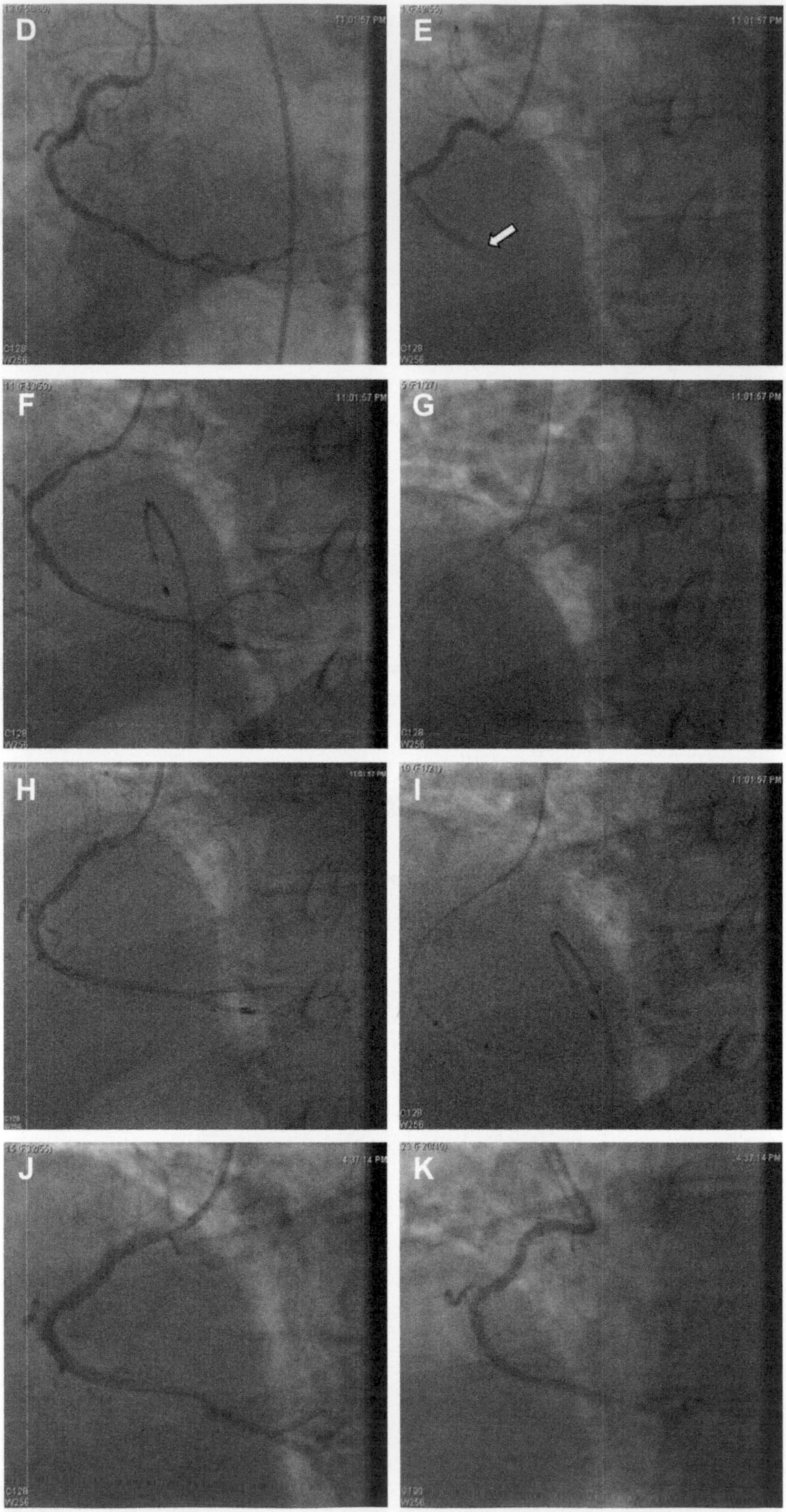

Fig. 15. *(continued)*

Box 14
Case 15 teaching highlights

Unless in situations with clearly no demonstrable thrombus by angiography, most STEMI lesions should be first approached with thrombectomy

Manual aspiration thrombectomy may serve as a default strategy

When stent thrombosis occurs, perform meticulous thrombectomy and be sure the vessel is appropriately sized

We are fairly liberal with our use of abciximab for STEMI interventions, and always use it if there is residual thrombus, a bifurcation lesion involving side-branch occlusion, or slow flow or incomplete reperfusion (persistent chest pain, <70% ST-segment resolution, <TIMI 3 flow, or inadequate myocardial perfusion).

None of these situations existed in this case, although some views suggested some haziness.

We postulated that the stent thrombosis occurred as a result of inadequate thrombus removal, which underscores the recurring theme in almost every case about the need to debulk STEMI lesions. This strategy must be the default, and exemptions should be made only in very straightforward cases, with no discernible thrombus by angiography.

The patient was brought back urgently to the laboratory and abciximab was added to his regimen. Meticulous thrombectomy was performed with the Angiojet. With these maneuvers, adequate flow was restored and the patient proceeded to have an uncomplicated hospital course and discharge.

Teaching highlights from case 15 are shown in **Box 14**.

SUMMARY

The illustrated cases and teaching highlights together with "The Ten Commandments for Short D2B Time STEMI Interventions" and the Mehta strategy for thrombus management are essential tools for STEMI interventions. The sole aim of this article is to focus on absolute and unequivocal strategies that we have used in the SINCERE database to abort the infarct, with rapid restoration (D2B time <90 minutes) of TIMI flow and myocardial perfusion.

REFERENCE

1. Mehta S, editor. Textbook of STEMI interventions. 2nd edition. Malvern (PA): HMP Communications, LLC; 2010.

STEMI Interventions

The European Perspective and Stent for Life Initiative

Ander Regueiro, MD[a,b], Javier Goicolea, MD[a,c], Antonio Fernández-Ortiz, MD, PhD[a,d], Carlos Macaya, MD, PhD[a,d], Manel Sabaté, MD, PhD[a,b,*]

KEYWORDS

• Stent for life • Primary angioplasty • Acute myocardial infarction • ST segment elevation • Networks

KEY POINTS

- STEMI networks coordinate resources to deliver the best care as soon as possible and thereby diminish mortality among this group of patients.
- Lessons learned from model countries should help set up an effective network. Primary percutaneous coronary intervention (pPCI) should be used for >70% of of ST segment elevation myocardial infarction (STEMI) patients with 24-hours-a-day, 7-days-a-week (24/7) services for pPCI procedures to cover the overall population.
- The Stent for Life (SFL) Initiative has the aim of supporting the implementation of the European Society of Cardiology (ESC) guidelines on management of STEMI patients and increasing access of patients to pPCI.

TREATMENT OF STEMI: FROM TECHNICAL AND PHARMACOLOGIC MANAGEMENT TO GLOBAL LOGISTIC APPROACH

Percutaneous coronary intervention (PCI), fibrinolytic treatment, or combinations of both are current strategies to treat patients with STEMI. pPCI is defined as percutaneous intervention in the setting of STEMI without previous or concomitant use of fibrinolytic treatment. Reperfusion therapy in STEMI patients is time dependent.[1] Survival benefit of fibrinolytic therapy is substantially higher if applied within the first 2 hours after the onset of symptoms.[2] Similarly, mortality benefit of pPCI is also time dependent.[3–5] When applied in a timely fashion, pPCI is able to reduce the risk of reinfarction and mortality compared with fibrinolyitic therapy.[6] Above all, pPCI, when performed in a timely fashion and by an experienced team, is the therapy of choice in patients with STEMI.[7,8] Transfer of patients from community hospitals, where pPCI is not available, to 24/7 pPCI hospitals is then crucial. Feasibility and safety of this strategy have been proved[9] as has the efficacy in terms of mortality reduction in patients presenting more than 3 hours after symptom onset.[9] As a rule, implementation of strategies to treat patients with pPCI according to guideline recommendations is associated with a significant improvement in clinical outcomes.[10] Several pharmacologic treatments, including antithrombotics, β-blockers, angiotensin-converting enzyme inhibitors, angiotensin receptor blockers, and aldosterone blockade, have also proved to increase survival when administered to patients with STEMI. As a result, in-hospital and 30-day

[a] Stent for Life Initiative, Spanish Society of Cardiology, Nuestra Señora de Guadalupe, # 5–7, Madrid 28028, Spain; [b] Cardiology Department, Thorax Institute, Hospital Clinic, c/Villarroel 170, Barcelona 08036, Spain; [c] Cardiology Department, 'Puerta de Hierro' Hospital, C/Manuel de Falla 1, Majadahonda, Madrid 28222, Spain; [d] Interventional Cardiology, Cardiovascular Institute, Clínico 'San Carlos' University Hospital, Madrid, Spain
* Corresponding author. Cardiology Department, Thorax Institute, Hospital Clínic, c/Villarroel 170, Barcelona 08036, Spain.
E-mail address: MASABATE@clinic.ub.es

Intervent Cardiol Clin 1 (2012) 559–565
http://dx.doi.org/10.1016/j.iccl.2012.06.008
2211-7458/12/$ – see front matter

mortality for STEMI has decreased dramatically over the past 30 years.[11–13]

In the real practice, however, not all STEMI patients benefit from the best treatment due to inadequate guideline implementation in daily practice or lack of access to the system.[14,15] Organizational strategies with the aim of implementing current guidelines and evidence-based treatment by improving patient care systems in and outside the hospital have proved, in qualitative and prospective studies, to decrease door-to-balloon time,[16,17] myocardial infarct size, hospital length of stay, total hospital costs,[18] and mortality.[19] In a survey including 365 hospitals, 6 strategies were significantly associated with a faster door-to-balloon time in a multivariate analysis. Those strategies included[20]

- Emergency physicians activating the catheterization laboratory
- Single call to a central page operator to activate the laboratory
- Emergency department activating the catheterization laboratory while patients are en route to the hospital
- Expecting staff to arrive in the catheterization laboratory within 20 minutes after being paged
- Having an attending cardiologist always on site
- Having staff in the emergency department and the catheterization laboratory use real-time data feedback

Moreover, transportation of patients by an emergency medical service (EMS) decreases system delay and mortality in STEMI patients treated with pPCI.[21] Prehospital ECG and further activation of catheterization laboratory is associated with a significantly shorter time to reperfusion,[22] and direct transfer from the field achieves door-to-balloon time of less than 90 minutes in 79.7% of patients in citywide protocols for pPCI.[23]

In summary, a systematic global approach that tackles both the logistic aspects and the clinical protocol is mandatory to successfully treat STEMI patients primarily with PCI as it is the most effective therapy.

STENT FOR LIFE INITIATIVE

Reperfusion Therapy in Europe

In 2008, the European Association of Percutaneous Cardiovascular Interventions (EAPCI) performed a survey at the country level to obtain a realistic, contemporary picture of how patients with STEMI were treated in different countries. Data were collected from 30 countries and the writing group was composed of members of national working groups and societies of interventional cardiology and selected experts known to be involved in the national registries.[15] Main conclusions were as follows:

- pPCI was the dominant strategy for STEMI patients in 16 of 30 countries and fibrinolytic therapy in 8 countries.
- Use of reperfusion (pPCI or fibrinolytic) varied from 37% to 93% of STEMI patients.
- Use of pPCI varied between 5% and 92% and the use of fibrinolytic therapy varied between 0% and 55% of all STEMI patients.
- On average, achievement of reperfusion was significantly lower (mean of 55%) in countries where fibrinolytic therapy was the dominant strategy.
- The mean population served by a single PCI center varied between 0.3 million and 1.1 million inhabitants.
- The time from onset of symptoms to first medical contact (FMC) varied between 60 and 120 minutes. The time from FMC to initiation of fibrinolytic therapy ranged from 30 to 110 minutes. Finally, the time from FMC to the initiation of PCI varied between 60 and 177 minutes.
- The overall in-hospital mortality varied between 4.2% and 13.5%. In patients with fibrinolytic therapy, it ranged from 3.5% to 14%. Mortality in patients treated with pPCI varied between 2.7% and 8%.
- Northern, Western, and Central Europe had well-developed pPCI networks whereas Southern Europe and the Balkans were still predominantly using fibrinolytic therapy. Lack of organized pPCI networks was associated with fewer patients overall receiving some form of reperfusion therapy. Moreover, the development of an acute myocardial infarction network was not related to the gross domestic product of the country.

Stent for Life Mission and Goals

Considering the indisputable scientific evidence and the inhomogeneity in the existing practice patterns resulting in tremendous inequalities in patient access to best treatment for STEMI,[24] Dr William Wijns together with Prof P. Widimský expressed at the ESC Board 2006–2008 the idea to organize a pan-European initiative to support the implementation of PCI in acute forms of coronary artery disease. In September 2008, at the first meeting of the "founding fathers," in Brussels, the name, *Stent for Life*, was proposed. The SFL

Initiative was launched by the EAPCI General Assembly during the ESC Annual Congress 2009 in Barcelona by a coalition of the EAPCI (a registered branch of the ESC) and EuroPCR. The partnering organizations are Eucomed, the ESC Working Group on Acute Cardiac Care, national cardiology societies, and/or national working groups for interventional cardiology. The SFL Initiative Executive Committee was initially constituted of Dr Wijns (cofounder and past president of the EAPCI), Prof Widimský (cofounder and past chair of SFL Initiative), Prof Carlo di Mario (past president of the EAPCI), Prof Jean Fajadet (cochairman and EAPCI president), and Prof Steen D. Kristensen (cochairman).

The mission of the SFL Initiative was to improve delivery of and patient access to the lifesaving indications of pPCI, thereby reducing the mortality and morbidity of patients suffering from acute coronary syndromes. The SFL Initiative is a unique European platform for interventional cardiologists, government representatives, industry partners, and patient groups to work together to help shape health care systems and medical practices and ensure that the majority of STEMI patients have equal access to pPCI.

Overall aims of SFL included the implementation of ESC guidelines on management of acute myocardial infarction in patients presenting persistent ST segment elevation; the identification of specific obstacles to the implementation of guidelines; and defining actions to make sure that the majority of STEMI patients in Europe have access to pPCI. Specific goals included defining the regions/countries with an unmet medical need in the optimal treatment of ACS and implementing an action program to increase patient access to pPCI where indicated. From the positive experiences of 5 countries, 3 realistic goals were defined to be implemented in the rest of the countries:

1. pPCI should be used for greater than 70% of all STEMI patients.
2. pPCI rates should reach more than 600 per million inhabitants per year.
3. Services for pPCI procedures should be offered 24/7 at invasive facilities to cover the overall STEMI population of the country.

Recommendations for Setting Up an Effective National pPCI Network

The following recommendations for setting up an effective national pPCI network were described, with the lessons learned from 5 European countries (Czech Republic, the Netherlands, Denmark, Austria, and Sweden), in which patient triage, prehospital management, and hospital networks were well developed.[25]

Public campaigns

Wide population knowledge about the key role of time in myocardial infarction symptoms and basic cardiopulmonary resuscitation with a unique national emergency phone number, is an important part of the process.

Emergency medical services

Experience demonstrated that nurses and paramedics can triage and transport STEMI patients with adequate training. EMS ambulances should be equipped to perform 12-lead ECG. ECG transmission may be decided locally. In countries with EMS staffed with physicians, the use of ECG transmission may be time consuming. If transmission of ECG is performed, transportation should not be delayed.

Networks and infrastructure

Development of regional networks, involving EMS, non-PCI, and PCI centers is necessary to implement pPCI services effectively. Regional networks should cover an area of approximately 0.5 million people; smaller areas create suboptimal effectiveness and larger areas may cause overload. All PCI centers should provide nonstop (24/7) services for pPCI, and non-PCI hospitals should have a qualified cardiologist available 24/7.

Transport and time delays

The primary transport of STEMI patients should always bypass the nearest non-PCI hospital or emergency department in the PCI center. Patients should be taken directly to a catheterization laboratory. Personal at the catheterization laboratory should be informed and activated immediately after STEMI diagnosis.

Catheterization Laboratory Staffing and Organization of Work

There are several approaches to catheterization laboratory staffing. In an economic approach, 1 cardiologist plus 1 nurse with additional staff (whenever necessary) coming from an ICU are paid outside regular working hours. An extended approach is represented by 1 cardiologist plus 1 trainee physician plus 2 nurses plus 1 technician. The number of personnel can be decided locally—with only 1 important point: at least 1 nurse should be present 24/7 to prepare the laboratory during the time when the interventional cardiologist is on the way. All personnel should arrive within 30 minutes from being called.

Financial aspects

Reimbursement does not seem to be a problem in fee-for-service systems. In government-run systems, professionals have succeeded in convincing politicians about the benefits for pPCI. Remuneration for staff needs to be set locally.

Coronary angiography after thrombolysis

Thrombolysis remains a viable alternative for regions with long transfer times to PCI centers. These patients should be transported to PCI centers, either for immediate angiography, if thrombolysis is unsuccessful, or if there is any doubt about its effect. As a rule, 100% of STEMI patients should be admitted to a PCI center within the first 24 hours.

High-risk non-ST elevation ACS

Patients with non-ST elevation acute myocardial infarction with ongoing or recurrent chest pain, signs of heart failure, cardiogenic shock, or significant arrhythmias should be transported to PCI centers in a similar manner to STEMI patients.

Political issues

Cooperation between cardiology societies, governments, health care financing organizations, hospitals, and EMS is effective in achieving the appropriate implementation of pPCI programs. Formalized national cardiology programs describing the recommendations on a national level may provide support to coordinate the effort of all stakeholders in this process.

Registries and quality control

National or regional acute coronary syndrome registries will help to further improve the system and will serve as a quality control tool. The importance of providing feedback with the data collected to every center and people involved in the process to define potential areas of improvement should be stressed.

Stent for Life: Implementation in Countries

Geographic expansion

Declaration of the SFL Initiative was signed at the ESC/EAPCI General Assembly on August 31, 2009. Initial pilot countries involved in the SFL Initiative were Bulgaria, France, Greece, Serbia, Spain, and Turkey. Egypt, Italy, and Romania joined in 2010 and Portugal in 2011 (**Fig. 1**). All country members expressed their interest in participating in the SFL Initiative and signed a declaration that effective actions were going to be taken to fulfill the mission of the SFL Initiative. Across Europe, national cardiac societies, working groups, and associations of interventional cardiology from 16 countries are currently active participants in the SFL Initiative.

Impact of Stent for Life Initiative on quality of care

Several local activities in the 10 target countries have been initiated since the SFL was launched in 2009.[26] Learning from the best-practice countries' experiences is keystone to developing action plans in SFL countries and building effective pPCI networks. Most SFLs have chosen to follow a regional approach in their management of STEMI and implementation of pPCI programs. Spain, Greece, France, and Turkey have chosen such a regional approach.[27] In Spain, there has been an increase in the population covered by STEMI network from 29% in 2008 to 39.2% at the beginning of 2012 and by the end of 2012 it is expected to increase up to 52%. Greece has succeeded in establishing pPCI networks in Attica and in the southwestern part of the country, increasing the pPCI rate to 20% compared with 8% in 2008. In Attica, which represents almost 50% of the total population, there has been an increase of 40%.[28] In Turkey, a pilot project with 18 regional STEMI networks was launched around the main PCI centers. The number of pPCIs performed per year has increased from 324 per million inhabitants in 2009 to 453 per million inhabitants in 2010.[28] Alternatively, Serbia is a good example of national approach. With strong support from government, a national program for the implementation of STEMI treatment guidelines was approved. Since joining the SFL, Serbia increased its annual number of pPCIs from 230 per million inhabitants to 337 in 2009 to 440 per million in 2010.[28] In several countries, intense training has been provided to EMS staff involved in the care of STEMI to increase the quality of prehospital care and decrease the system's time delay.[26]

ACT NOW. SAVE A LIFE: public awareness campaign

All countries have reported the lack of public knowledge of the signs and symptoms of an acute coronary syndrome and, more importantly, the lack of knowledge on what to do if symptoms appear. This is reflected by the usual time delays caused by patients before contacting the system and the low rate of patients who arrive at the hospital through EMS. To address this issue, the SFL Initiative developed a public awareness campaign and is currently coordinating its implementation in countries/regions where a pPCI network is already established. The ACT NOW. SAVE A LIFE campaign has been rolled out in Bulgaria, Portugal, Spain, and Turkey. This campaign is aimed at improving the delivery of, and patient access to, the life-saving treatment of pPCI, educating patients to act quickly and to call the

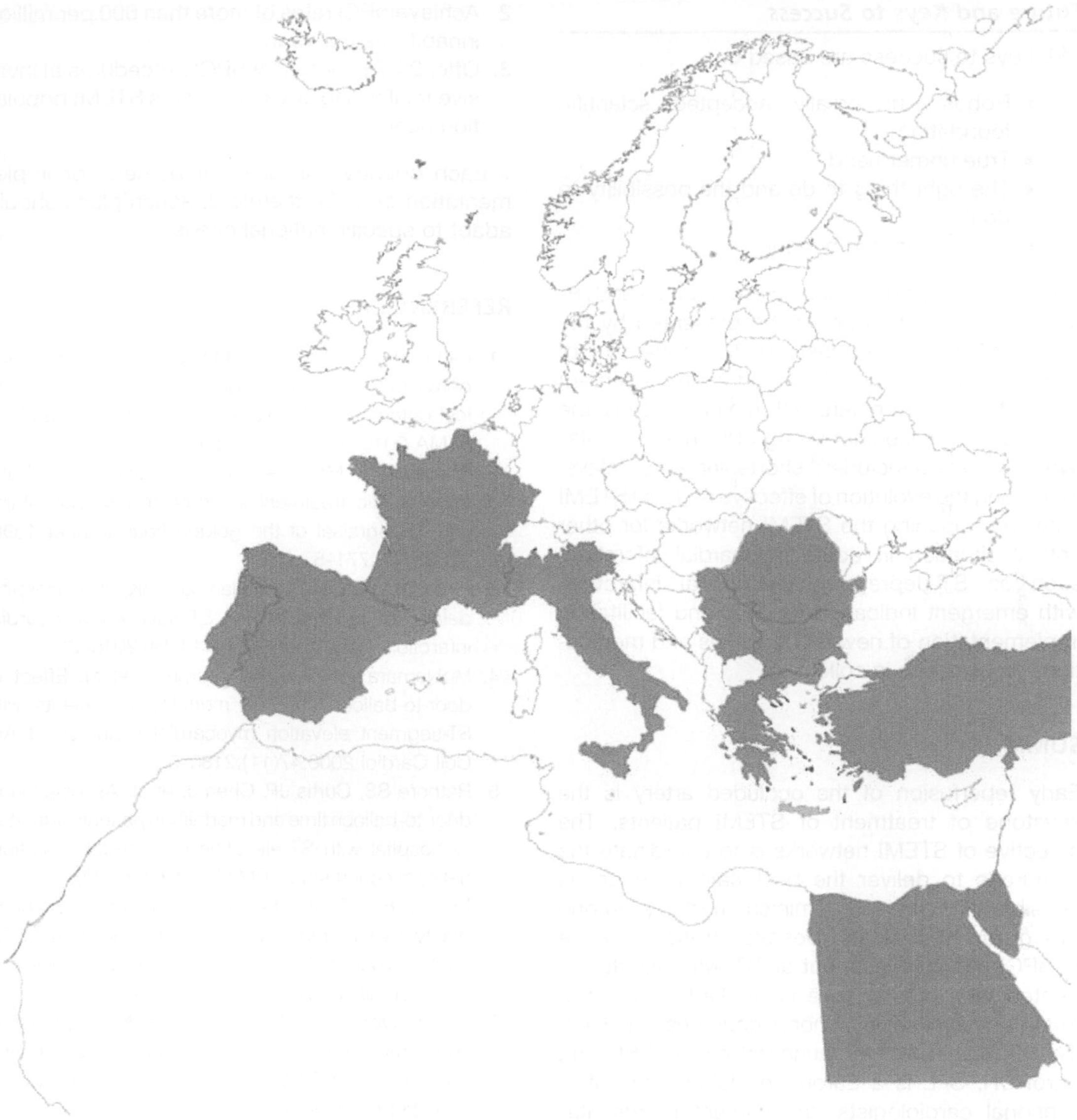

Fig. 1. The SFL Initiative is currently supported by 10 national cardiac societies and/or working groups or associations of interventional cardiology, including those from Bulgaria, Egypt, France, Greece, Italy, Portugal, Romania, Serbia, Spain, and Turkey.

unique national emergency phone number to be transferred by ambulance to a pPCI center, bypassing the nearest hospital without pPCI facilities. The campaign will be based in the 4 following messages:

1. Know the signs.
2. Act quickly.
3. Call emergency services.
4. Receive treatment.

The impact of ACT NOW. SAVE A LIFE campaign will be measured and a case study published thereafter.

Collaboration between Stent for Life and Women in Innovations

Women in Innovations (WIN) is currently affiliated with both the EAPCI and the Society for Cardiovascular Angiography and Interventions. WIN's mission is to address gender disparities in cardiovascular care and professionalism through education, research, professional development, and innovation. The collaboration has just begun; so far, SFL/WIN has launched a patient and provider education Web site and gathers data from both groups for further study about heart disease in women in Spain.

Future and Keys to Success

SFL keys to success are based on

- Robust, universally accepted scientific foundation
- True unmet need
- The right thing to do and the possibility to do it
- Leadership and support

A detailed report describing the situation of STEMI treatment in Europe will be presented by the ESC Congress in August 2012. Irrespective of these results, SFL should aim at an improvement in qualitative parameters with maintenance of the quantitative phase (increasing pPCI use). Qualitative parameters include[29] shortening time delays; facilitating the evolution of effective regional STEMI networks; opening the STEMI networks for other critical situation in acute myocardial infarction, such as ST-depression myocardial infarction, with emergent indication for PCI; and facilitating implementation of new technologies and medications as evidence is collected.

SUMMARY

Early reperfusion of the occluded artery is the keystone of treatment of STEMI patients. The objective of STEMI networks is to coordinate the resources to deliver the best care as soon as possible and thereby diminish mortality among this group of patients. Despite strong evidence of pPCI effectiveness, not all STEMI patients are treated with pPCI. There is marked variation in treatment availability among countries. In 2008, the SFL Initiative was launched by the ESC and EuroPCR. SFL is a European platform for interventional cardiologists, government representatives, industry partners, and patient groups that aims to improve the delivery of care and patient access to pPCI. The SFL Initiative has 2 key objectives:

1. Define the regions with an unmet medical need in the optimal treatment of acute coronary syndrome.
2. Implement an action plan to increase patient access to pPCI.

Since SFL was launched, 10 countries (Bulgaria, Egypt, France, Greece, Italy, Portugal, Romania, Serbia, Spain, and Turkey) have joined the SFL Initiative after an invitation to participate and 3 targets were set:

1. Increase the use of pPCI to more than 70% among all STEMI patients.
2. Achieve pPCI rates of more than 600 per million inhabitants per year.
3. Offer 24/7 services for pPCI procedures at invasive facilities to cover a region's STEMI population need.

Each country has different barriers for implementation of pPCI; therefore, action plans should adapt to specific national needs.

REFERENCES

1. Lambert L, Brown K, Segal E, et al. Association between timeliness of reperfusion therapy and clinical outcomes in ST-elevation myocardial infarction. JAMA 2010;303(21):2148–55.
2. Boersma E, Maas AC, Deckers JW, et al. Early thrombolytic treatment in acute myocardial infarction: reappraisal of the golden hour. Lancet 1996; 348(9030):771–5.
3. Pinto DS, Kirtane AJ, Nallamothu BK, et al. Hospital delays in reperfusion for ST-elevation myocardial infarction. Circulation 2006;114(19):2019–25.
4. McNamara RL, Wang Y, Herrin J, et al. Effect of door-to-balloon time on mortality in patients with ST-segment elevation myocardial infarction. J Am Coll Cardiol 2006;47(11):2180–6.
5. Rathore SS, Curtis JP, Chen J, et al. Association of door-to-balloon time and mortality in patients admitted to hospital with ST elevation myocardial infarction: national cohort study. BMJ 2009;338:b1807.
6. Keeley EC, Boura JA, Grines CL. Primary angioplasty versus intravenous thrombolytic therapy for acute myocardial infarction: a quantitative review of 23 randomised trials. Lancet 2003;361(9351):13–20.
7. Van de Werf F, Bax J, Betriu A, et al. Management of acute myocardial infarction in patients presenting with persistent ST-segment elevation. Eur Heart J 2008;29(23):2909–45.
8. Kushner FG, Hand M, Smith SC Jr, et al. 2009 focused updates: ACC/AHA guidelines for the management of patients with ST-elevation myocardial infarction (updating the 2004 guideline and 2007 focused update) and ACC/AHA/SCAI guidelines on percutaneous coronary intervention (updating the 2005 guideline and 2007 focused update) a report of the American College of Cardiology Foundation/American Heart Association Task Force on Practice Guidelines. J Am Coll Cardiol 2009; 54(23):2205–41.
9. Widimský P, Budešínský T, Voráč D, et al. Long distance transport for primary angioplasty vs immediate thrombolysis in acute myocardial infarction. Eur Heart J 2003;24(1):94–104.
10. Kalla K, Christ G, Karnik R, et al. Implementation of guidelines improves the standard of care. Circulation 2006;113(20):2398–405.

11. Gibson CM, Pride YB, Frederick PD, et al. Trends in reperfusion strategies, door-to-needle and door-to-balloon times, and in-hospital mortality among patients with ST-segment elevation myocardial infarction enrolled in the National Registry of Myocardial Infarction from 1990 to 2006. Am Heart J 2008; 156(6):1035–44.
12. Rosamond WD, Chambless LE, Heiss G, et al. Twenty-two year trends in incidence of myocardial infarction, CHD mortality, and case-fatality in four US communities, 1987 to 2008. Circulation 2012; 125(15):1848–57.
13. Smolina K, Wright FL, Rayner M, et al. Determinants of the decline in mortality from acute myocardial infarction in England between 2002 and 2010: linked national database study. BMJ 2012;344:d8059.
14. Peterson ED, Bynum DZ, Roe MT. Lessons learned from the CRUSADE National Quality Improvement Initiative. Curr Cardiol Rep 2008;10(4):285–90.
15. Widimsky P, Wijns W, Fajadet J, et al. Reperfusion therapy for ST elevation acute myocardial infarction in Europe: description of the current situation in 30 countries. Eur Heart J 2010;31(8):943–57.
16. Bradley EH, Roumanis SA, Radford MJ, et al. Achieving door-to-balloon times that meet quality guidelines: how do successful hospitals do it? J Am Coll Cardiol 2005;46(7):1236–41.
17. Bradley EH, Curry LA, Webster TR, et al. Achieving rapid door-to-balloon times. Circulation 2006;113(8):1079–85.
18. Khot UN, Johnson ML, Ramsey C, et al. Emergency department physician activation of the catheterization laboratory and immediate transfer to an immediately available catheterization laboratory reduce door-to-balloon time in ST-elevation myocardial infarction. Circulation 2007;116(1):67–76.
19. Jernberg T, Johanson P, Held C, et al. Association between adoption of evidence-based treatment and survival for patients with ST-elevation myocardial infarction. JAMA 2011;305(16):1677–84.
20. Bradley EH, Herrin J, Wang Y, et al. Strategies for reducing the door-to-balloon time in acute myocardial infarction. N Engl J Med 2006;355(22): 2308–20.
21. Terkelsen CJ, Sørensen JT, Maeng M, et al. System delay and mortality among patients with STEMI treated with primary percutaneous coronary intervention. JAMA 2010;304(7):763–71.
22. Curtis JP, Portnay EL, Wang Y, et al. The pre-hospital electrocardiogram and time to reperfusion in patients with acute myocardial infarction, 2000–2002: findings from the National Registry of Myocardial Infarction-4. J Am Coll Cardiol 2006;47(8):1544–52.
23. Le May MR, So DY, Dionne R, et al. A citywide protocol for primary PCI in ST-segment elevation myocardial infarction. N Engl J Med 2008;358(3):231–40.
24. Widimsky P, Fajadet J, Danchin N, et al. "Stent 4 Life" targeting PCI at all who will benefit the most. A joint project between EAPCI, Euro-PCR, EUCOMED and the ESC Working Group on Acute Cardiac Care. EuroIntervention 2009;4(5):555–7.
25. Knot J, Widimsky P, Wijns W, et al. How to set up an effective national primary angioplasty network: lessons learned from five European countries. EuroIntervention 2009;5(3):299, 301–9.
26. Laut KG, Kaifoszova Z, Kristensen SD. Status of stent for life initiative across Europe. J Cardiovasc Med (Hagerstown) 2011;12(12):856–9.
27. Kristensen SD, Fajadet J, Di Mario CD, et al. Implementation of primary angioplasti in Europe: stent for life initiative progress report. EuroIntervention 2012; 8:35–42.
28. Kaifoszova Z, Widimsky P. Increasing the penetration of primary angioplasty in Europe. Eur Cardiol 2012;8(1):3.
29. Widimsky P, Kristensen SD. Stent for life initiative: where are we standing and where are we going?. Acute Cardiovascular Care. Eur Heart J 2012;1(1): 48–9.

Lessons Learned from the Ottawa Regional STEMI Program

Michel R. Le May, MD*, Melissa S.K. Blondeau, BSc

KEYWORDS

• STEMI • Primary angioplasty • Pharmacoinvasive strategy • Acute myocardial infarction

KEY POINTS

- Availability of a prehospital ECG is critical for early identification of ST-segment elevation myocardial infarction (STEMI) patients.
- Trained paramedics can identify STEMI patients in the field and directly transfer these patients to a percutaneous coronary intervention (PCI)-capable hospital for primary PCI. This process shortens the door-to-balloon time.
- Empowering emergency medicine physicians to activate the code STEMI without consultation with a cardiologist is required when patients are transferred from non-PCI–capable hospitals to a PCI center.
- Incorporating a pharmacoinvasive strategy for community hospitals in which transfer for primary PCI is not an option improves clinical outcomes.
- Standardization is the key to a successful STEMI program: it allows the process to move more quickly and more efficiently. It reduces the likelihood of errors in the medication prescribed to patients and leads to faster reperfusion.

Primary PCI has become the dominant strategy for the treatment of STEMI when rapid access to a catheterization facility is available. In communities where primary PCI is not feasible, a pharmacoinvasive strategy has become a recommended option. At the University of Ottawa Heart Institute (UOHI), a care delivery model has been developed in which primary PCI and pharmacoinvasive strategies are applied for an entire region. This article reviews the lessons learned in setting up and maintaining a regional STEMI program.

USING EVIDENCE-BASED MEDICINE TO OBTAIN CONSENSUS

In the province of Ontario, Canada, the government has created 14 local health integration networks (LHINs) to plan, integrate, and fund local health services in each region. The UOHI is a tertiary cardiac center located in the city of Ottawa. The UOHI works in collaboration with 16 other hospitals within the Champlain LHIN for the purposes of delivering cardiac care to a geographic area of approximately 1.2 million people. All of the region's cardiac catheterization laboratories are located at this designated cardiac center. Within the context of the LHIN, a care delivery model has been developed to improve access to this specialized cardiac center to ensure timely reperfusion for patients with STEMI. The model uses systematic primary PCI for patients within the metropolitan area and a pharmacoinvasive approach for patients presenting to community hospitals outside the metropolitan area. This regional model was an outgrowth of

On behalf of the Ottawa Interventional Group.
None of the authors has a conflict of interest in connection with this article.
Department of Medicine, Division of Cardiology, University of Ottawa Heart Institute, 40 Ruskin Street, Ottawa, Ontario K1Y 4W7, Canada
* Corresponding author.
E-mail address: mlemay@ottawaheart.ca

Intervent Cardiol Clin 1 (2012) 567–582
http://dx.doi.org/10.1016/j.iccl.2012.06.012
2211-7458/12/$ – see front matter

a citywide STEMI program, because primary PCI became the standard of care in May of 2005 for the city of Ottawa.

In 2003, 2 landmark studies[1,2] that compared primary PCI to fibrinolysis established primary PCI as the dominant strategy because it reduces important clinical events, such as death, stroke, and reinfarction. Also, at the UOHI, compared with fibrinolytic therapy, primary PCI was shown a cost-saving strategy.[3] The combination of clinical efficiency and cost savings of primary PCI compared with fibrinolysis became a valuable argument in convincing hospital administrators of the need for change.

Before July 2004, patients presenting with STEMI within the UOHI region were managed on a case-by-case basis, because there was no existing program defining the standards of practice. Fibrinolytic therapy was by far the dominant strategy for managing STEMI patients in non-PCI–capable hospitals. Patients who presented to a non-PCI–capable hospital were immediately transferred to the PCI center only if the administration of fibrinolytic therapy was contraindicated. They likewise were transferred if rescue PCI were required because of failed fibrinolytic therapy or if they were enrolled in a clinical trial that mandated immediate transfer. The usual practice was for an emergency medicine physician to consult with the on-site hospital cardiologist. If there was a need to transfer a patient to the PCI center, it was also the practice to discuss the case with the receiving interventionalist, who authorized the transfer and alert the catheterization team. Finally, a significant proportion of patients did not receive any reperfusion therapy because of relative contraindications to fibrinolytic therapy (such as advanced age or prior stoke) and because access to primary PCI was limited. STEMI patients visiting Ottawa emergency departments between 2002 and 2004—prior to initiation of the STEMI program—experienced a 10% mortality rate, representing an increase over previous years.

In January 2004, recruitment was completed in the CAPITAL AMI study.[4] The results of this trial subsequently showed that a pharmacoinvasive strategy was better than a fibrinolysis-alone approach. In hindsight, this fibrinolytic-based trial paved the way for the early deployment of the STEMI system. The CAPITAL AMI design led to developing transfer protocols between the city hospitals because patients who were assigned to the tenecteplase-facilitated PCI arm required immediate transfer from the local emergency department to the PCI center. In addition, the study fostered a good relationship with the Ottawa Base Hospital and the Ottawa Paramedic Service. This strong working relationship with the emergency medical service (EMS) led to a collaborative effort to evaluate the ability of paramedics to interpret ECG in the field.

With the timely completion of the CAPITAL AMI trial, evidence provided by the DANAMI-2 trial[1] and Keeley and colleagues' quantitative review of 23 randomized trials,[2] we became convinced that primary PCI should become the dominant reperfusion strategy for management of STEMI within the city boundaries and that a pharmacoinvasive strategy should be applied to community hospitals within our region where rapid transfer for primary PCI is not be possible.

The first step in developing a STEMI program, the goal of which is improved survival outcomes, was to obtain a general consensus among all stakeholders that primary PCI should become the dominant strategy for the entire city.

A general meeting was organized in spring 2004 and the directors of the local emergency departments and representatives of the Base Hospital and EMS, as well as cardiologists, nurse coordinators, and the chief executive officers of each hospital, were invited. As part of the initial agenda, the evidence supporting primary PCI over fibrinolytic therapy was reviewed, emphasizing the better survival outcomes with primary PCI and the relevance to survival advantage of short door-to-balloon times. STEMI is a medical emergency in which minutes to reperfusion strongly correlate with survival, and delays in door-to-balloon times are associated with increased mortality.[5–7] Each 30 minutes of added delay increases the relative risk of 1-year mortality by 7.5%.[7] The 2004 American College of Cardiology (ACC)/American Heart Association (AHA) guidelines strongly recommended that a door-to-balloon time of less than 90 minutes be achieved in patients managed with primary PCI. The use of evidence-based medicine gave credibility to the task, and the logistic steps to make the STEMI system work followed.

There was a need to change the fundamental approach to STEMI management, and this required a complete re-engineering of the protocols and pathways for delivering STEMI care. From the beginning, the project required the development of new ambulance transport protocols and changes to physician referral patterns. Because the paramedics were successfully trained at interpreting the ECG in STEMI patients, it was agreed that the first phase of the program would feature a paramedic-referred pathway (ie, prehospital triage). The Ontario Ambulance Act stipulates that, unless otherwise directed by a communications officer, the ambulance driver should transport patients to the closest medical facility that can provide the necessary care. It was essential that for each participating hospital approval be obtained from the medical staff and the chief executive officer to allow the ambulance units to bypass the city's emergency departments and transport patients directly to the PCI centers. The first phase of the STEMI program was officially launched on July 1, 2004.

EMS PLAYS A PIVOTAL ROLE

Most studies of the prehospital management of STEMI have involved physicians accompanying the ambulance crew or receiving ECG transmissions at the Base Hospital. Before initiation of the STEMI program, it was determined that trained paramedics could accurately identify STEMI on prehospital ECGs and contribute to strategies that shorten time to reperfusion.[8] The Ottawa paramedics received supplementary classroom training that focused on the interpretation of ECGs for STEMI. They were then certified for this skill after passing a written examination. The performance of the paramedics in identifying STEMI on the ECG resulted in a sensitivity of 95%, a specificity of 96%, a positive predictive value of 82%, and a negative predictive value of 99%.[8] These results strongly influenced the decision to include paramedics in the first phase of the STEMI program, because paramedics were skilled at identifying STEMI as having real potential for reducing delays to reperfusion. Patients with onset of symptoms of less than or equal to 12 hours and greater than or equal to 1-mm ST-segment elevation in greater than or equal to 2 contiguous limb leads or greater than or equal to 2 mm in greater than or equal to 2 contiguous precordial leads on the prehospital 12-lead ECG were considered eligible for direct transfer from the field to PCI receiving centers.

In July 2004, paramedics trained at interpreting the ECG began to independently triage patients in the field and refer patients with STEMI directly to the receiving centers for primary PCI. In addition, paramedics routinely gave aspirin and nitroglycerine at the scene to patients with symptoms of ischemia. Using a dedicated STEMI line, the paramedics alerted the central operator at the PCI center of the impending arrival of a patient. The farthest distance the Ottawa ambulances traveled from dispatch to the receiving PCI center was 37 miles. Because this project was initiated as a pilot, patients with absent vital signs, severe hemodynamic instability, or left bundle branch block were excluded and transported to the nearest hospitals. As the program matured over the ensuing years, paramedics were later instructed to transport patients with cardiogenic shock directly to the PCI centers whenever medically feasible.

The initial experience with EMS providers at independently triaging patients for STEMI and directly transferring them to heart centers was encouraging.[9] Among 108 consecutive patients directly transferred from the field by EMS providers, the median door-to-balloon time was 63 minutes, and this was associated with a low in-hospital mortality of 1.9%.

EMPOWER THE EMERGENCY MEDICINE PHYSICIAN

In the second phase of the regional STEMI program, a protocol was initiated by which all patients presenting to the city's 4 emergency departments were to be immediately transferred to the PCI centers for primary PCI. Successful implementation of this step required that the emergency medicine physicians be empowered with the authority to activate the catheterization laboratory without consulting a cardiologist. As of May 1, 2005, it became policy to refer to the PCI centers all STEMI patients within the city boundaries presenting with primary PCI. The following criteria have been used in the emergency departments for referring patients for primary PCI: onset of symptoms of less than or equal to 12 hours and at least 1-mm ST-segment elevation in 2 or more contiguous leads on the 12-lead ECG. The emergency medicine physician activates the code STEMI by simply calling the ambulance dispatch to arrange transfer. Immediately on departure from the community hospital, the paramedics notify the central operator at the receiving PCI center of the impending arrival of a STEMI patient.

HAVE A DEDICATED AREA TO ASSESS THE ARRIVING STEMI PATIENT: THE STEMI ROOM

Concern was initially expressed that the possible lack of available beds at the receiving center would limit access to and delay transfer of STEMI patients. To address this concern, a dedicated room was provided. In the room was a fully monitored bed for the exclusive assessment of arriving STEMI patients, ensuring that a bed was always available at the time of admission. Hence, once the paramedics announces an incoming STEMI patient, the receptionist activates the code STEMI, prompting members of the cardiology team to assemble in the STEMI room located in proximity to the catheterization laboratories. The team consists of cardiology staff, residents, and nurses. Signs are posted in the heart center to guide the paramedics to the STEMI room.

When a patient arrives in the STEMI room, a brief exchange of critical information takes place between the paramedics and the medical staff. The index ECG and medications are reviewed, a targeted history and physical examination completed, and patient consent obtained. It is a process that usually takes no more than 5 to 10 minutes. This step is important and ensures patient safety, because 5 patients to date have been identified with aortic dissection at the time of evaluation. A STEMI assessment tool has been created that the admitting physician uses to quickly capture all relevant data prior to cardiac catheterization (**Fig. 1**).

After this pit stop, patients are taken immediately to the catheterization laboratory. During off-hours, an additional 10 to 20 minutes' delay may occur while waiting for the arrival of the on-call staff; coronary care unit nurses assist with patients before transfer to the catheterization laboratory. In high-volume centers, such as the UOHI, the availability of the STEMI room facilitates the logistics of triaging patients and ensures proper assessment and preparation of patients for primary PCI. It allows the medical team to verify the information provided by the paramedics, perform a targeted history and physical examination of patients, and ensure that STEMI protocol medication has been given. After a few minutes of assessment, the patients are brought to the catheterization laboratory.

STANDARDIZATION

The efficiency of a STEMI program is measured in minutes. Among 43,801 patients referred for primary PCI who were enrolled in the National Cardiovascular Data Registry, any delay to reperfusion after hospital arrival was associated with a higher mortality, even in patients with door-to-balloon times of less than 90 minutes.[10] Therefore, every attempt should be made to shorten door-to-balloon times, and no door-to-balloon time is short enough. The 2009 ACC/AHA focus update on STEMI guidelines recommended that the emphasis on door-to-balloon time should be "as soon as possible" rather than a specific 90-minute benchmark.[11]

To achieve the fastest door-to-balloon time for each patient, it is critical that all logistic barriers be addressed. One of the most important aspects of setting up a successful STEMI program is implementing well-defined protocols and pathways (ie, standardization). **Fig. 2** highlights the protocol, which can be displayed as a poster in an emergency department or placed on a hospital Web site. With slight modifications, the 6 strategies proposed by Bradley and colleagues[12] to reduce door-to-balloon time have been implemented:

1. Emergency medicine physicians are permitted to activate the catheterization laboratory without consulting a cardiologist.
2. A single call to a central page operator is used to activate the catheterization laboratory.
3. Paramedics interpret the prehospital ECG without transmitting the tracing to the emergency department and independently triage patients in the field.
4. During off-hours, the staff in the catheterization laboratory is ready to start the case within 30 minutes of the code being activated.
5. A cardiology resident, providing on-site 24-hours-a-day/7-days-a-week (24/7) service at the receiving PCI center, assesses patients immediately on arrival.
6. Prompt feedback is provided to the emergency department by direct phone call and quality assurance reports.

Whether patients are referred for primary PCI directly from the field or from a sending hospital, it is always the paramedic crew that notifies the central page operator of the impending arrival of a STEMI patient. The emergency department physicians do not need to call the heart center unless there is a specific complication that needs to be discussed. Crew members use a preset number on their cell phones to call the receiving center and announce an incoming STEMI patient. A receptionist receives the call on a dedicated STEMI line and activates the code STEMI. On arrival at the receiving center, paramedics take the patient immediately to the STEMI room for further assessment.

Standing orders embedded within the code STEMI protocol include giving patients, in advance of a PCI procedure, chewable aspirin (160 mg), oral clopidogrel (600 mg), and unfractionated heparin (60 U/kg; maximum 4000 U) administered intravenously. In the past, these medications were given in the emergency department of the sending hospital; currently, paramedics administer aspirin in the field, and the other medications are given in the STEMI room. Because of the recently published mortality benefits associated with the use of ticagrelor,[13] clopidogrel is planned to be replaced with this new antiplatelet agent for patients referred for primary PCI. Since the completion of the ASSIST trial,[14] glycoprotein IIb/IIIa platelet receptor inhibitors are no longer used before cardiac catheterization in patients referred for primary PCI. This is because patients given high-dose clopidogrel and then treated with heparin plus eptifibatide, compared with heparin alone, experienced unimproved clinical outcomes and more bleeding complications. Also, in light of the results from the

UNIVERSITY OF OTTAWA HEART INSTITUTE
INSTITUT DE CARDIOLOGIE DE L'UNIVERSITÉ D'OTTAWA

TARGETED HISTORY AND PHYSICAL FOR STEMI ASSESSMENT

Date (yyyy/mm/dd): Time:

Patient history:
Age: ______ Sex: ____
Chief complaint:

Initial Patient Presentation:
❑ Ambulance: ❑ Field to cath lab ❑ Field to Emergency Department
❑ Self Transport
❑ Inpatient
Initial Hospital:

Time of onset of symptoms:

History of Present Illness

Medications given:

	YES	NO	UNKNOWN
ASA	❑	❑	❑
Clopidogrel/Prasugrel/Ticagrelor	❑	❑	❑
Heparin	❑	❑	❑
Lytics given:	❑	❑	❑

If yes, Date (yyyy/mm/dd): Time:

Previous Home Medications

Cardiac Risk Factors:

	YES	NO	UNKNOWN
a) Hypertension	❑	❑	❑
b) Diabetes Mellitus	❑	❑	❑
i. *Oral agents*	❑	❑	❑
ii. *Insulin*	❑	❑	❑
c) * Family History	❑	❑	❑
d) Smoking	❑	❑	❑
e) Dyslipidemia	❑	❑	❑

* ***Immediate family member less than 60 years old with coronary disease.***

Physical Exam
General Appearance: ______
Level of Consciousness: ______
HR: ______ BP: (R) ______ (L) ______ JVP: ______
Chest: ______
S1: ______ S2: ______ S3: ______ S4: ______
Murmur: ______
Abdomen: ______
Extremities:

Pulses:	Femoral Rt	Femoral Lt	Radial Rt	Radial Lt	Allen's Rt	Allen's Lt
Normal						
Anormal						

Previous Cardiovascular History:

	YES	NO	UNKNOWN
a) Angina	❑	❑	❑
b) CHF	❑	❑	❑
c) Peripheral Artery Disease	❑	❑	❑
d) MI Year: ______	❑	❑	❑
e) PCI Year: ______	❑	❑	❑
f) CABG Year: ______	❑	❑	❑
g) Stroke Year: ______	❑	❑	❑
h) TIA Year: ______	❑	❑	❑
History of Significant Bleeding	❑	❑	❑
Upcoming Procedures (Surgery, biopsy, etc)	❑	❑	❑

Qualifying ECG (check 1 only):
Anterior ST ↑ (V1-V6): ______
Lateral ST ↑ (I, AVL): ______
Inferior ST ↑ (II, III, AVF): ______
New LBBB: ______
Ventricular paced rhythm: ______
Other:

Past Medical / Social History

Assessment:

	YES	NO	UNKNOWN
STEMI	❑	❑	❑

If no, give reason: ______
Killip Class 1 2 3 4
I - No evidence of CHF
II - Crackles/Rales in less than ½ lung field, S3, ↑ JVP
III - Crackles/Rales in more than ½ lung field-pulmonary edema
IV - Cardiogenic Shock

Plan:

	YES	NO
Consent Obtained		
Primary PCI	❑	❑
Pharmacoinvasive	❑	❑
Other (Specify):	❑	❑

Allergies:

	YES	NO	UNKNOWN
Contrast Dye	❑	❑	❑
Other:			

Printed name: Signature:

HEA 207 (03/2012) 1-CHART 2-REFERRAL HOSPITAL

Fig. 1. This STEMI assessment forms helps physicians at the PCI receiving center with gathering key data elements before cardiac catherization. (*Courtesy of* University of Ottawa Heart Institute; with permission.)

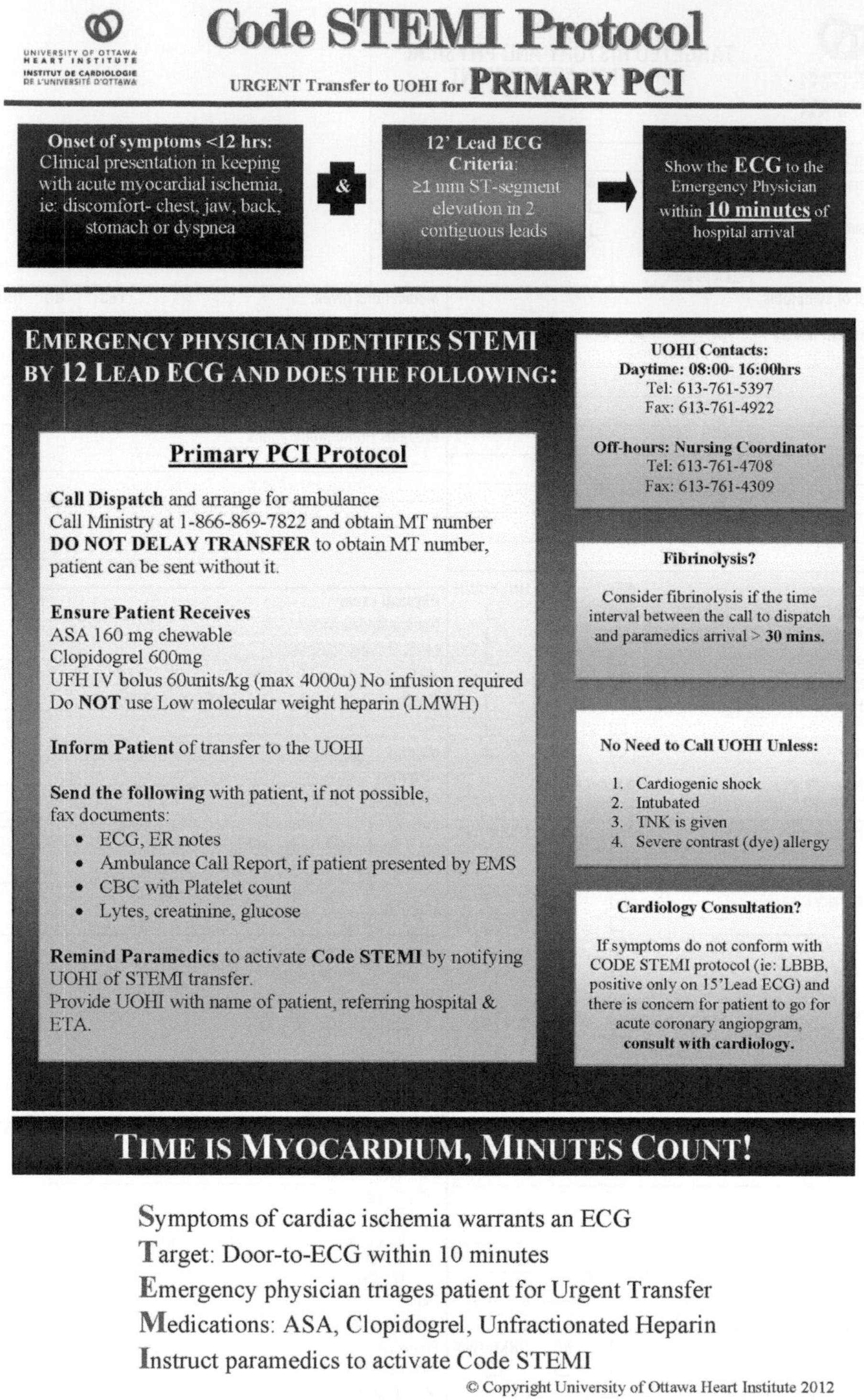
UNIVERSITY OF OTTAWA HEART INSTITUTE
INSTITUT DE CARDIOLOGIE DE L'UNIVERSITÉ D'OTTAWA
Code STEMI Protocol
URGENT Transfer to UOHI for PRIMARY PCI
Onset of symptoms <12 hrs: Clinical presentation in keeping with acute myocardial ischemia, ie: discomfort- chest, jaw, back, stomach or dyspnea
&
12' Lead ECG Criteria: ≥1 mm ST-segment elevation in 2 contiguous leads
Show the ECG to the Emergency Physician within 10 minutes of hospital arrival
EMERGENCY PHYSICIAN IDENTIFIES STEMI BY 12 LEAD ECG AND DOES THE FOLLOWING:
Primary PCI Protocol
Call Dispatch and arrange for ambulance
Call Ministry at 1-866-869-7822 and obtain MT number
DO NOT DELAY TRANSFER to obtain MT number, patient can be sent without it.
Ensure Patient Receives
ASA 160 mg chewable
Clopidogrel 600mg
UFH IV bolus 60units/kg (max 4000u) No infusion required
Do NOT use Low molecular weight heparin (LMWH)
Inform Patient of transfer to the UOHI
Send the following with patient, if not possible, fax documents:
• ECG, ER notes
• Ambulance Call Report, if patient presented by EMS
• CBC with Platelet count
• Lytes, creatinine, glucose
Remind Paramedics to activate Code STEMI by notifying UOHI of STEMI transfer.
Provide UOHI with name of patient, referring hospital & ETA.
UOHI Contacts:
Daytime: 08:00- 16:00hrs
Tel: 613-761-5397
Fax: 613-761-4922
Off-hours: Nursing Coordinator
Tel: 613-761-4708
Fax: 613-761-4309
Fibrinolysis?
Consider fibrinolysis if the time interval between the call to dispatch and paramedics arrival > 30 mins.
No Need to Call UOHI Unless:
1. Cardiogenic shock
2. Intubated
3. TNK is given
4. Severe contrast (dye) allergy
Cardiology Consultation?
If symptoms do not conform with CODE STEMI protocol (ie: LBBB, positive only on 15'Lead ECG) and there is concern for patient to go for acute coronary angiopgram, consult with cardiology.
TIME IS MYOCARDIUM, MINUTES COUNT!
Symptoms of cardiac ischemia warrants an ECG
Target: Door-to-ECG within 10 minutes
Emergency physician triages patient for Urgent Transfer
Medications: ASA, Clopidogrel, Unfractionated Heparin
Instruct paramedics to activate Code STEMI
© Copyright University of Ottawa Heart Institute 2012

Fig. 2. UOHI code STEMI protocol for urgent transfer to PCI center for primary PCI. Posters are printed of the primary PCI protocol, which are distributed to all the local emergency departments. Some of the hospitals also post the protocol on their Web sites. (*Courtesy of* University of Ottawa Heart Institute; with permission.)

HORIZONS-AMI trial,[15] use of glycoprotein IIb/IIIa platelet receptor inhibitors in the laboratory has been significantly curtailed; bivalirudin alone is preferred, started at the beginning of the PCI and continued at renal doses for 2 hours after the procedure. Prolonging bivalirudin for 2 hours after the PCI in the setting of STEMI may reduce the risk of acute stent thrombosis without losing the benefits of bivalirudin in lowering bleeding.[16]

REPATRIATION AND FALSE-POSITIVE STEMI IDENTIFICATIONS

Since the inception of the program, the rate of false-positive STEMIs associated with paramedics identifying patients in the prehospital setting has ranged from 10% to 15%. The rate of false-positive STEMI identifications for emergency medicine physicians referring STEMI patients has averaged slightly higher, 15% to 20%. Causes for false-positive identification have included left bundle branch block, ventricular paced rhythm, left ventricular hypertrophy, early repolarization abnormalities, pericarditis, myocarditis, previous STEMI with persistent ST-segment elevation and Takotsubo cardiomyopathy.

Because of the limited bed capacity of the receiving center, the stakeholders agreed that patients could be repatriated by the sending hospitals to maximize use of resources: specifically, patients with a false-positive diagnosis could be transferred back to the referring emergency department for further evaluation, and STEMI patients, once stable, could be transferred to the cardiology service of the referring hospital after PCI. In practice, this repatriation agreement has been used mostly for false-positive STEMI identifications because the majority of patients treated with primary PCI have been admitted and discharged home from the PCI center.

THE ROLE OF A STEMI COORDINATOR AND THE IMPORTANCE OF DATA COLLECTION

A STEMI coordinator is a valuable and indispensable asset to any STEMI program. This person is responsible for collecting and entering patient data into the database. The coordinator troubleshoots logistic issues relating to the day-to-day operation of the program and ensures that it continues to function smoothly. The coordinator helps update the STEMI procedure manual, which is provided for the house staff in our institution at the beginning of their training. This manual highlights the logistics of the STEMI program and reviews the relevant scientific literature.

Providing feedback is important to improving and sustaining the program. The coordinator prepares report cards on the performance of the paramedics and the emergency medicine physicians. The ambulance call reports have been essential for measuring critical time intervals. These reports provide feedback on key quality indicators that help monitor the program's effectiveness. The time stamp on the qualifying ECG performed in the prehospital setting or in the emergency department is used to calculate the ECG-to-balloon intervals. The door-to-balloon time is defined as the time elapsed between arrival at the first hospital and the first balloon inflation or first use of another therapeutic interventional device, such as thrombectomy aspiration catheter. In cases referred directly from the field, the first hospital is the receiving center.

In 2008, the results of the first full year of operation of the citywide primary PCI program were published, describing 344 consecutive STEMI patients referred for primary PCI. Guideline door-to-balloon times were achieved more often when trained paramedics independently triaged and transported patients directly to the PCI center than when patients were referred from emergency departments.[17]

STEMI CLINICS

Before hospital discharge, STEMI patients are routinely screened for participation in cardiac rehabilitation and smoking cessation programs and, within 4 weeks of discharge, patients meet for clinical follow-up with the interventional cardiologists who performed their procedures. This provides an opportunity for the cardiologists to review symptoms and compliance with medications as well as address any concerns raised by patients. **Fig. 3** depicts the STEMI clinic tool that was developed. This tool has been found useful in focusing the visit on relevant clinical issues and capturing key elements for the database.

EXPANDING A STEMI PROGRAM SHOULD BE DONE GRADUALLY

It was decided that the program be gradually expanded to provide optimal reperfusion to all patients presenting with STEMI in UOHI region. The experience gained from establishing the citywide program was valuable. Because some hospitals were beyond the reach of acceptable reperfusion times with primary PCI, a referral cutoff of 40 miles from any PCI center was established. This allowed approximately 30 to 45 minutes for an ambulance to transfer a patient from the farthest

STEMI Follow Up Clinic Physician Sheet

STEMI Follow-Up Clinic

Appointment: *(Circle one)* ☐ 1 month ☐ 6-12 months

Date of Appointment: ______ Date of STEMI: ______

Name of Patient: ______ MRN #: ______

Family Doctor: ______ Cardiologist: ______

History

______

______

Present Smoker: ☐ Yes ☐ No

______

Events since Discharge

Re-hospitalization: ☐ Yes ☐ No   Hospital: OHI ☐ Yes ☐ No
Other: ______

Cardiac: ☐ Yes ☐ No   Non-Cardiac:
i. PCI ☐ Yes ☐ No   Reason: ______
ii. CABG ☐ Yes ☐ No
iii. Stroke ☐ Yes ☐ No
iv. Other: ______

Medications

Class	Name of Medication	Dose
Antiplatelet	Aspirin (ASA)	☐ 81mg ☐ 325mg
Antiplatelet	Clopidogrel Ticagrelor (BRILINTA) Prasugrel (EFFIENT) Other:	
Beta Blocker		
ACE Inhibitors		
ARB		
Statins		
Other Lipid Lowering Agents		
Coumadin		
Diuretics		
Amiodarone		
Others		

Other Medications:

 1

Fig. 3. STEMI follow-up clinic tool used by physicians at 1-month and 6–12-month visits. This tool helps with focusing the visit on relevant clinical issues and capturing key elements for the database. (*Courtesy of* University of Ottawa Heart Institute; with permission.)

hospital. **Fig. 4** is a map displaying the 9 hospitals identified as primary PCI sending centers and the relative distance of these hospitals to the receiving center. By applying the same principles for the 5 community hospitals located on the outskirts of the city, a model of care was developed that provides 24/7 systematic primary PCI for approximately 1 million people within the region.

STEMI Follow Up Clinic Physician Sheet

Exam

BP: ____/____mmHg HR: __________bpm

Lungs: ____________________

Cardiac: ____________________

Other Physical Findings: ____________________

____

Assessment

CCS Angina Class 0☐ 1☐ 2☐ 3☐ 4☐

(NYHA) CHF 1☐ 2☐ 3☐ 4☐

LV Function:

1 Month Follow-Up (complete the following question)

A. Did patient have evaluation of LV EF at initial admission? ☐ Yes ☐ No

i. MUGA ☐
ii. ECHO ☐
iii. Cath ☐
iv. Other: __________

6-12 Month Follow-up (complete the following question)

A. Has LVEF been evaluated in previous visit(s)? ☐ Yes ☐ No

B. Did patient receive an ICD? ☐ Yes ☐ No

Next Follow Up Appointment:

Please book next follow-up appointment with myself ☐ or with Dr. __________ in __________ mos.

Date of Appointment: __________ Time: __________

Dictated: ☐ **Yes** ☐ **No** **Physician's Signature:** __________

 2

Fig. 3. (*continued*).

Fig. 5 illustrates the annual growth in the number of patients with confirmed STEMI referred via the primary PCI pathway. In 2011, a total of 502 confirmed STEMI patients were referred to the PCI center and managed by 7 interventional cardiologists.

All patients were included in the database regardless of language barrier, atypical presentation, cardiac arrest, shock, or any factor that could have led to longer times to reperfusion. **Table 1** compares the baseline demographics of a total

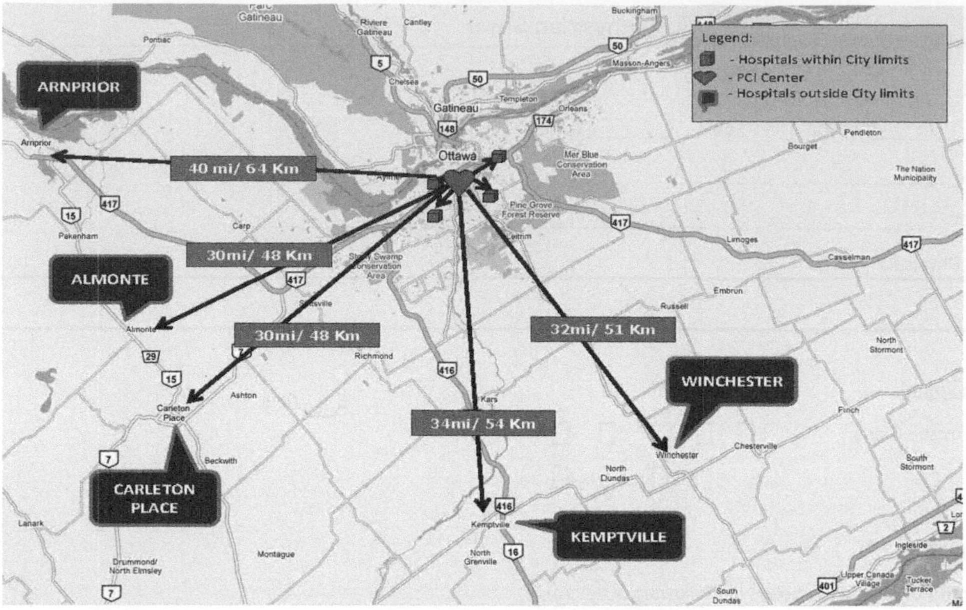

Fig. 4. Map of community hospitals participating in the primary PCI pathway. The map shows the location of the 5 hospitals beyond the city of Ottawa boundaries that were gradually added to the program. By May 2009, all hospitals within 40 miles of the UOHI were officially participating in the regional primary PCI Program.

of 2483 STEMI-confirmed patients who were referred between July 2004 and April 2011 for primary PCI by the paramedics (37%) with patients referred by the emergency departments (63%). More than 99% of patients underwent immediate catheterization and more than 93% PCI.

Critical time intervals for these patients are displayed in **Table 2**. Reperfusion times were consistently shorter in patients referred by the paramedics compared with patients referred by

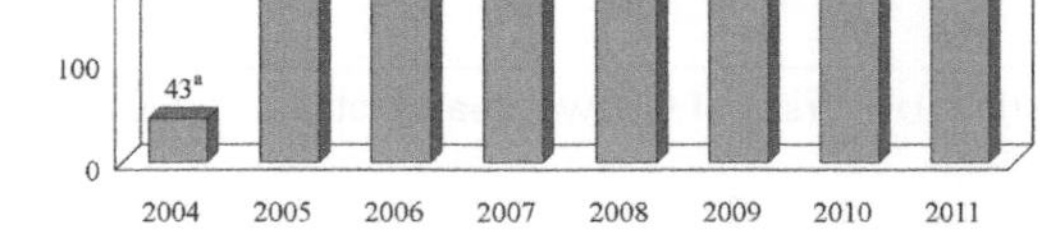

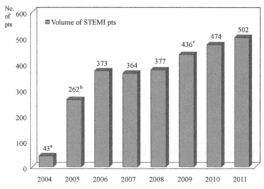

Fig. 5. The volume of confirmed STEMI patients referred yearly for primary PCI since the start of the program. [a] First phase: includes only patients referred directly to the PCI center from the field by the EMS. [b] Second phase: in May 2005, the program expanded to include the city hospitals. [c] Third phase: expansion of the program was complete by 2009 and now includes 9 referring hospitals.

the emergency departments. The median door-to-balloon time was shorter in patients referred directly from the field by the paramedics (66 minutes; interquartile range 42–82) compared with patients needing interhospital transfer (120 minutes; interquartile range 97–151; *P*<.001). The cumulative percentage of door-to-balloon time intervals as a function of time is depicted in **Fig. 6**. Door-to-balloon times of less than 90 minutes were achieved in 83% of patients transferred directly from the field by the paramedics and in 18% of patients transferred from the emergency departments (*P*<.001). Door-to-balloon times of less than 120 minutes were achieved in 95% of patients transferred from the field and in 50% of patients transferred from the emergency departments (*P*<.001). These results are encouraging when considering the shortening of door-to-balloon intervals over the years. Among 4278 patients enrolled in the National Registry of Myocardial Infarction who, between January 1999 and December 2002, were transferred for primary PCI from a noncatheterization hospital to a PCI-capable center, the median total door-to-balloon time was 180 minutes, with only 4.2% of patients treated within 90 minutes.[18]

Recent analyses from randomized trials[19] and from registry data[20] suggest that primary PCI remains superior to fibrinolysis, even when a time delay related to PCI extends up to 110 and 114 minutes, respectively. The 2008 European STEMI

Table 1
Baseline demographics

Patient Characteristic	EMS-Referred (n = 927)	ED-Referred (n = 1556)	*P* Value
Age, y	62.5 ± 13.7	61.9 ± 13.3	0.32
Male gender, %	72.3	72.2	0.96
Hypertension, %	46.7	48.9	0.30
Diabetes mellitus, %	13.9	19.5	0.0003
Current smoker, %	41.9	41.1	0.73
History of dyslipidimia, %	41.9	40.2	0.41
Prior myocardial infarction, %	14.4	13.2	0.39
Prior angioplasty, %	9.7	9.6	0.94
Prior bypass surgery, %	3.8	3.8	1.00
Anterior myocardial infarction, %	39.3	40.7	0.50
Heart rate, beats per minute	76.2 ± 17.6	78.6 ± 21.4	0.005
Systolic blood pressure, mm Hg	129.2 ± 25.3	139.6 ± 30.9	<0.0001
Diastolic blood pressure, mm Hg	77.2 ± 15.7	81.7 ± 18.8	<0.0001
Killip			<0.0001
Class 1, %	85.8	86.4	
Class 2, %	11.7	7.3	
Class 3, %	0.7	1.9	
Class 4, %	1.8	4.4	
Height, cm	171.1 ± 9.6	171.3 ± 9.6	0.57
Weight, kg	79.9 ± 16.9	82.1 ± 18.6	0.004
Creatinine clearance, mL/min	72.1 ± 21.6	73.3 ± 31.5	0.31
Catheterization performed, %	99.4	99.0	0.50
PCI performed, %	94.1	92.7	0.22
Multivessel disease, %	55.2	56.4	0.59

Plus-minus values are means ± SD.
Abbreviation: ED, emergency department.

Table 2
Critical time intervals (min)

Interval	EMS-Referred (n = 927)	ED-Referred (n = 1556)	*P* Value
Onset of symptoms to arrival at first hospital			0.005
Median	87	104	
Interquartile range	61–152	56–228	
Onset of symptoms to balloon			<0.0001
Median	158	241	
Interquartile range	121–222	175–380	
ECG-to-balloon			<0.0001
Median	90	107	
Interquartile range	67–111	87–132	
Door-to-balloon			<0.0001
Median	66	120	
Interquartile range	42–82	97–151	

Abbreviation: ED, emergency department.

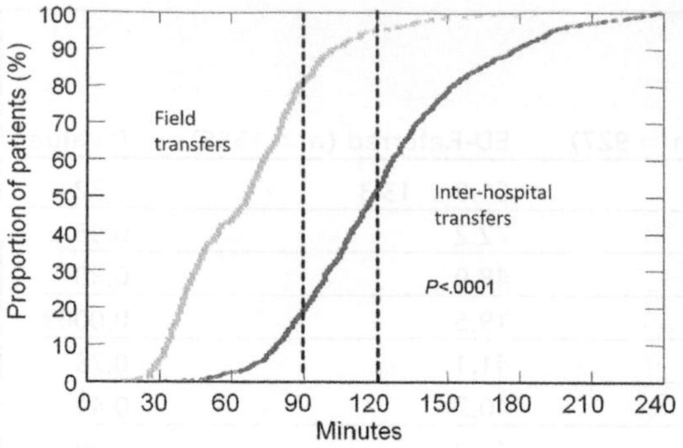

Fig. 6. The quantile plot displays the cumulative percent of door-to-balloon time intervals as a function of time for 2483 STEMI patients referred to the UOHI for primary PCI between July 2004 and April 2011. Door-to-balloon times of less than 90 minutes were achieved in 83% of patients who were transferred directly from the field and in 18% of patients who were transferred from emergency departments; door-to-balloon times of less than 120 minutes were achieved in 95% of patients transferred from the field and in 50% of patients transferred from emergency departments.

guidelines now recommend that balloon inflation be performed within 120 minutes of first medical contact.[21] The 2011 updated ACC/AHA PCI guidelines recommend as a systems goal that patients with STEMI receive primary PCI within 90 minutes of first medical contact in a PCI-capable hospital and within 120 minutes in a non-PCI–capable hospital.

It could be argued that more centers equipped with catheterization laboratories are needed to reduce the delays associated with interhospital transfer. Studies indicate, however, that mortality is significantly lower when primary PCI procedures are performed in high-volume centers by high-volume operators.[22–24] Time to treatment from

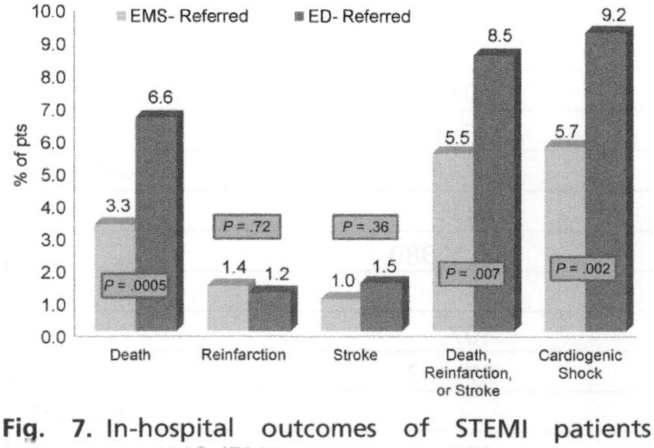

Fig. 7. In-hospital outcomes of STEMI patients referred by EMS (EMS-referred) and the emergency department physicians (ED-referred). Clinical events were significantly lower in the patients referred directly from the field by EMS.

symptom onset is also faster in high-volume centers compared with low-volume centers.[24]

In-hospital events in the patients are shown in **Fig. 7**. Mortality was 3.3% for patients referred directly from the field and 6.6% for patients transferred from the emergency departments ($P = .005$). Mortality totals 5.4% for all patients enrolled in the STEMI program since 2004. The incidence of cardiogenic shock developing during the hospitalization was lower in patients referred by the paramedics compared with patients transferred from the emergency departments: 6.0% versus 9.9% ($P = .003$). The rates of reinfarction and stroke were low and comparable in the 2 groups. A multivariate logistic regression analysis to determine whether the paramedic referral pathway is an independent predictor for survival is needed.

USE A PHARMACOINVASIVE STRATEGY WHEN PRIMARY PCI IS NOT READILY AVAILABLE

Several recently published trials have shown that STEMI patients treated with fibrinolysis should be routinely transferred to a PCI center for intervention within 24 hours of presentation.[4,25–30] An early invasive strategy after fibrinolytic therapy restores coronary flow in patients who do not clinically achieve reperfusion, in patients who develop recurrent symptoms after apparent initial success with fibrinolysis, and in patients with a persistently occluded coronary artery, who otherwise would not have been identified based on symptoms or ST-segment changes. The CAPITAL AMI study[4] showed that in patients presenting with high-risk STEMI, tenecteplase plus immediate angioplasty reduced the risk of recurrent ischemic events compared with tenecteplase alone and was not associated with an increase in major bleeding complications. Results were confirmed by the larger TRANSFER AMI study.[27] In addition, in a pooled meta-analysis of pharmacoinvasive trials, early routine PCI after fibrinolysis significantly reduced reinfarction and recurrent ischemia at 1 month, with no significant increase in adverse bleeding events compared with standard therapy, and the benefits of early PCI persisted at 6-month to 12-month follow-up.[31]

In light of these results, protocols were developed that use a pharmacoinvasive strategy for STEMI patients presenting to community hospitals where long transfer delays prevent timely reperfusion with primary PCI. By 2009, all these community hospitals were included in the regional STEMI program. **Fig. 8** displays the hospitals where the pharmacoinvasive approach is used and the

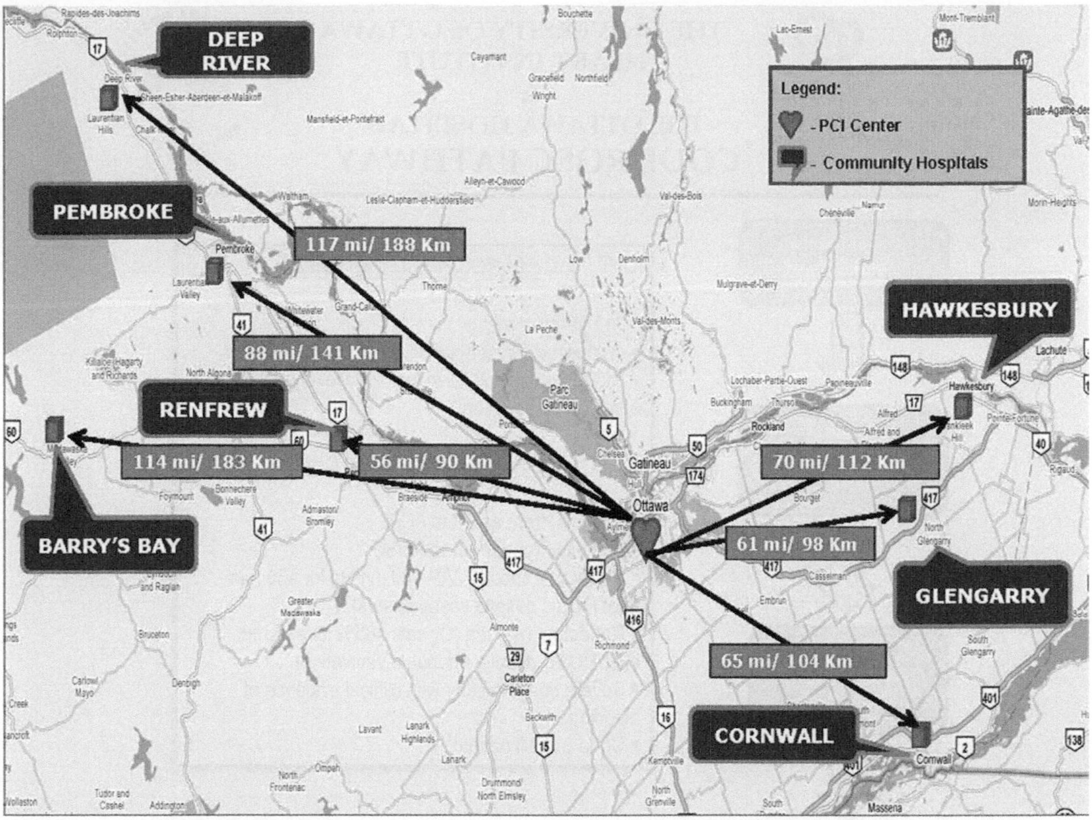

Fig. 8. Map of community hospitals participating in the pharmacoinvasive strategy. All patients with STEMI treated with fibrinolytic therapy in these community hospitals are immediately transferred to the PCI center. It is UOHI's policy to perform cardiac catheterization within 24 hours on all of these patients and immediately if rescue is needed.

distance away from the cardiac center. The CAPITAL AMI inclusion criteria were initially used to identify high-risk STEMI patients for a lyse and ship strategy. It was decided later, however, that all STEMI patients treated with fibrinolysis could benefit from transfer to the cardiac center because some patients who were initially classified as low risk experience significant clinical events during admission at the community hospital. It is currently our policy to perform cardiac catherization within 24 hours on all STEMI patients treated initially with fibrinolytic therapy regardless of symptoms.

CARDIAC ARREST PROGRAMS WORK WELL WITH STEMI PROGRAMS

In 2002, 2 clinical trials provided evidence that lowering the body temperature of comatose post-cardiac arrest patients to 32°C to 34°C increased survival and improved neurologic outcome.[32,33] Since then, the AHA and the International Liaison Committee on Resuscitation have endorsed the use of therapeutic hypothermia as part of the standard patient care for this population of patients. Data from our STEMI database also seem to support the use of therapeutic hypothermia and highlight the need for a standardized program for cardiac arrest patients. The authors have recorded a survival rate of 69% for comatose STEMI patients with return of spontaneous circulation (ROSC) treated with therapeutic hypothermia and primary PCI (data presented at the American Heart Association [AHA] 2010 Scientific Sessions, Chicago, Illinois). Among the survivors, 89% were discharged to their home. These preliminary results are encouraging and have given insights for the need of standardized protocols and customized pathways for all cardiac arrest patients.

The recent global momentum to develop centers of excellence for postcardiac arrest and/or cardiogenic shock patients is prompting the development of expanded multidisciplinary programs with standardized protocols for the management of these patients. In September 2011, the UOHI initiated a code ROSC program in conjunction

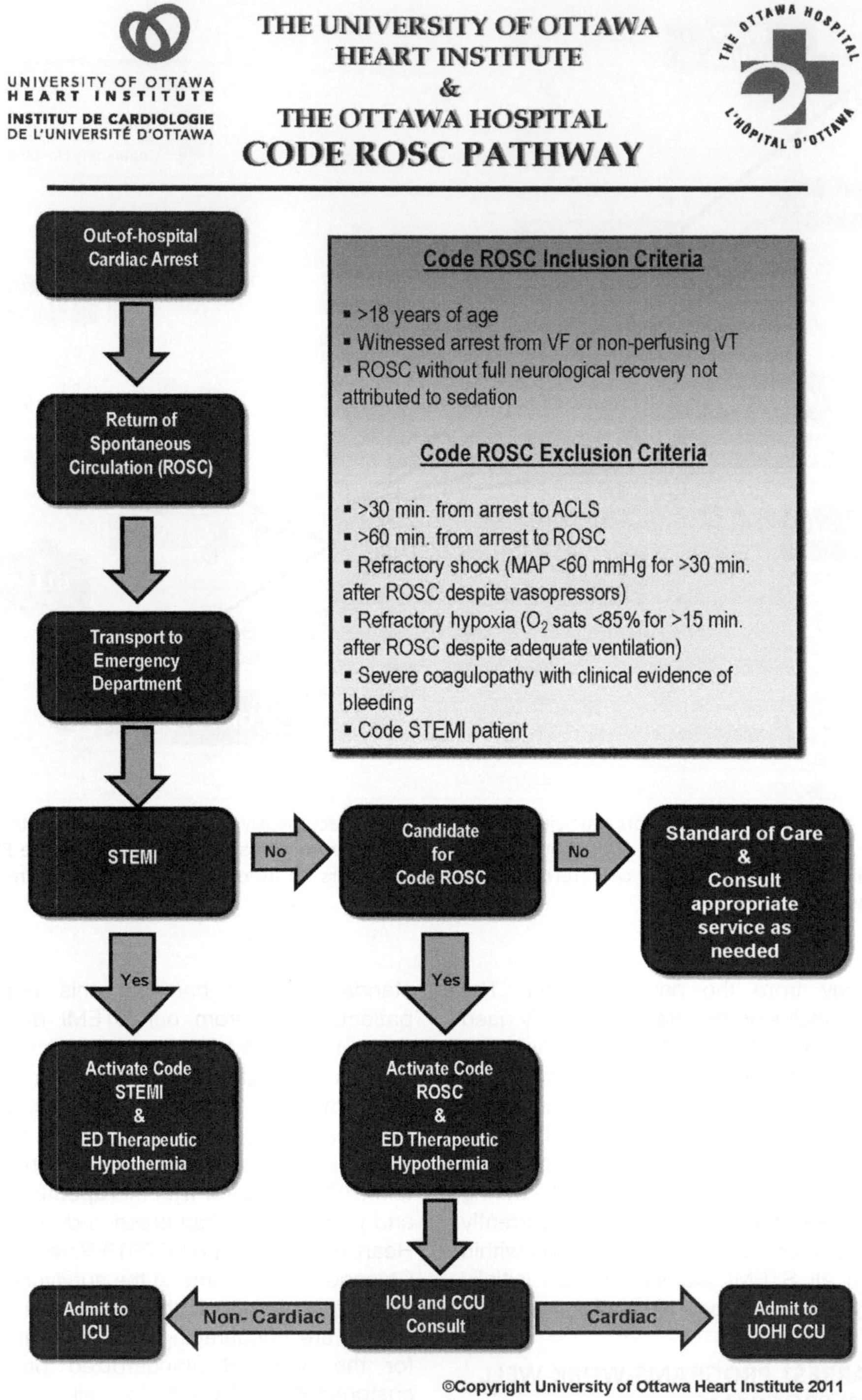

Fig. 9. The UOHI have developed a code ROSC protocol for comatose patients after a cardiac arrest with the collaboration of the UOHI and the Ottawa Hospital. The program was officially initiated in September 2011. (*Courtesy of* University of Ottawa Heart Institute; with permission.)

with the Ottawa Hospital (**Fig. 9**). Expanding and refining the code ROSC program to a wider network of hospitals will allow for the development of additional protocols and for a larger number of cardiac arrest patients to be transported promptly to a specialized center. The authors believe this project will strongly benefit from the lessons learned from the regional STEMI program and that this project has the definite potential to have an impact on the health care system.

SUMMARY

The authors and colleagues have previously shown that a citywide systematic application of primary PCI using standardized protocols is feasible.[17] This report reviews how a STEMI system was initially established and how it has continued to grow and become a fully regionalized STEMI program. It highlights the critical role of trained paramedics in identifying patients with STEMI in the field and directly transferring them to a designated cardiac center for primary PCI. The data presented relating to the primary PCI pathway were collected in a real-world setting in which all patients presenting with STEMI were considered for primary PCI. Results suggest that survival may be significantly improved when these trained paramedics bypass the nearest hospitals and refer patients to dedicated cardiac center. It also emphasizes the need to incorporate a pharmacoinvasive strategy for community hospitals in which transfer for primary PCI is not an option because travel distances are prohibitive for this latter strategy. Finally, it indicates that cardiac arrest programs need to be developed and can be integrated with STEMI systems to provide optimal care for all patients.

ACKNOWLEDGMENTS

We thank all the paramedics and their management team for their commitment and enthusiasm. They are responsible for the success of the STEMI program. We are also indebted to our staff working in the catheterization laboratories for their important contribution.

REFERENCES

1. Andersen HR, Nielsen TT, Rasmussen K, et al. A comparison of coronary angioplasty with fibrinolytic therapy in acute myocardial infarction. N Engl J Med 2003;349(8):733–42.
2. Keeley EC, Boura JA, Grines CL. Primary angioplasty versus intravenous thrombolytic therapy for acute myocardial infarction: a quantitative review of 23 randomised trials. Lancet 2003;361(9351):13–20.
3. Le May MR, Davies RF, Labinaz M, et al. Hospitalization costs of primary stenting versus thrombolysis in acute myocardial infarction: cost analysis of the Canadian STAT Study. Circulation 2003;108(21):2624–30.
4. Le May MR, Wells GA, Labinaz M, et al. Combined angioplasty and pharmacological intervention versus thrombolysis alone in acute myocardial infarction (CAPITAL AMI study). J Am Coll Cardiol 2005;46(3):417–24.
5. Berger PB, Ellis SG, Holmes DR Jr, et al. Relationship between delay in performing direct coronary angioplasty and early clinical outcome in patients with acute myocardial infarction: results from the global use of strategies to open occluded arteries in Acute Coronary Syndromes (GUSTO-IIb) trial. Circulation 1999;100(1):14–20.
6. Cannon CP, Gibson CM, Lambrew CT, et al. Relationship of symptom-onset-to-balloon time and door-to-balloon time with mortality in patients undergoing angioplasty for acute myocardial infarction. JAMA 2000;283(22):2941–7.
7. De Luca G, Suryapranata H, Ottervanger JP, et al. Time delay to treatment and mortality in primary angioplasty for acute myocardial infarction: every minute of delay counts. Circulation 2004;109(10):1223–5.
8. Le May MR, Dionne R, Maloney J, et al. Diagnostic performance and potential clinical impact of advanced care paramedic interpretation of ST-segment elevation myocardial infarction in the field. CJEM 2006;8(6):401–7.
9. Le May MR, Davies RF, Dionne R, et al. Comparison of early mortality of paramedic-diagnosed ST-segment elevation myocardial infarction with immediate transport to a designated primary percutaneous coronary intervention center to that of similar patients transported to the nearest hospital. Am J Cardiol 2006;98(10):1329–33.
10. Rathore SS, Curtis JP, Chen J, et al. Association of door-to-balloon time and mortality in patients admitted to hospital with ST elevation myocardial infarction: national cohort study. BMJ 2009;338:b1807.
11. Kushner FG, Hand M, Smith SC Jr, et al. 2009 focused updates: ACC/AHA guidelines for the management of patients with ST-elevation myocardial infarction (updating the 2004 guideline and 2007 focused update) and ACC/AHA/SCAI guidelines on percutaneous coronary intervention (updating the 2005 guideline and 2007 focused update) a report of the American College of Cardiology Foundation/American Heart Association Task Force on Practice Guidelines. J Am Coll Cardiol 2009;54(23):2205–41.
12. Bradley EH, Herrin J, Wang Y, et al. Strategies for reducing the door-to-balloon time in acute myocardial infarction. N Engl J Med 2006;355(22):2308–20.
13. Wallentin L, Becker RC, Budaj A, et al. Ticagrelor versus clopidogrel in patients with acute coronary syndromes. N Engl J Med 2009;361(11):1045–57.
14. Le May MR, Wells GA, Glover CA, et al. Primary percutaneous coronary angioplasty with and without eptifibatide in ST-segment elevation myocardial infarction: a safety and efficacy study of integrilin-

facilitated versus primary percutaneous coronary intervention in ST-segment elevation myocardial infarction (ASSIST). Circ Cardiovasc Interv 2009; 2(4):330–8.
15. Stone GW, Witzenbichler B, Guagliumi G, et al. Bivalirudin during primary PCI in acute myocardial infarction. N Engl J Med 2008;358(21):2218–30.
16. Anderson PR, Gogo PB, Ahmed B, et al. Two hour bivalirudin infusion after PCI for ST elevation myocardial infarction. J Thromb Thrombolysis 2011;31(4):401–6.
17. Le May MR, So DY, Dionne R, et al. A citywide protocol for primary PCI in ST-segment elevation myocardial infarction. N Engl J Med 2008;358(3):231–40.
18. Nallamothu BK, Bates ER, Herrin J, et al. Times to treatment in transfer patients undergoing primary percutaneous coronary intervention in the United States: National Registry of Myocardial Infarction (NRMI)-3/4 analysis. Circulation 2005;111(6):761–7.
19. Betriu A, Masotti M. Comparison of mortality rates in acute myocardial infarction treated by percutaneous coronary intervention versus fibrinolysis. Am J Cardiol 2005;95(1):100–1.
20. Pinto DS, Kirtane AJ, Nallamothu BK, et al. Hospital delays in reperfusion for ST-elevation myocardial infarction: implications when selecting a reperfusion strategy. Circulation 2006;114(19):2019–25.
21. Van de WF, Bax J, Betriu A, et al. Management of acute myocardial infarction in patients presenting with persistent ST-segment elevation: the Task Force on the Management of ST-Segment Elevation Acute Myocardial Infarction of the European Society of Cardiology. Eur Heart J 2008;29(23):2909–45.
22. Canto JG, Every NR, Magid DJ, et al. The volume of primary angioplasty procedures and survival after acute myocardial infarction. National Registry of Myocardial Infarction 2 Investigators. N Engl J Med 2000;342(21):1573–80.
23. Magid DJ, Calonge BN, Rumsfeld JS, et al. Relation between hospital primary angioplasty volume and mortality for patients with acute MI treated with primary angioplasty vs thrombolytic therapy. JAMA 2000;284(24):3131–8.
24. Vakili BA, Kaplan R, Brown DL. Volume-outcome relation for physicians and hospitals performing angioplasty for acute myocardial infarction in New York state. Circulation 2001;104(18):2171–6.
25. Armstrong PW. A comparison of pharmacologic therapy with/without timely coronary intervention vs. primary percutaneous intervention early after ST-elevation myocardial infarction: the WEST (Which Early ST-elevation myocardial infarction Therapy) study. Eur Heart J 2006;27(13):1530–8.
26. Bohmer E, Hoffmann P, Abdelnoor M, et al. Efficacy and safety of immediate angioplasty versus ischemia-guided management after thrombolysis in acute myocardial infarction in areas with very long transfer distances results of the NORDISTEMI (NORwegian study on DIstrict treatment of ST-Elevation Myocardial Infarction). J Am Coll Cardiol 2010;55(2):102–10.
27. Cantor WJ, Fitchett D, Borgundvaag B, et al. Routine early angioplasty after fibrinolysis for acute myocardial infarction. N Engl J Med 2009;360(26):2705–18.
28. Di Mario C, Dudek D, Piscione F, et al. Immediate angioplasty versus standard therapy with rescue angioplasty after thrombolysis in the Combined Abciximab REteplase Stent Study in Acute Myocardial Infarction (CARESS-in-AMI): an open, prospective, randomised, multicentre trial. Lancet 2008; 371(9612):559–68.
29. Fernandez-Aviles F, Alonso JJ, Castro-Beiras A, et al. Routine invasive strategy within 24 hours of thrombolysis versus ischaemia-guided conservative approach for acute myocardial infarction with ST-segment elevation (GRACIA-1): a randomised controlled trial. Lancet 2004;364(9439):1045–53.
30. Scheller B, Hennen B, Hammer B, et al. Beneficial effects of immediate stenting after thrombolysis in acute myocardial infarction. J Am Coll Cardiol 2003;42(4):634–41.
31. Borgia F, Goodman SG, Halvorsen S, et al. Early routine percutaneous coronary intervention after fibrinolysis vs. standard therapy in ST-segment elevation myocardial infarction: a meta-analysis. Eur Heart J 2010;31(17):2156–69.
32. Mild therapeutic hypothermia to improve the neurologic outcome after cardiac arrest. N Engl J Med 2002;346(8):549–56.
33. Bernard SA, Gray TW, Buist MD, et al. Treatment of comatose survivors of out-of-hospital cardiac arrest with induced hypothermia. N Engl J Med 2002; 346(8):557–63.

Setting Up a Population-Based Program to Optimize ST-Segment Elevation Myocardial Infarction Care

Orlando Rodríguez-Vilá, MD, MMS[a,b,*],
Miguel A. Campos-Esteve, MD[c]

KEYWORDS

- STEMI-PCI • STEMI systems of care • Myocardial infarction

KEY POINTS

- Timely reperfusion therapy in ST-segment elevation myocardial infarction (STEMI) saves lives.
- Optimization of processes to reduce door-to-balloon times at percutaneous coronary intervention (PCI) hospitals requires teamwork, collaboration, and continuous quality improvement efforts.
- Both access to reperfusion therapy as well as its timeliness can be maximized for a population only by integrating an advanced emergency medical services (EMS) system with the capability for prehospital diagnosis and triage into the process of STEMI care, even in geographically challenged areas.
- A STEMI system of care should be custom designed, taking into consideration local constraints and incorporating to various degrees direct transfer for primary PCI or combinations of pharmacologic and mechanical reperfusion strategies.
- Challenges ahead include minimizing the patient-related delay and promoting the use of EMS as the point of entry into the STEMI system of care in order to minimize total ischemia time.

INTRODUCTION: THE EVOLUTION OF ST-SEGMENT ELEVATION MYOCARDIAL INFARCTION SYSTEMS OF CARE

One hundred years ago, Herrick described coronary thrombosis as the mechanism of acute myocardial infarction.[1] In 1977, Reimer and colleagues[2] showed the time-sensitive nature of myocardial damage after a coronary occlusion. Further understanding and angiographic proof of the cause and timing of coronary thrombosis in the early hours of acute myocardial infarction became available in the landmark study by DeWood and colleagues in 1980.[3] The incremental value of earlier reperfusion relative to the onset of symptoms and the nonlinear relationship between treatment delay and clinical benefit was subsequently well established.[4,5] The applicability and superiority of primary angioplasty compared with intravenous (IV) thrombolysis resulted in its gradual widespread acceptance over the last 25 years.[6,7] Since 2004, the American College of Cardiology (ACC)/American Heart Association (AHA) practice guidelines as well as the European Society of Cardiology (ESC) practice guidelines recommended primary angioplasty for

[a] Cardiac Catheterization Laboratories, Cardiology Section, VA Caribbean Healthcare System, 10 Casia Street, San Juan 00921, Puerto Rico; [b] Cardiac Catheterization Laboratories, Auxilio Mutuo Hospital, 735 Ponce de Leon, Suite 503, Torre Medical Auxilio Mutuo, Hato Rey 00917, Puerto Rico; [c] Cardiac Catheterization Laboratories, Pavia Hospital, 1462 Asia Street, Santurce 00909, Puerto Rico
* Corresponding author. Cardiac Catheterization Laboratories, Cardiology Section, VA Caribbean Healthcare System, 10 Casia Street, San Juan 00921, Puerto Rico.
E-mail address: orodriguezvila@yahoo.com

Intervent Cardiol Clin 1 (2012) 583–597
http://dx.doi.org/10.1016/j.iccl.2012.06.009
2211-7458/12/$ – see front matter Published by Elsevier Inc.

the treatment of acute myocardial infarction when performed by experienced operators in less than 90 minutes from first medical contact (defined by time of contact with emergency medical services [EMS] or time of arrival to any emergency room) and when the expected percutaneous coronary intervention (PCI)-related delay is less than 60 minutes.[8,9] Furthermore, contemporary studies have shown that system delays that result in failure to adhere to these guideline-recommended times to reperfusion increase mortality.[10,11]

The proven feasibility and efficacy of timely reperfusion with primary PCI (PPCI) in ST-segment elevation myocardial infarction (STEMI) fueled the impetus for the development of STEMI systems of care over the last decade to help extend the limited reach of this therapy and thus optimize its effectiveness.[12,13] The early European experience with the primary angioplasty in patients transferred from general community hospitals to specialized PTCA units with or without emergency thrombolysis (PRAGUE-2) and Danish multicenter randomized study on fibrinolytic therapy versus acute coronary angioplasty in acute myocardial infarction (DANAMI-2) trials showed a superiority of transfer for primary angioplasty compared with thrombolysis at the non-PCI–capable hospital.[14,15] An early model of regional STEMI system of care was successfully implemented in Vienna.[16] In North America, initial skepticism because of geographic challenges and limitations with the EMS system was superseded by the pioneering work in Boston, Minneapolis, Durham, Rochester, and Ottawa that established proof of concept of the feasibility of implementing STEMI systems of care even in geographically challenging areas.[17–21] All of these events enhanced the interest in developing STEMI systems of care and STEMI-receiving center (SRC) networks.[22,23] In the United States, the swift national response to the quality initiatives by the ACC (*D2B An Alliance for Quality*) and the AHA (*Mission Lifeline*) coupled with the data-harnessing power of the ACC National Cardiovascular Data Registry (NCDR) showed how quality improvement can be accomplished in a dramatic fashion in such a short period of time across all of the United States.[24] In Europe, the recently launched *STENT for Life* initiative aims to promote the spread of systems of care across countries that have yet to formally establish these.[25]

Despite this success, most regions within the United States and across the world have yet to establish regional systems of care. The dramatic operational changes that must occur for the development of a STEMI system of care may encounter barriers that impede its ignition or progress. This lag is even more evident when one examines the global landscape. In Europe, there is marked heterogeneity in reperfusion strategy, ranging from advanced PPCI centers and regional STEMI systems of care to areas where the predominant strategy is thrombolysis.[26] In a recent survey in 19 countries in Africa, Latin America, and the Middle East, IV streptokinase was the most common reperfusion strategy and 39% received no reperfusion therapy.[27] Most countries in Asia are at a similarly underdeveloped stage in terms of STEMI systems of care. As cardiovascular disease remains the principal cause of mortality, awareness of the global cardiovascular epidemic has become an increasing priority and a call for social responsibility.[28]

The dramatic success of the *Mission Lifeline* and *D2B An Alliance for Quality* initiatives along with the commitment of thousands of health care providers across the United States to improve STEMI systems of care should serve as a trigger to extend this know-how to the rest of the world. However, the success of a global application of proven processes is governed by local circumstances. There is extensive information on the organizational framework and process implementation tools and guides available from the early *Guidelines Applied in Practice* project and the ACC *D2B Alliance* and the AHA *Mission Lifeline*.[29] This article synthesizes the available accumulated evidence that supports the implementation of STEMI systems of care on a citywide, regional, or nation-wide population-based scale and provides practical insights into the process, derived in part from the authors' experience with setting up a national STEMI-PCI network in Puerto Rico.

SETTING UP A STEMI PROGRAM FROM THE GROUND UP

Step 1: Getting Started

As monumental as it may first seem, all it takes is 1 committed individual to begin the chain reaction of quality improvement in STEMI. The first step in setting up a STEMI system of care is making it a priority and accepting the challenge. A committed physician champion (or nurse champion) is an essential catalyst at all phases of the project. This individual has 3 initial tasks:

1. *Evaluate the current strengths and limitations of the hospital and system of care.*
   As a minimum, a STEMI-PCI program requires 24/7 catheterization laboratory support from staff and interventional cardiologists. If not already available, staffing issues or on-call arrangements may be needed to provide the service on and off hours. No STEMI-PCI program can mature by on-hours STEMI-PCI only. There needs to be an evolution to the culture of racing against the clock

with each STEMI. Other challenges that PCI hospitals may initially face include an inadequate emergency department (ED) triage process or outdated referral or consulting patterns that introduce process inefficiency. Limitations may also involve a crippled, ineffective, or poorly integrated EMS system. Examining the current relationship status with surrounding non-PCI–capable hospitals is also warranted. This is the time to begin to identify barriers and opportunities. As described later, highly effective integrated work with EMS and STEMI referral centers is essential for a successful STEMI system of care.

2. *Identify and persuade the stakeholders to buy in to the project.*
   Although an individual may be a catalyst through leadership and tenacity, success in setting up a STEMI program depends on the willful commitment of all stakeholders. These stakeholders include the catheterization laboratory staff, emergency room (ER) staff, nursing, EMS system, hospital administrators, and quality department. Ideally, the physician champion and the rest of the core leadership group may gather stakeholders together to make the case for why it is so important to establish a STEMI program and STEMI system of care. At the top of the list is saving lives. However, along with better outcomes, cost savings are to be expected by virtue of lower length of stay, faster return to work, better left ventricular function, and less need for defibrillators, all of which affect the hospital, the payers, and society. Decision-analytical models of projected cost-effectiveness of primary angioplasty showed cost savings compared with thrombolytic therapy and a cost of $12,000/quality-adjusted life year saved compared with no intervention.[30] Additional benefits include prestige to the institution, more patient referrals, improved job satisfaction for the staff, and the gratification that comes with serving a higher purpose beyond the self.
3. *Establish institutional and regional working groups*.
   A STEMI quality management (QM) committee within a hospital must be organized and led by the physician champion. The first key player should be the STEMI coordinator, ideally an enthusiastic individual with clinical, research, or quality assurance experience, who should be assigned to lead the supervision and execution of tasks and work closely with the physician champion. Leaders from the ED, nursing, administration, and quality office, among others within this committee, are expected to meet at regular intervals to lead the implementation of proven door-to-balloon reduction measures as well as to develop innovative approaches that may best serve the local realities. This group is also expected to review all STEMI-PCI cases and provide both feedback and solutions. Barriers to care may be easily identified and solutions may be quickly proposed when both the field worker and the decision maker sit at the same table.

   These leaders must in turn inspire others who participate in the STEMI chain of survival of STEMI-PCI to feel vested in the project.[31] Particularly important within a hospital is that the system be decentralized in a way that every member feels part of the process and of the outcome and shares the reward. Teamwork within small units such as within the ED, within the catheterization laboratory staff, within the coronary care unit staff, and within the paramedic community is essential. Moreover, the concept of disciplined collaboration among units may be applied to define the optimal environment for a new STEMI-PCI program to thrive.[32] A concept adopted from the business literature, disciplined collaboration may be characterized by 3 qualities:

   1. Collaboration is not the same as teamwork. Teamwork occurs within units of work (ie, ER registered nurses [RNs]), whereas collaboration is among different units (ER and catheterization laboratory RNs working together).
   2. Collaboration not for the sake of collaboration but for better results. This collaboration requires well-defined and common goals (such as door-to-balloon time and mortality) and a mechanism to measure these before, during, and after implementation.
   3. Collaboration benefits from decentralization. One must let the people own a chunk of the work and of the results and rewards.

   Besides the institutional working group, the physician champion and core institutional leadership should reach out to the clinical and administrative leadership of potential STEMI referral hospitals in their catchment area and, more importantly, to the leadership of the EMS system(s). This regional working group focuses on the broader agenda of prehospital management described later and is a vital link in setting up a STEMI system of care. Topics to be addressed by this working group include prehospital electrocardiogram (ECG) acquisition, interpretation, and transmission, transfer protocols, door-in door-out strategies, and prehospital catheterization laboratory activation among others, as discussed later. This working group is the forum for operational wish lists to be discussed, viable solutions found, and agreements reached.

Step 2: Executing the Plan

To the extent that minimizing delay to treatment from the onset of the STEMI is the goal, a successful and efficient STEMI system of care must address the 3 core intervals of time to reperfusion: patient delay, hospital transport delay, and hospital-related delay.[33] Translating these intervals into organizational processes yields the 3 pillars of setting up a successful STEMI system of care at any population scale, chronologically listed in **Table 1**. In regards to the sequence of organization and implementation, efforts should proceed in reverse order, as described later.

First pillar: PCI hospital-related/door-to-balloon time

Early efforts to evaluate and optimize the timely execution of STEMI-PCI identified the value of prospective process implementation and continuous quality improvement in the 1990s.[34] Successful strategies accumulated over time and helped shape our current understanding of how to optimize STEMI care.[35,36]

As mentioned earlier, meeting the basic capability to perform 24/7 timely PCI interventions in patients arriving with STEMI is a requirement. The next step is first to implement process improvement interventions that contribute to minimizing door-to-balloon times consistently, coupled with a strategy of data monitoring and continuous quality improvement of processes. In addition, depending on the institutional characteristics, experience, and PCI volume, a concurrent process improvement effort may be directed toward promoting optimal evidence-based STEMI-PCI strategies among the institution's interventional cardiologists.

a. *ACC door-to-balloon reduction criteria:* Seven elements were originally described that favorably affect door-to-balloon times in high-performing institutions.[37,38] In addition, institutions may consider implementing complementary processes with these 7 elements, which they find may help in their specific situation. These processes should be constructed in standardized protocols and algorithms in the ED and catheterization laboratory. In drafting these processes, one should be reminded that simplicity and ease of use are the keys to compliance.
   1. *ER physician activates the catheterization laboratory.*

      Once a STEMI is confirmed by accepted standard clinical and ECG criteria, either at the ED or before hospital, the ability of the ED physician to activate the on-call team is not only time-saving but also empowering. The responsible ED physician must have a protocol-based simple algorithm to follow in every case. This strategy does not preclude direct physician-to-physician conversation for a debriefing of the case as the interventional cardiologists makes his/her way in. STEMI alert activation further upstream by paramedics has been evaluated and shown to have both pros and cons, including more false-positive activations and cancellations.[39,40] In addition, once the team is activated, the physician may initiate the standardized pre-PCI

Table 1
Three process pillars of a STEMI system of care

Delay Interval Source	Targets (Focus)	Process Pillar
Patient	Patient education Access to EMS	Early symptoms recognition of suspected STEMI and rapid activation of the EMS system as point of entry into the STEMI system of care
Hospital transport	EMS system: • Prehospital triage • Interhospital transfer	An advanced EMS system that integrates prehospital ECG and triage with standard transfer and door-in door-out protocols to STEMI referral hospitals and established transport protocols to SRCs coupled with prehospital catheterization laboratory activation and criteria for ED bypass
PCI hospital-related	Door-to-balloon time	Optimal standardized door-to-balloon reducing processes at the SRCs (PCI-capable hospitals) integrated seamlessly with the EMS system and STEMI referral hospitals coupled with a continuous quality improvement effort

pharmacotherapy and the nurse in charge should begin the preprocedure preparation, which involves preparing the access area, placing leads and defibrillator pads, and getting the patient ready for transfer to the catheterization laboratory on command.

2. *Single-call system for activating the catheterization laboratory*.
   A process by which the emergency room physician can activate the cardiac catheterization laboratory on-call team by placing a single telephone call to a central operator is one of the proven time-saving strategies. In turn, the central operator or ED clerk responsible for "activating" the on-call team should do so via a group paging system or an alternative automated simultaneous cellphone calls that may be set up by the hospital's communications department or by commercial providers such as Liveprocess or Sendwordnow.[41,42] Having a hospital operator or ED clerk individually and sequentially contact each team member introduces unnecessary delay and should be discouraged. Important in this step is to have a reply verification system of call-back requirement to ensure that all members of the team are activated and on their way. Failure to receive confirmation from any team member within 5 minutes should prompt another call via the same single-call system and via an alternate individual line such as cell phone or beeper. Failure to contact or receive confirmation by 10 minutes of the original call should prompt direct contact to the back-up team member for the individual. This process and time sequence should be clearly delineated in writing along with the appropriate training to the hospital operator and catheterization laboratory on-call staff. Mock STEMI drills can be coordinated to test these processes and identify flaws early in the program implementation, as well as to help maintain group skills in lower-volume SRCs.[43]
3. *STEMI-PCI team expected in with 20 to 30 minutes.*
   The philosophy of "drop what you are doing and go" must be instilled in the on-call team. Additional education or reinforcement may be needed as well as explicit expectations and monitoring to ensure compliance. Geographic constraints on meeting this time frame should be examined. In addition, local processes may include a dedicated parking space closest to the catheterization laboratory access for use during off-hours activations. Complementary strategies include cross-training of ER or intensive care unit nursing staff to bridge the transition of care from the ED to the catheterization laboratory and accelerate patient readiness while the on-call catheterization laboratory team arrives. Processes 2 and 3 are aimed at the goal of transferring the patient to the cardiac catheterization laboratory within 30 minutes from activation of the STEMI alert.[35] This goal gains relevance when one considers that almost two-thirds of patients with STEMI are treated during off hours, which is in turn associated with a delay in patients treated with PPCI.[44]
4. *Data monitoring and prompt feedback to ER and catheterization laboratory staff*.
   Key to continuous quality improvement are data collection and prompt feedback. Either participation in the ACC-sponsored ACTION Registry or using a custom data collection form, demographic, clinical, angiographic, procedural, in-hospital outcomes and time interval data must be prospectively collected, inspected, and aggregated for analysis and discussions at the QM committee meetings. Auditing and troubleshooting door-to-balloon times is essential to identify subtle barriers, find solutions, and formalize nonpunitive accountability for the process.[45] To accomplish this goal, a commonly feasible alternative is to recruit the support of the hospital's quality department staff or research staff, if applicable, who are familiar with data extraction and the rigors of accurate data collection. Prompt feedback may take a variety of forms. Ideally, the more personal and timely (<24–48 hours), the better. ED physicians may appreciate a call from the interventional cardiologist at the end of the case to relate the outcome and point out any positive or negative aspects observed about the care. ED nurses or paramedics who bring the patient into the catheterization laboratory may be thrilled to be invited to watch long enough to see the culprit lesion. Such intimacy with the STEMI can be a powerful incentive to promote buying in to the process and foster empowerment and empathy.
5. *Senior management support and organizational environment that fosters and sustains organizational change directed at improving door-to-balloon time*.
   The benefits of a successful STEMI-PCI program, including faster care, lower length of stay, better outcomes, and increased prestige and referrals are easy to pinpoint to hospital administrators. Their involvement

and buy-in from step 1 are key. Their decision-making power and their unique perspectives may bring to the table creative solutions to barriers that may not have surfaced among clinicians alone. It is therefore imperative that representatives from the senior management participate regularly at the STEMI-PCI program QM committee meetings. In addition, senior management commitment that is visible and tangible in their operational support and highlighting of outcomes data more effectively influences the hospital culture of change.[36]

6. *Team-based approach from ambulance to balloon, within a culture of continuous quality improvement*.

   A well-defined unifying goal and owning a part of the success are essential elements of the disciplined collaboration that can foster the sustainability of process improvement, as detailed earlier. Successful organizations have identified having "an explicit goal of reducing door-to-balloon time" as one of the keys to their success.[36] Effective and timely feedback that fosters communication has been identified as key in the long-term postimplementation phase.[46] The ongoing role of the QM committee cannot be overemphasized. Tools to help sustain the gain is the current focus of the original *D2B An Alliance for Quality* campaign of the ACC.[47]

7. *Use of prehospital ECG to activate the catheterization laboratory*.

   The benefit of the prehospital ECG for triage and catheterization laboratory activation was recognized early on and has been validated in multiple studies.[38,48] This topic is discussed later.

b. *Optimal STEMI procedure:* Evidence-based best practices in STEMI intervention have accumulated over the last decade. The organizational structure that promotes improvement in STEMI processes may also be used to promote among interventional cardiologists a consistent evidence-based approach to the STEMI procedure. Wide heterogeneity in the execution of an optimal STEMI-PCI procedure may exist among operators within an institution and among institutions within a region.

   Early on, we identified this variability as a potential limitation of our broader STEMI-PCI process campaign. For this reason, we incorporated a best practices curriculum among interventional operators, which included case reviews, lectures, visual aids, and one-on-one discussion led by the physician champion to promote the application of well-established best practices during STEMI procedures.[49] These practices include using bivalirudin as a PCI anticoagulant to reduce bleeding compared with using unfractionated heparin (UFH) plus a glycoprotein (GP) IIb/IIIa antagonist, using prasugrel instead of clopidogrel or clopidogrel 600 mg instead of 300 mg load to reduce stent thrombosis, approaching the thrombus-laden lesion with thrombectomy first to improve perfusion, and avoiding a nonculprit vessel intervention during a STEMI-PCI to avoid an excess mortality risk. These data of STEMI procedure patterns are also collected prospectively and reviewed as part of the same quality improvement strategy.

   PCI hospitals that are early in the planning and implementation phase of a STEMI system of care may benefit from using this more comprehensive educational and systems improvement approach that encompasses both the STEMI procedure as well as the STEMI process.

Second pillar: integrated EMS system and STEMI referral hospitals

The prehospital phase of STEMI is perhaps the most complex in terms of possible algorithms and the one that may have the most influence on prereperfusion delays. Both the speed of the initial response to STEMI symptoms and the point of entry into the STEMI system of care are determined by the patient. On the other hand, a successful STEMI system of care depends on an operational EMS infrastructure that is integrated into a closely tied network of STEMI referral hospitals and STEMI receiving center(s) in order to establish a STEMI diagnosis early, make prehospital triage decisions, and expedite transport within a STEMI-PCI center "catchment area" or within a whole region or country, as depicted in **Fig. 1**.[43] Depending on clinical and geographic variables, the prehospital phase may include STEMI diagnosis, prehospital thrombolysis, transport to a non-PCI center en route to a PCI center, or bypassing non-PCI centers. The complexity of the decision flow is shown in **Fig. 2** and the rationale for a custom-built scheme tailored to local realities is elaborated later.

There are 2 broad categories of patients who do not present directly to a PCI hospital (where PPCI is the treatment of choice): (1) those who enter into the system of care either via the EMS system or (2) those who enter into the system via self-transport to a non-PCI hospital.

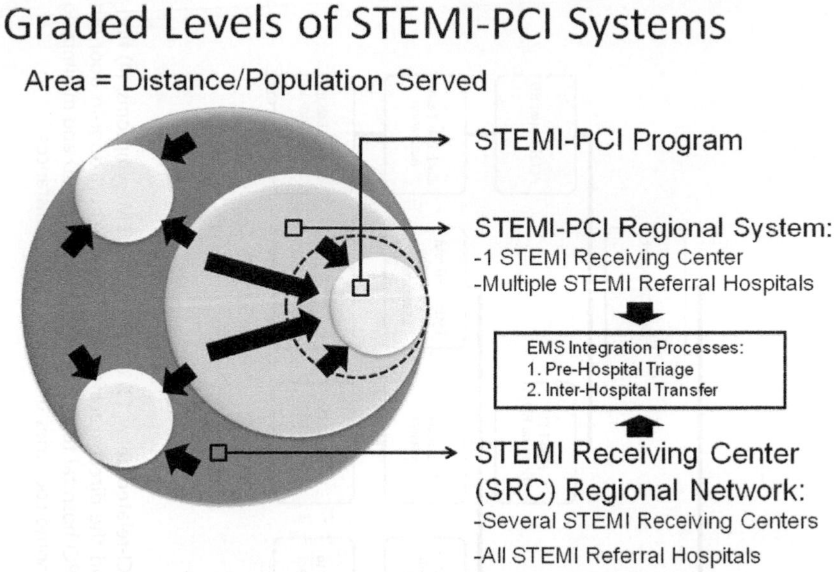

Fig. 1. STEMI-PCI programs consist of 1 PCI-capable hospital with 24/7 STEMI-PCI capability, represented in the white circle with the surrounding immediate catchment area in the dotted circle. The 2 larger circles represent the catchment area that includes multiple STEMI referral hospitals for 1 SRC (STEMI-PCI regional system) or the larger catchment area of all STEMI referral hospitals in a region that refer to several SRCs.

a. *Prehospital STEMI diagnosis and triage: entry via the EMS system*

Over the last 2 decades in the United States, roughly 5% to 60% of patients with STEMI access the system of care via EMS, although this figure may be lower in other countries.[50,51]

It is well established that patients who enter via the EMS system experience shorter delays in hospital arrival from the onset of symptoms as well as faster reperfusion in both door-to-balloon and door-to-needle time than those who self-transport to the ED.[51] Moreover, the feasibility and efficacy of integrating prehospital ECGs has been shown among well-developed regional STEMI systems of care in the United States.[52]

Many challenges exist in the prehospital phase. Data from the NCDR in regions with top-performing hospitals show that 40% of patients with STEMI do not benefit from entry via EMS transport.[51] The approach to this cohort that self-transports to non-PCI centers is discussed later. Among those who do enter via EMS, only a few undergo a prehospital ECG, ranging from less than 10% in the National Registry of Myocardial Infarction experience to 27% in the NCDR Action Registry.[53,54] In addition, even when an ECG can be performed, barriers to prehospital STEMI diagnosis may interfere with an optimal process. These barriers include paramedic training in accurate ECG diagnosis and interference related to wireless transmission to an SRC ED either because of technological limitations or because of geographic and signal constraints.[43]

Different STEMI systems of care models have tailored solutions to both their constraints and their advantages in regards to prehospital care. For example, in the French and Vienna systems, ambulances are staffed with physicians who are capable of making both ECG diagnosis and triage decisions.[16,55] In the Ottawa model, prehospital STEMI diagnosis effectively relies on trained paramedics.[19] In the absence of capability for reliable wireless transmission, combining the paramedic training with the ECG computer algorithm has been applied successfully.[56,57] Other systems rely on 100% wireless transmission with either on-call cardiologists or the SRC emergency room.[58,59] In all scenarios, developing clear and standardized criteria and algorithms for appropriate catheterization laboratory team activation according to both classic STEMI presentations as well as STEMI equivalents such as true posterior, new left bundle branch block, suspected left main occlusion will simplify decision making, save time, spare false activations, and avoid missed STEMIs.[60]

In addition to establishing the STEMI diagnosis early and facilitating prehospital catheterization laboratory activation, the prehospital ECG

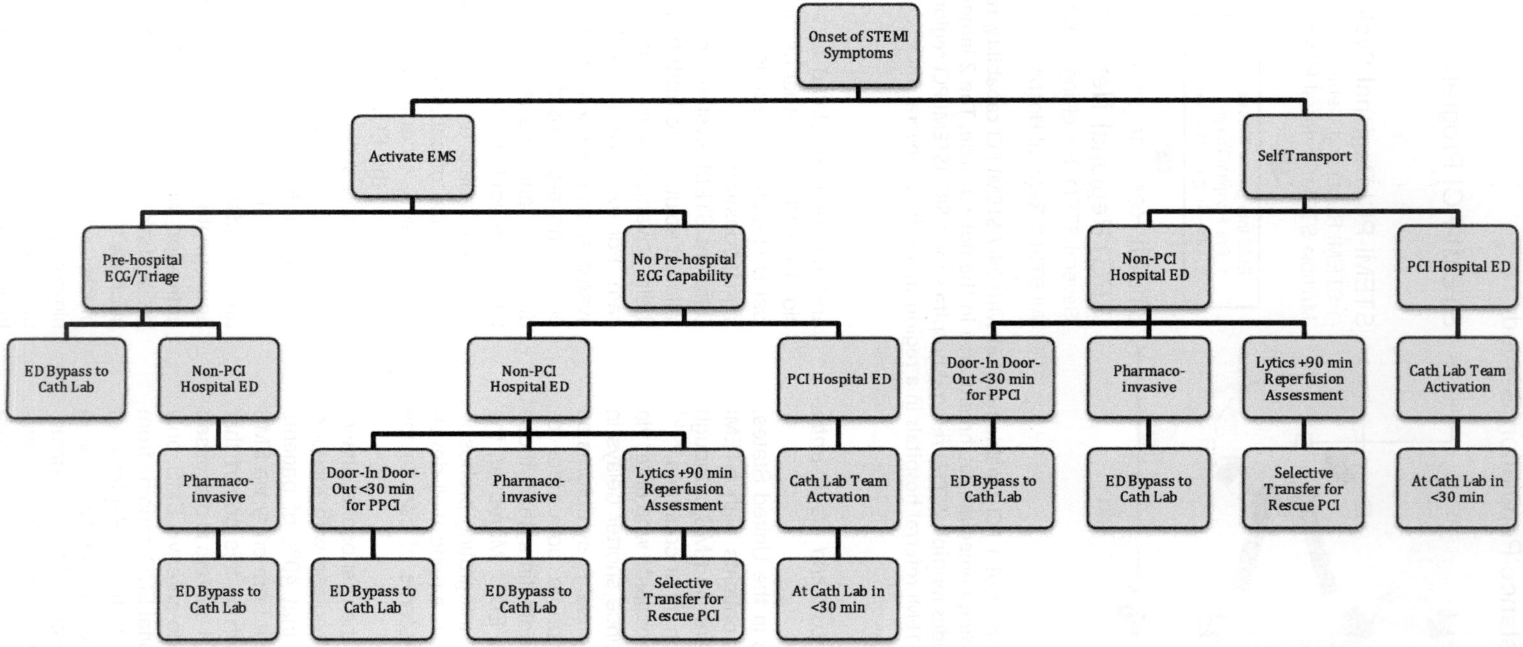

Fig. 2. STEMI system of care possible care decision flow depending on (1) distance from SRC, (2) anticipated PCI-related delay, (3) duration of STEMI symptoms, (4) fibrinolysis risk assessment, and (5) STEMI risk assessment. The prehospital ECG/triage, the pharmacoinvasive, and the direct transfer for PCI with short door-in door-out strategy all would involve activation of the catheterization laboratory team before the patient arrives at the PCI hospital to allow for bypassing the ED and minimizing the door-to-balloon time. Prehospital fibrinolysis, which is not included in this care flow, may be feasible in some countries under certain circumstances.

allows for early triage of patients with suspected STEMI. However, considering that only 5% of patients with chest pain transported by EMS end up having a STEMI, transferring all patients with chest pain via ambulance to an SRC would tip the balance and overburden the PCI hospitals.[61]

b. *SRC protocols: entry via a non-PCI hospital*
Formerly known as non-PCI centers or spoke centers, the STEMI referral hospital is one that does not offer PPCI but that is integrated into a STEMI system of care with the capability to approach a patient with STEMI who presents within 12 hours from the onset of STEMI symptoms in 3 possible strategies supported by current guidelines.[9,62]

1. *IV thrombolysis with door-to-needle time less than 30 minutes.*
This strategy may be best suited for hospitals with long (>1 hour) transfer times to an SRC, especially if the onset of STEMI symptoms is less than 3 hours, although current guidelines leave this decision open to clinician assessment and weighted factors.[8] Next in the decision algorithm is whether to immediately initiate transfer to an SRC for planned PCI (pharmacoinvasive strategy) or reserve transfer for the absence of reperfusion and need for rescue PCI. A common denominator of the pharmacoinvasive strategy discussed later and its efficacy and safety is that the timing of PCI after thrombolytic therapy in randomized trials is between 2 and 24 hours. The so-called facilitated PCI defined as half-dose or full-dose thrombolytic with or without GPIIb/IIIa antagonist and routine immediate transfer (within 2 hours) has been associated with worse or similar outcomes.[63,64] On the other hand, assessment of clinical reperfusion after fibrinolytic therapy followed rescue PCI if failure to reperfuse is suspected is a core element of the lytic strategy.[65] Similarly, standard protocols for transfer criteria and logistics should be in place at any STEMI referral center that administers thrombolytics.

2. *Pharmacoinvasive strategy.*
Also suited for hospitals with long or intermediate (>96.5 km [60 miles] or > 1 hour) transfer delays, a strategy of IV thrombolysis and routine transfer for PCI has been evaluated in patients within 12 hours if there is a STEMI and at least 1 high-risk feature. In the CARESS-in-AMI trial, the combination of half-dose reteplase and abciximab followed by immediate transfer for PCI (performed on average 2.3 hours after thrombolysis) was superior to expectant therapy with transfer only for rescue PCI.[66] Similarly, the TRANSFER-AMI trial found benefit of using full-dose IV thrombolysis followed by routine transfer for PCI (on average 3.9 hours after thrombolysis) compared with thrombolysis and rescue PCI.[67] A meta-analysis of trials comparing routine early PCI with standard therapy after thrombolysis for STEMI showed lower reinfarction and recurrent ischemia with routine PCI.[68] A pharmacoinvasive strategy using half-dose thrombolytic (most commonly tenecteplase) and immediate transfer for PCI in patients presenting to non-PCI hospitals more than 60 miles from an SRC compared favorably, with similar survival to the cohort who underwent PPCI directly from within a 96.5-km (60-mile) radius, with median door-to-balloon times of 122 minutes and 62 minutes, respectively.[69]

3. *Immediate transfer for PPCI.*
Immediate transfer for PPCI in a mature and well-orchestrated STEMI system of care achieving the guideline-recommended first-medical-contact-to-balloon time of less than 90 minutes in most patients has been shown to be feasible.[52] However, in patients who arrive at a non-PCI hospital, the decision whether to administer fibrinolytic therapy or transfer immediately for a PPCI strategy at an SRC depends on the PCI-related delay (door-to-balloon time–door-to-needle time), the time from the onset of symptoms, STEMI risk, and fibrinolytic risk.[8,62] In general, shorter (<3 hours) duration of symptoms and longer (>60 minutes) total transfer time for PPCI may favor fibrinolysis. In an analysis of randomized trials of PPCI versus fibrinolysis, a PCI-related delay (defined as the door-to-balloon time minus the door-to-needle time) greater than 1 hour negated the survival benefit of PPCI over lytic therapy.[70] Similarly, using data from the National Registry of Myocardial Infarction, Pinto and colleagues showed that clinical equipoise between the two strategies occurred at a PCI-related delay of close to two hours in both the complete registry cohort and in a propensity-matched cohort.[71,72] The effect of the PCI-related delay on mortality is also variable and dependent on patient characteristics such as age, infarct location and duration of symptoms. For example, in younger

patients (<65 years) presenting early (<2 hours) after the onset of symptoms of an anterior STEMI showed clinical equipoise of both strategies when the PCI-related delay exceeded only 40 minutes.[71] Therefore, the benefit of an immediate transfer for PPCI depends on a reliable EMS transport system and processes at the STEMI referral center aimed at keeping the door-in door-out interval less than 30 minutes and the first-medical-contact-to-balloon time at less than 90 minutes.[73]

Since 2008 and 2009, the ESC and the ACC/AHA guidelines have given a pharmacoinvasive strategy a class IIa indication with a level of evidence B.[9,62] Regardless of the strategy used, it is vital that all STEMI referral centers use the same standardized and simple decision algorithm in order to minimize heterogeneity in decision making, which introduces delays.[74] As mentioned earlier, a delay from first hospital presentation to the second PCI hospital of door-in door-out of more than 30 minutes has been shown to be associated with worse outcomes.[73] EMS processes have been described as associated with lower door-in door-out delays, including the availability of prehospital ECG and paramedic interpretation, use of local ambulances for transfers, and keeping the patient on the EMS stretcher while an ECG is performed at the first hospital when a prehospital ECG is not available.[75]

Direct planning between the SRC and their referral centers to agree on ideal and viable processes is essential for its success. Typically, the setup should include a no-questions-asked policy of the receiving center to accept patients with STEMI. Steps that include verification of bed availability, insurance coverage, or accepting physician only introduce delay to the process. Similarly, simplifying the pretransfer treatment algorithm improves efficiency. Current guidelines support the administration of aspirin, clopidogrel load, and UFH (60 U/kg up to 4000 units) to all patients with STEMI.[8,76] This simple algorithm may be complemented by a pharmacoinvasive approach with half-dose or full-dose thrombolysis and immediate transfer in hospitals more than 60 miles or 1 hour from the SRC. Given the lack of evidence of their efficacy, adding an upstream GPIIb/IIIa inhibitor is not helpful and only adds complexity and delay.

Standardizing this protocol across the STEMI referral centers in close coordination with the SRC yields optimal results within regions and across regions.[52] Early in the process, it is recommended to pilot test the STEMI system of care, starting with 1 STEMI referral hospital to gain experience and iron out difficulties. Thereafter, extending the process to other referral hospitals is increasingly smoother. In areas where competition among PCI hospitals is a factor, careful planning, sometimes incorporating the advice of a neutral mediator, consultation with health or legal authorities, and written agreements may be required to consolidate a preconceived STEMI system of care into a functional unit.

Third pillar: patient response: the ultimate challenge on total ischemic time

The sum of time from the onset of coronary occlusion to the onset of symptoms, to recognition and appropriate reaction by the patient is where most of the delay in STEMI care occurs, precisely during the most critical golden-hour period.[5,77] In cases with brief delays, myocardial infarction can be aborted.[78] However, in acute coronary syndrome, patient-related median delays from the onset of symptoms range from 1.5 to 6 hours in the United States and a variety of factors have been implicated.[79]

The limited use of the EMS system as point of entry further compounds the problem. Only by choosing the EMS system as the point of entry are benefits of prehospital diagnosis, triage to SRCs and its effect on reducing door-to-balloon time taken advantage of. Therefore, interventions that promote recognition of STEMI symptoms and activation of the EMS system may represent an area of opportunity for systems improvement. In the large REACT (Rapid Early Action for Coronary Treatment) trial, an 18-month multilevel intervention in 20 US cities had no effect on patient delay from symptom onset to hospital arrival but did result in a relative 20% increase in the appropriate use of the EMS system as point of entry.[80]

Access into a STEMI system of care via the EMS system may also be the most cost-effective strategy to improve overall access to STEMI-PCI. Using registry data and computer modeling, Concannon and colleagues estimated the actual access to PPCI of all STEMI patients at 30.4% (down from the theoretical 80% of patients who live within one hours of a PCI center), when factors such as frequency of arrival at a non-PCI hospital, time of day, and 24/7 STEMI-PCI availability were entered into the model.[81] In this study, the greater the proportion of patients who entered the system of care via EMS, the more the cost savings when compared with a strategy of building more PCI-capable hospitals.

The difficulty in estimating the potential benefit or impact of a STEMI system of care is also determined by the ability of STEMI registries to capture

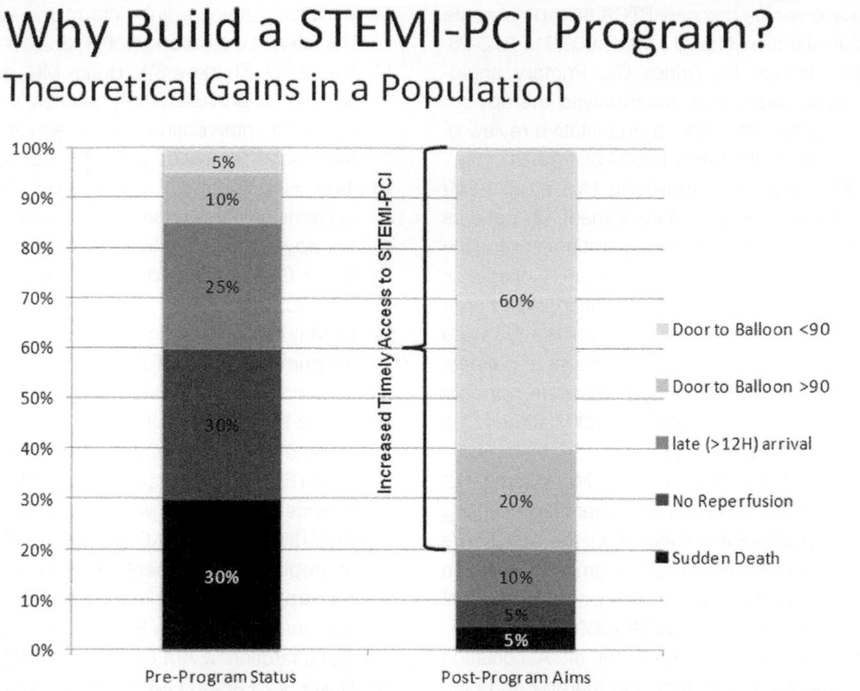

Fig. 3. The theoretic absolute change in the possible outcomes of all STEMI cases that may occur in a population before and after a program to optimize STEMI care.

all patients with STEMI. Unless uniform and broad criteria are used, this figure may be grossly underestimated.[82] By raising awareness of STEMI symptoms, speeding the patient response, maximizing the use of the EMS system, and optimizing the prehospital triage phase, the impact of a STEMI system of care may be larger than expected. As theoretically pictured in **Fig. 3**, such an ideal STEMI system of care may shift late-presenters, victims of sudden cardiac death, and those treated with long delays to most patients in whom the total ischemia time and the risk of death are reduced dramatically.

Until we know better, patient education on early recognition and appropriate response to suspected STEMI must be incorporated at all levels of patient education from the physician's office to hospital discharge planning. Interventions aimed at optimizing the use of an advanced EMS system with capability for prehospital diagnosis and triage are also imperative.

SUMMARY

Remarkable progress has been made over the last 3 decades in the care of STEMI. The evolution of PPCI into the growing concept of STEMI systems of care improves outcomes and saves lives. We have reached a point at which STEMI systems of care can be made feasible within cities, regions, or countries. Specific organizational processes, strategies, and tools have been developed and shared to allow for the dissemination of successful STEMI systems of care and the relentless pursuit of the ideal system. The next challenge is to help promote the development of STEMI systems of care across the world. Anyone and everyone in the STEMI chain of life can make a difference. Why not start today?

REFERENCES

1. Herrick JB. Clinical features of sudden obstruction of the coronary arteries. JAMA 1912;59:2015.
2. Reimer KA, Lowe JE, Rasmussen MM, et al. The wavefront phenomenon of ischemic cell death. Myocardial infarct size vs. duration of coronary occlusion in dogs. Circulation 1977;56:786–94.
3. DeWood MA, Spores J, Notske R, et al. Prevalence of total coronary occlusion during the early hours of transmural myocardial infarction. N Engl J Med 1980;303:897–902.
4. Vermeer F, Simoons ML, Bär FW, et al. Which patients benefit most from early thrombolytic therapy with intracoronary streptokinase? Circulation 1986; 74:1379–89.
5. Boersma E, Maas AC, Deckers JW, et al. Early thrombolytic treatment in acute myocardial infarction: reappraisal of the golden hour. Lancet 1996;348:771–5.
6. O'Neill WW, Timmis GC, Bourdillon PD, et al. A prospective randomized clinical trial of intracoronary

streptokinase versus coronary PTCA therapy of acute myocardial infarction. N Engl J Med 1986;314:812–28.
7. Keeley EC, Boura JA, Grines CL. Primary angioplasty versus intravenous thrombolytic therapy for acute myocardial infarction: a quantitative review of 23 randomised trials. Lancet 2003;361:13–20.
8. Antman EM, Anbe DT, Armstrong PW, et al. ACC/AHA guidelines for the management of patients with ST-Elevation myocardial infarction—executive summary: a report of the American College of Cardiology/American Heart Association Task Force on Practice Guidelines (writing committee to revise the 1999 guidelines for the management of patients with acute myocardial infarction) [Erratum appears in Circulation 2005;111:2013–4, 2007;115:e411.]. Circulation 2004;110:e82–292.
9. Van deWerf F, Bax J, Betriu A, et al. Management of acute myocardial infarction in patients presenting with persistent ST-segment elevation: the Task Force on the Management of ST-Segment Elevation Myocardial Infarction of the European Society of Cardiology. Eur Heart J 2008;29:2909–45.
10. Lambert L, Brown K, Segal E, et al. Association between timeliness of reperfusion therapy and clinical outcomes in ST-elevation myocardial infarction. JAMA 2010;303:2148–55.
11. Terkelsen CJ, Sorensen JT, Maeng M, et al. System delay and mortality among patients with STEMI treated with primary percutaneous coronary intervention. JAMA 2010;304:763–71.
12. Henry TD, Atkins JM, Cinningham MS, et al. ST-segment elevation myocardial infarction: recommendations on triage of patients to heart attack centers. Is it time for a national policy for the treatment of ST-segment elevation myocardial infarction? J Am Coll Cardiol 2006;47:1339–45.
13. Jacobs AK, Antman EM, Ellrodt G, et al. Recommendation to develop strategies to increase the number of ST-segment elevation myocardial infarction patients with timely access to primary percutaneous coronary intervention. The American Heart Association's Acute Myocardial Infarction (AMI) Advisory Working Group. Circulation 2006;113:2152–63.
14. Widimsky P, Groch L, Zelizko M, et al. Multicentre randomized trial comparing transport to primary angioplasty vs. immediate thrombolysis vs. combined strategy for patients with acute myocardial infarction presenting to a community hospital without a catheterization laboratory: the PRAGUE study. Eur Heart J 2000;21:823–31.
15. Andersen HR, Nielsen TT, Rasmussen K, et al, DANAMI-2 investigators. A comparison of coronary angioplasty with fibrinolytic therapy in acute myocardial infarction. N Engl J Med 2003;349:733–42.
16. Kalla K, Christ G, Karnik R, et al. Implementation of guidelines improves the standard of care. The Viennese registry on reperfusion strategies in ST-elevation myocardial infarction (Vienna STEMI Registry). Circulation 2006;113:2398–405.
17. Henry TD, Sharkey SW, Burke MN, et al. A regional system to provide timely access to percutaneous coronary intervention for ST-elevation myocardial infarction. Circulation 2007;116:721–8.
18. Ting HH, Rihal CS, Gersh BJ, et al. Regional systems of care to optimize timeliness of reperfusion therapy for ST-elevation myocardial infarction. The Mayo Clinic STEMI protocol. Circulation 2007;116:729–36.
19. Le May MR, So DY, Dionne R, et al. A citywide protocol for primary PCI in ST-segment elevation myocardial infarction. N Engl J Med 2008;358:231–40.
20. Moyer P, Feldman J, Cannon CP, et al. Implications of the mechanical (PCI) vs. thrombolytic controversy for STEMI on the organization of EMS: the Boston experience. Crit Pathw Cardiol 2004;3:53–61.
21. Waters RE II, Singh KP, Roe MT, et al. Rationale and strategies for implementing community-based transfer protocols for primary percutaneous coronary intervention for acute ST-segment elevation myocardial infarction. J Am Coll Cardiol 2004;43:2153–9.
22. Rokos IC, Larson DM, Henry TD, et al. Rationale for establishing regional ST-elevation myocardial infarction receiving centre (SRC) networks. Am Heart J 2006;152:661–7.
23. Jacobs AK, Antman EM, Faxon DP, et al. Development of systems of care for ST-elevation myocardial infarction patients. Executive summary. Circulation 2007;116:217–30.
24. Krumholz HM, Herrin J, Miller LE, et al. Improvements in door-to balloon time in the United States, 2005 to 2010. Circulation 2011;124:1038–45.
25. Available at: http://www.pcronline.com/stentforlife/_news_pr_2009.php. Accessed September 26, 2011.
26. Widimsky P, Wijns W, Fajadet J, et al. Reperfusion therapy for ST elevation acute myocardial infarction in Europe: description of the current situation in 30 countries. Eur Heart J 2010;31:943–57.
27. The ACCESS Investigators. Management of acute coronary syndromes in developing countries: acute coronary events–a multinational survey of current management strategies. Am Heart J 2011;162:852–9.
28. Fuster V, IOM (Institute of Medicine). Promoting cardiovascular health in the developing world: a critical challenge to achieve global health. Washington, DC: The National Academies Press; 2010.
29. Montoye CK, Eagle KA. An organizational framework for the AMI ACC-GAP™ Project. J Am Coll Cardiol 2005;46:1B–29B.
30. Lieu TA, Gurley RJ, Lundstrom RJ, et al. Projected cost-effectiveness of primary angioplasty for acute myocardial infarction. J Am Coll Cardiol 1997;30:1741–50.
31. Ornato JP. The ST-segment elevation myocardial infarction chain of survival. Circulation 2007;116:6–9.

32. Hansen MT. Collaboration. How leaders avoid the traps, create unity and reap big results. Boston: Harvard Business Press; 2009.
33. Weaver WD. Time to thrombolytic treatment: factors affecting delay and their influence on outcome. J Am Coll Cardiol 1995;25:3S–9S.
34. Caputo RP, Ho KK, Stoler RC, et al. Effect of continuous quality improvement analysis on the delivery of primary percutaneous transluminal coronary angioplasty for acute myocardial infarction. Am J Cardiol 1997;79:1159–64.
35. Bradley EH, Roumanis SA, Radford MJ, et al. Achieving door-to-balloon times that meet quality guidelines: how do successful hospitals do it? J Am Coll Cardiol 2005;46:1236–41.
36. Bradley EH, Curry LA, Webster TR, et al. Achieving rapid door-to-balloon times. How top hospitals improve complex systems. Circulation 2006;113:1079–85.
37. Bradley EH, Herrin J, Wang Y, et al. Strategies for reducing the door-to-balloon time in acute myocardial infarction. N Engl J Med 2006;355:2308–20.
38. Krumholz HM, Bradley EH, Nallamothu BK, et al. A campaign to improve the timeliness of primary percutaneous intervention. Door-to-Balloon: an alliance for quality. JACC Cardiovasc Interv 2008;1: 97–104.
39. Ting HH, Krumholz HM, Bradley EH, et al. Implementation and integration of prehospital ECGs into systems of care for acute coronary syndrome. A scientific statement from the American Heart Association Interdisciplinary Council on Quality of Care and Outcomes Research, Emergency Cardiovascular Care Committee, Council on Cardiovascular Nursing, and Council on Clinical Cardiology. Circulation 2008;118:1066–79.
40. Garvey JL, Monk L, Granger CB, et al. Rates of cardiac catheterization cancellation for ST-segment elevation myocardial infarction after activation by emergency medical services or emergency physicians. Results from the North Carolina catheterization laboratory activation registry. Circulation 2012;125:308–13.
41. Liveprocess. Available at: http://www.liveprocess.com/. Accessed April 6, 2012.
42. Sendwordnow. Available at: http://www.sendwordnow.com/. Accessed April 6, 2012.
43. Moyer P, Ornato JP, Brady WJ, et al. Development of systems of care for ST-elevation myocardial infarction patients. The emergency medical services and emergency department perspective. Circulation 2007;116:e43–8.
44. Magdi DJ, Wang Y, Herrin J, et al. Relationship between time of day, day of week, timeliness of reperfusion, and in-hospital mortality for patients with acute ST-segment elevation myocardial infarction. JAMA 2005;294:803–12.
45. Ward MR, Lo ST, Herity NA, et al. Effect of audit on door-to-inflation times in primary angioplasty/stenting for acute myocardial infarction. Am J Cardiol 2001;87:336–8.
46. Nestler DM, Noheria A, Haro LH, et al. Sustaining improvement in door-to-balloon time over 4 years: the Mayo Clinic ST-elevation myocardial infarction protocol. Circ Cardiovasc Qual Outcomes 2009;2:508–13.
47. American College of Cadiology Door to Balloon Alliance. Available at: http://www.d2balliance.org/. Accessed March 29, 2012.
48. Canto JG, Rogers WJ, Bowlby LJ, et al. The prehospital electrocardiogram in acute myocardial infarction: is its full potential being realized? National Registry of Myocardial Infarction 2 Investigators. J Am Coll Cardiol 1997;29:498–505.
49. Rodriguez-Vila O, Martinez H, Campos MA, et al. Improving quality in STEMI-PCI beyond the door-to-balloon time: rationale for a collaborative model to standardize evidence-based practices in STEMI-PCI. Indian Heart J 2011;63:67–74.
50. Canto JG, Zalenski RJ, Ornato JP, et al. Use of emergency medical services in acute myocardial infarction and subsequent quality of care. Observations from the National Registry of Myocardial Infarction 2. Circulation 2002;106:3018–23.
51. Mathews R, Peerson ED, Li S, et al. Use of emergency medical service transport among patients with ST-segment elevation myocardial infarction. Findings from the National Cardiovascular Data Registry Acute Coronary Treatment Intervention Outcomes Network Registry–Get With the Guidelines. Circulation 2011;124:154–63.
52. Rokos IC, French WJ, Koenig WJ, et al. Integration of pre-hospital electrocardiograms and ST-elevation myocardial infarction receiving center (SRC) networks. Impact on door-to-balloon times across 10 independent regions. JACC Cardiovasc Interv 2009;2:339–46.
53. Curtis JP, Portnay EL, Wang Y, et al. The pre-hospital electrocardiogram and time to reperfusion in patients with acute myocardial infarction, 2000–2002: findings from the National Registry of Myocardial Infarction-4. J Am Coll Cardiol 2006;47:1544–52.
54. Diercks DB, Kontos MC, Chen AY, et al. Utilization and impact of pre-hospital electrocardiograms for patients with acute ST-segment elevation myocardial infarction: data from the NCDR (National Cardiovascular Data Registry) ACTION (Acute Coronary Treatment and Interventions Outcomes Network) Registry. J Am Coll Cardiol 2009;53:161–6.
55. Danchin N, Coste P, Ferrieres J, et al. Comparison of thrombolysis followed by broad use of percutaneous coronary intervention with primary percutaneous coronary intervention for ST-segment elevation acute myocardial infarction: data from the French registry on acute ST-elevation myocardial infarction (FAST-MI). Circulation 2008;118:268–76.
56. Nestler DM, White RD, Rihal CS, et al. Impact of prehospital electrocardiogram protocol and immediate

cardiac catheterization team activation for patients with ST-elevation myocardial infarction. Circ Cardiovasc Qual Outcomes 2011;4:640–6.
57. Mixon TA, Suhr E, Caldwell G, et al. Retrospective description and analysis of consecutive catheterization laboratory ST-segment elevation myocardial infarction activations with proposal, rationale, and use of a new classification scheme. Circ Cardiovasc Qual Outcomes 2011;5:62–9.
58. Dhruva VN, Abdelhadi SI, Anis A, et al. ST-Segment Analysis Using Wireless Technology in Acute Myocardial Infarction (STAT-MI) trial. J Am Coll Cardiol 2007;50:509–13.
59. Sanchez-Ross M, Oghlakian G, Maher J, et al. The STAT-MI (ST-Segment Analysis Using Wireless Technology in Acute Myocardial Infarction) trial improves outcomes. JACC Cardiovasc Interv 2011;4:222–7.
60. Rokos IC, French WK, Mattu A, et al. Appropriate cardiac cath lab activation: optimizing electrocardiogram interpretation and clinical decision-making for acute ST-elevation myocardial infarction. Am Heart J 2010;160:995–1003.
61. Weaver WD, Eisenberg MS, Martin JS, et al. Myocardial infarction triage and intervention project-phase I: patient characteristics and feasibility of prehospital initiation of thrombolytic therapy. J Am Coll Cardiol 1990;15:925–31.
62. Kushner FG, Hand M, Smith SC, et al. 2009 Focused Updates: ACC/AHA guidelines for the management of patients with ST-elevation myocardial infarction (updating the 2004 guideline and 2007 focused update) and the ACC/AHA/SCAI guidelines on percutaneous coronary intervention (updating the 2005 guideline and 2007 focused update). J Am Coll Cardiol 2009;54:2205–41.
63. Assessment of the Safety and Efficacy of a New Treatment Strategy with Percutaneous Coronary Intervention (ASSENT-4 PCI) Investigators. Primary versus tenecteplase-facilitated percutaneous coronary intervention in patients with ST-segment elevation acute myocardial infarction (ASSENT-4 PCI): randomized trial. Lancet 2006;367:569–78.
64. Ellis SG, Tendera M, de Belder MA, et al. Facilitated PCI in patients with ST-elevation myocardial infarction. N Engl J Med 2008;358:2205–17.
65. Carver A, Rafelt S, Gershlick AH, et al, REACT investigators. Longer-term follow up of patients recruited to the REACT (Rescue Angioplasty Versus Conservative Treatment or Repeat Thrombolysis) trial. J Am Coll Cardiol 2009;54:118–26.
66. Di Mario C, Dudek D, Piscione F, et al. Immediate angioplasty versus standard therapy with rescue angioplasty after thrombolysis in the Combined Abciximab REteplase Stent Study in Acute Myocardial Infarction (CARESS-in-AMI): an open, prospective, randomized, multicentre trial. Lancet 2008;371:559–68.
67. Cantor WJ, Fitchett D, Borgundvaag B, et al. Routine early angioplasty after fibrinolysis for acute myocardial infarction. N Engl J Med 2009;360:2705.
68. Borgia F, Goodman SG, Halvorsen S, et al. Early routine percutaneous coronary intervention after fibrinolysis vs. standard therapy in ST-segment elevation myocardial infarction: a meta-analysis. Eur Heart J 2010;31:2156–69.
69. Larson DM, Duval S, Sharkey SW, et al. Safety and efficacy of a pharmaco-invasive reperfusion strategy in rural ST-elevation myocardial infarction patients with expected delays due to long-distance transfers. Eur Heart J 2012;33(10):1232–40.
70. Nallamothu BK, Bates ER. Percutaneous coronary intervention versus fibrinolytic therapy in acute myocardial infarction: is timing (almost) everything? Am J Cardiol 2003;92:824–6.
71. Pinto DS, Kirtane AJ, Nallamothu BK, et al. Hospital delays in reperfusion for ST-elevation myocardial infarction. Implications when selecting a reperfusion strategy. Circulation 2006;114:2019–25.
72. Pinto DS, Frederick PD, Chakrabarti AK, et al. Benefit of transferring ST-segment elevation myocardial infarction patients for percutaneous coronary intervention compared with administration of onsite fibrinolytic declines as delays increase. Circulation 2011;124:2512–21.
73. Wang TY, Nallamothu BK, Krumholz HM, et al. Association of door-in to door-out time with reperfusion delays and outcomes among patients transferred for primary percutaneous coronary intervention. JAMA 2011;305:2540–7.
74. Miedema MD, Ndwell MC, Duval S, et al. Causes of delay and associated mortality in patients transferred with ST-segment elevation myocardial infarction. Circulation 2011;124:1636–44.
75. Glickman SW, Lytle BL, Ou FS, et al. Care processes associated with quicker door-in-door-out times for patients with ST elevation myocardial infarction requiring transfer. Results from a statewide regionalization program. Circ Cardiovasc Qual Outcomes 2011;4:383–8.
76. Dangas GD, Caixeta A, Mehran R, et al. Frequency and predictors of stent thrombosis after percutaneous coronary intervention in acute myocardial infarction. Circulation 2011;123:1745–56.
77. Gersh BJ, Stone GW, White HD, et al. Pharmacological facilitation of primary percutaneous coronary intervention for acute myocardial infarction. Is the slope of the curve the shape of the future? JAMA 2005;293:979–86.
78. Lamfers EJ, Hooghoudt TH, Uppelschoten A, et al. Effect of prehospital thrombolysis on aborting acute myocardial infarction. Am J Cardiol 1999;84:928–30.
79. Moser DK, Kimble LP, Alberts MJ, et al. Reducing delay in seeking treatment by patients with acute coronary syndrome and stroke. A scientific statement from the American Heart Association Council

on Cardiovascular Nursing and Stroke Council. Circulation 2006;114:168–82.

80. Luepker RV, Raczynski JM, Osganian S, et al. Effect of a community intervention on patient delay and emergency medical service use in acute coronary heart disease. The Rapid Early Action for Coronary Treatment (REACT) Trial. JAMA 2000; 284:60–7.

81. Concannon TW, Kent DM, Normand SL, et al. Comparative effectiveness of ST-segment elevation myocardial infarction regionalization strategies. Circ Cardiovasc Qual Outcomes 2010;3:506–13.

82. Campbell AR, Satran D, Larson DM, et al. ST-elevation myocardial infarction. Which patients do quality assurance programs include? Circ Cardiovasc Qual Outcomes 2009;2:648–55.

The Critical Imperative

Prehospital Management of the Patient with ST-Elevation Myocardial Infarction

David A. Hildebrandt, RN, EMT-P[a], David M. Larson, MD[b,c,*], Timothy D. Henry, MD[a,c]

KEYWORDS

• STEMI • Emergency medical services • Prehospital • 12-Lead ECG

KEY POINTS

- Depending on where one lives, a wide variety of combinations of emergency medical services levels of care exist in the United States.
- Prehospital acquisition of a 12-lead electrocardiogram is a key factor to reduce time to treatment in the patient with ST-elevation myocardial infarction.
- Paramedics can reliably acquire and interpret 12-lead electrocardiogram results for the patient with ST-elevation myocardial infarction and activate the cardiac catheterization laboratory with a high degree of accuracy.
- Prehospital fibrinolysis is rarely used in the United States because primary percutaneous coronary intervention has become the preferred method of reperfusion.

CASE STUDY

On a cold, early spring morning, Marvin, a 57-year-old man, develops chest pain while working on his farm. Marvin lives on a dairy farm 10 miles outside of a rural community of 14,000, located 60 miles west of a large urban center. He summons his wife, who then dials 911. Within 5 minutes, county sheriff deputies arrive and administer oxygen. Eleven minutes after the 911 call, paramedics arrive and begin their assessment. Marvin explains that he has no medical history but had a father and uncle who died of heart disease in their 60s. He complains of chest pain that radiates down his left arm. He is immediately given 325 mg of aspirin and sublingual nitroglycerin 0.4 mg, vital signs are taken, and a prehospital 12-lead electrocardiogram (ECG) (PHECG) is obtained that reveals significant ST-elevation in the inferior leads, II, III, and aVF, and reciprocal changes are present (**Fig. 1**A). Emergency medical services (EMS) personnel immediately transport the patient, with lights and siren, to the local hospital. En route, they notify the receiving hospital that they have a 57-year-old man with ST-elevation myocardial infarction (STEMI) and request that the helicopter be dispatched. Following an 8-minute on-scene time and 12-minute transport time, Marvin arrives at the hospital, where the emergency department (ED) staff and a helicopter crew are awaiting his arrival. Marvin is wheeled into the ED, remains on the ambulance stretcher, and is quickly interviewed by the emergency physician, as his PHECG is confirmed as STEMI. He receives a loading dose of 600 mg of oral clopidogrel and 4000 U of intravenous heparin, blood is drawn for lab work, and a call is made to the Minneapolis Heart Institute at Abbott-Northwestern Hospital in Minneapolis,

[a] Department of Research, Minneapolis Heart Institute Foundation at Abbott-Northwestern Hospital, 920 East 28th Street, Suite 100, Minneapolis, MN 55407, USA; [b] Department of Emergency Medicine, Ridgeview Medical Center, 500 South Maple Street, Waconia, MN 55387, USA; [c] University of Minnesota Medical School, Minneapolis, MN, USA
* Corresponding author. Department of Emergency Medicine, Ridgeview Medical Center, 500 South Maple Street, Waconia, MN 55387.
E-mail address: dlarsonmd@visi.com

Intervent Cardiol Clin 1 (2012) 599–608
http://dx.doi.org/10.1016/j.iccl.2012.07.001

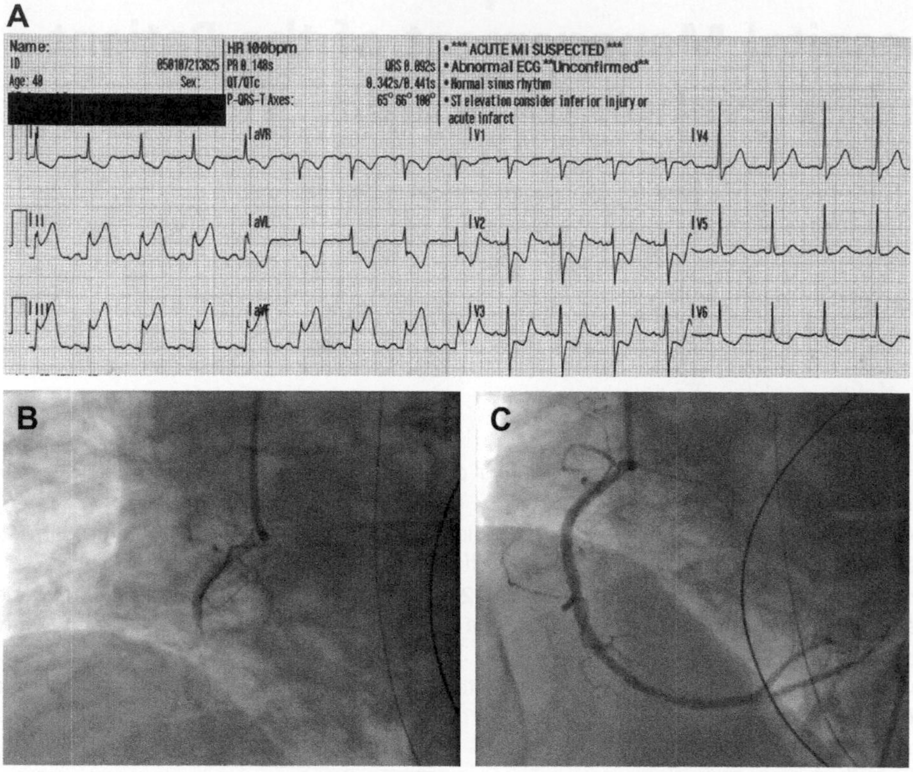

Fig. 1. (*A*) PHECG obtained by EMS personnel, showing inferior STEMI, and EMS request that helicopter be dispatched to meet them at referring hospital. (*B*) Pre-PCI angiogram, showing 100% occlusion of mid–right coronary artery. (*C*) Post-PCI angiogram. Mid–right coronary arteryocclusion now opened, stent placed, and patient has Thombolysis in Myocardial Infarction flow 3.

MN, USA, to declare a Level One STEMI. He is moved from the ambulance stretcher to the flight stretcher and immediately taken to the helipad and flown the 30 minutes to Minneapolis. His door-in, door-out time at the local community hospital doors was 12 minutes. While in flight, his lab results, a 1-page demographics sheet, and a copy of the PHECG were faxed to Abbott-Northwestern Hospital by the community hospital staff and reviewed by the receiving cardiology team. As the helicopter lands on the rooftop of Abbott-Northwestern Hospital, hospital security staff meets the flight team and escorts them to the elevator and then immediately to the cardiac catheterization laboratory (CCL), where the cardiac team is waiting. The patient is quickly interviewed by the admitting cardiologist while the team preps him for his emergent angiogram. The angiogram reveals a 100% occluded mid–right coronary artery with Thombolysis in Myocardial Infarction 0 flow (see **Fig. 1**B). Within 15 minutes of his arrival at the percutaneous coronary intervention (PCI)-capable hospital, the lesion is opened with successful PCI. After the procedure, he has Thombolysis in Myocardial Infarction 3 flow to the coronary artery and his heart attack is aborted (see **Fig. 1**C). He is admitted to the intensive care unit and is discharged from the hospital 3 days later.

Marvin's case is an example of a systems approach to STEMI care. Although he lives in a rural area more than 60 miles from a PCI-capable hospital, his total time from arrival at the initial non–PCI-capable hospital to "artery open" was 57 minutes, and his time from first medical contact (ie, paramedics) to open artery was 77 minutes, both of which are well below the total door-to-balloon (D2B) time goal of less than 120 minutes for transferred patients.

INTRODUCTION

For patients who present with symptoms of cardiac ischemia of less than 24 hours with persistent ST-segment elevation or new left bundle-branch block, the immediate goal is to restore coronary flow and myocardial tissue perfusion as soon as possible. Primary PCI is the preferred reperfusion strategy if it can be performed in a timely manner by experienced providers (D2B time <120 minutes for transferred patients with STEMI and <90 minutes for patients with STEMI presenting to a PCI-capable hospital). Excellent prehospital care is essential to achieve timely reperfusion in STEMI patients.[1] In 2006, the National Heart Attack Alert Program of the National Heart, Lung, and Blood Institute, a division of the National Institutes of Health, recommended widespread implementation of PHECG as a key component to STEMI care systems.[2] Current American Heart Association (AHA)/American College of Cardiology (ACC) STEMI guidelines and AHA scientific statements also recommend implementation and integration of the PHECG.[3,4] Prehospital care is delivered by EMS systems, which include emergency medical dispatchers (EMDs), first responders (FRs), and ambulance response. There is considerable variation in the training and capabilities of the EMS providers in the United States depending on their location (ie, rural vs urban) and local jurisdictions. In this article, we review the key components of prehospital care of the patient with STEMI and the various levels of training and capabilities of EMS providers. Not only is EMS critical in the initial evaluation and transport of the patients, but it also plays an important role in interhospital transfers. Unfortunately, 40% to 50% of patients with STEMI in the United States do not use the EMS system but instead drive or are driven to the initial hospital by private vehicle.[5,6] We will discuss the critical role of EMS as part of STEMI systems of care.

COMPONENTS OF PREHOSPITAL CARE AND THE EMS SYSTEM

The 911 system is currently available to greater than 95% of the US population.[3] Most calls to 911 are answered by law enforcement or public safety officials responsible for operating 911 centers. Dispatchers may have very limited medical training, but some systems have dispatchers who are trained as an emergency medical technician (EMT) or as an EMD. Dispatchers operate according to standardized protocols. In addition to sending appropriate emergency units to a scene of a medical emergency, the dispatcher acts as the true "first responder" and is the first one to have contact with a patient or 911 caller. As part of their standardized protocols, many dispatch centers can give prearrival instructions that at times may be lifesaving for 911 callers. For example, callers can be instructed on how to perform cardiopulmonary resuscitation (CPR) in the event of cardiac arrest while awaiting the arrival of an EMS unit, or, in some protocols, the patient with chest pain can be instructed to take an aspirin as recommended in AHA/ACC guidelines.[1]

There are several different levels of competency and training standards for EMS personnel. The federal government currently has standard curricula developed by the National Highway Traffic Safety Administration for 4 different levels of EMS training: the emergency medical responder (EMR) (often known as the FR), the EMT, the advanced EMT (AEMT), and the paramedic (http://www.nhtsa.gov/people/injury/ems/emsscope.pdf) (**Table 1**). The National Registry of Emergency Medical Technicians (www.nremt.org) serves as a national board that follows federal training curricula and certifies providers according to their training levels. Although these standards and curricula exist, many states have their own regulations for each level of certification and variances, and not all states recognize the National Registry of Emergency Medical Technicians as their standard for training.

EMRs have minimal medical training, but they are able to initiate immediate lifesaving care to critical patients who access the EMS system. Their skill level provides them with basic life support (BLS) capabilities until a higher level of personnel arrives. The EMR is generally capable of administering first aid, oxygen, and CPR and can operate an automated external defibrillator (AED).

The EMT has more training than the EMR and is able to provide basic emergency care including transport of patients who access the EMS system. EMTs possess the skills and knowledge needed to use basic equipment that could be found on an ambulance (first aid, splinting, and CPR equipment and the AED are examples). In addition, the EMT is allowed to assist the patient with their own medications, give a diabetic oral glucose, and administer aspirin to a patient with chest pain. To minimize time to lifesaving treatment, most communities have FRs who are dispatched the same time as the ambulance but generally arrive before the ambulance and are able to initiate this lifesaving care. The FR may be trained at either the EMR or EMT level and is often a law enforcement member, firefighter, or, in some rural areas, local volunteer.

A level above the EMT is the AEMT. AEMTs receive medical training at a complex fundamental depth, including BLS to advanced life support (ALS). The AEMT is able to perform skills such as, but not limited to, intravenous line insertion and administration of sublingual nitroglycerin, subcutaneous injections, and nebulized medications. It should be noted that some states have variances that allow EMTs who are under medical direction (whether verbal or standing orders) to perform some of these listed skills.

The highest level of training recognized by the NHTSA is the paramedic. The paramedic is an

Table 1
Example of EMS skill set capabilities based on training level

	EMR	EMT	AEMT	Paramedic
Basic first aid skills	X	X	X	X
CPR	X	X	X	X
Basic airway management	X	X	X	X
Endotracheal intubation				X
Autoinjector medication administration	X	X	X	X
Assist patient with administration of their own medications	X	X	X	X
Administer physician-approved over-the-counter medications such as aspirin for chest pain		X	X	X
Administer sublingual nitroglycerin			X	X
Administer IV fluid infusion			X	X
Perform peripheral IV insertion			X	X
Perform intraosseous insertion			X	X
Administration of IV medications and IV drip lines				X
ACLS trained				X
Thrombolytic initiation				X
AED use	X	X	X	X
Manual defibrillation/cardioversion and transcutaneous pacing				X
12-Lead ECG acquisition		X	X	X
Interpretation of 12-lead ECG				X

Abbreviations: ACLS, advanced cardiac life support; AED, automated external defibrillator; IV, intravenous.

allied health professional who has undergone complex and comprehensive medical training from a nationally accredited paramedic program. Many paramedics possess an associate or 4-year degree. The paramedic is able to perform BLS and ALS and skills such as intubation, manual defibrillation/cardioversion, and chest decompression. Cardiology training includes assessment, medications, cardiac diseases, advanced cardiac life support, and ECG rhythm interpretation. The most recent version (2007) of the paramedic standards and curricula now include 12-lead ECG findings and interpretation (http://www.nhtsa.gov/people/injury/ems/emsscope.pdf).

Depending on where one lives, EMS configurations include a wide combination of EMS care available. Rural areas usually have BLS–capable ambulances provided by either community volunteers or municipal services. Many of the ambulance responders are basic EMTs and have the assistance of the EMR. Some rural areas are served by neighboring metropolitan ALS units. In some cases, rural EMS systems are able to call for "ALS intercepts." In this setting, the BLS unit responds to the scene, and if a higher level of care is warranted, the EMS unit may request a helicopter or ALS ground unit to the scene. In an ALS ground unit intercept, care is initiated and transport to the hospital is started with the ALS unit meeting the ambulance en route, jumping on board the BLS-capable ambulance, and then assisting with ALS care.

Urban and suburban EMS responses also have considerable variation. Nearly all metropolitan areas are provided with ALS (paramedic coverage) capability. Ambulance teams may consist of 2 paramedics, 1 paramedic and 1 EMT, or any other combination of providers that allows the unit to be ALS capable. EMS in these areas may be provided by paid fire department personnel, private EMS system personnel, or hospital-based or third-party EMS personnel. The FR unit is often a police and/or fire unit. Some metropolitan areas use a "2-tiered" response system in which the 911 call is screened and both a BLS unit and an ALS unit are sent to the scene. If ALS is unnecessary, the BLS unit can cancel the responding ALS unit. In contrast to many European countries, physicians are not present on ambulances in the prehospital setting in the United States.

Helicopter EMS (HEMS) has been used since the 1970s and is now available in most regions of the United States. These air critical care units respond to both trauma and medical emergencies and play an important role for small, rural critical access hospitals by providing transport of patients with STEMI to PCI-capable centers. When minutes count, helicopters can reduce the time of transport from the referring to the receiving hospital, or reduce time even further by responding directly to a scene and providing transport directly to a tertiary center. An Ohio study demonstrated potential time savings from first medical contact to balloon time when ground EMS units requested a helicopter to the scene for direct transport of the patient with STEMI to a PCI-capable center, rather than transport to a local hospital with subsequent transfer.[7] Median first medical contact to balloon time was 160 minutes for transfers initiated by the referring hospitals, 112 minutes for transfer of patients with STEMI by HEMS directly from the scene of the patient with STEMI, and 113 minutes for HEMS hospital rendezvous after ground EMS initiation of transfer. In contrast, a study from North Carolina reported treatment times for patients with STEMI transported by air were not faster than if they were transferred by ground.[8] This is likely related to both availability and "systems" issues. As in Ohio, HEMS has been a critical component of the "Minneapolis Heart Institute Level One MI" regional STEMI system (**Fig. 2**).[9,10]

Often, actual transport time by helicopter from the referring hospital to the receiving hospital may be shorter than ground ambulance transport time, but ground transport may be faster within a certain distance if transport is initiated immediately rather than waiting for a responding helicopter. Even if ground transport may be faster, however, hospitals may wait for the ALS care provided by HEMS personnel if the transporting ambulance is not ALS capable. HEMS may consist of any combination of a registered nurse, paramedic, respiratory therapist, or, in some cases, a physician.

Prehospital ECG

In its 2010 International Consensus on Cardiopulmonary Resuscitation and Emergency Cardiovascular Care Science with Treatment Recommendations Acute Coronary Syndromes report, the International Liaison Committee on Resuscitation states that, "The acquisition of a PHECG is essential for identification of patients with STEMI before hospital arrival and should be used in conjunction with pre-arrival hospital notification and concurrent activation of the catheter laboratory."[11] EMS units provide a major improvement in time to treatment when a PHECG can be obtained at first medical contact. Unfortunately, not all EMS units have the capability or equipment required to acquire a PHECG. Acquisition of a PHECG is much more common in the urban/suburban areas than in rural areas. A 2006 *Journal of Emergency Medical Services* 200-city study reported that 90.6% of America's 200 largest cities have 12-lead capabilities, and in a subsequent 2009 study of America's 200 largest cities, 58% of EMS systems had a protocol in place to guide patient transport to an appropriate cardiac center.[12,13]

With the availability of the PHECG to identify a patient with STEMI, a variety of protocols that allow paramedics to communicate the PHECG findings to a receiving hospital have been developed. The PHECG can be transmitted to the receiving hospital, where it is read by the emergency physician and/or the cardiologist, thus allowing activation of the CCL team for the patient with STEMI. Alternatively, paramedics can be trained to interpret the PHECG and activate the CCL team without physician interpretation of the 12-lead ECG. For example, in Minneapolis/St. Paul, paramedics are allowed to activate the CCL from the field if the 12-lead computer algorithm reports STEMI and the paramedic agrees with the reading in a patient with ischemic symptoms (chest pain or dyspnea). This does not include patients with left bundle-branch block (**Fig. 3**).

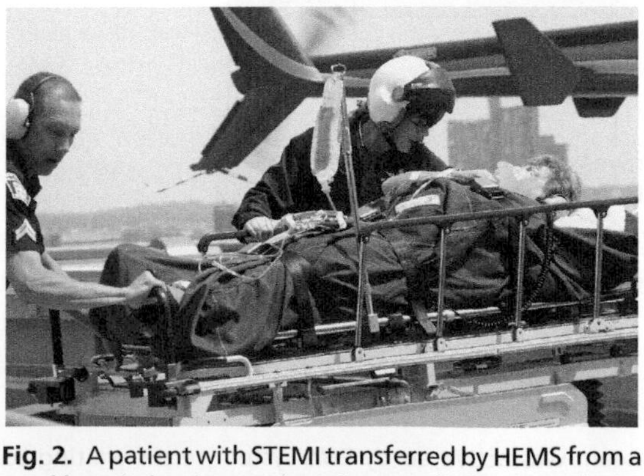

Fig. 2. A patient with STEMI transferred by HEMS from a rural hospital arrives at the Minneapolis Heart Institute.

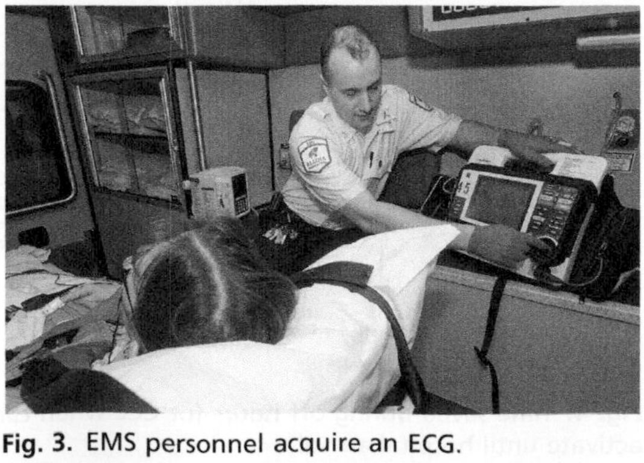

Fig. 3. EMS personnel acquire an ECG.

Studies report a decrease in D2B times of 15 to 20 minutes as a result of PHECG acquisition, and an even more substantial reduction occurs when the CCL team is activated in the field as a result of the PHECG.[4] The earlier the PHECG is performed and the CCL team is activated at the PCI-capable hospital, the faster is the D2B time. This is especially true during after-hours and on the weekends, when most CCL teams are not in-house. Prehospital activation allows "parallel processing" so the CCL team staff and the patient are simultaneously en route to the PCI-capable hospital, thus reducing D2B times (**Fig. 4**). Prehospital activation during the workday also has benefits for scheduling and treatment time. Some systems have recently allowed paramedics with field-activated patients who have STEMI to go directly to the CCL if the team is ready, thus bypassing the ED. For example, in Boston, Massachusetts, USA, paramedics bypass the ED when they believe they have a patient with a "definite" STEMI and stop in the ED for triage when they have a patient with a "possible" STEMI.[3]

Many studies show that paramedics can activate the CCL in the patient with STEMI with a high degree of accuracy. A study of 14 PCI-capable hospitals in North Carolina reported that of 3973 activations (29% by EMS personnel and 71% by emergency physicians) during a 1-year period, 85% of CCL activations were appropriate, and in 76.9% of the appropriate activations, the patient received PCI. Of the 15% inappropriate activations, 4.6% were ECG reinterpretations initially activated by an emergency physician and 6% were initially activated by EMS personnel. The other 4.3% of the inappropriate activations occurred in patients who were not CCL candidates.[14]

An additional study with urban/suburban US paramedics demonstrated a high degree of accuracy in diagnosing STEMI. Paramedics were given 5 brief scenarios with an associated 12-lead ECG and were asked to determine whether the 12-lead ECG demonstrated STEMI and if they would activate the CCL. For the STEMI diagnosis, sensitivity was 92.6% (95% confidence interval 88.9%–95.1%) and specificity was 85.4% (79.7%–89.8%). When asked if they would activate, the CCL sensitivity was 88.3% (83.8%–91.3%) and specificity was 88.3% (83.0%–92.2%). False activation occurred in only 8.1% (5.4%–12.0%) of cases.[15]

Unfortunately, frequently rural EMS and most BLS services do not have the equipment or training to acquire and transmit a PHECG. This is largely due to the cost of both training and equipment. In an effort to improve STEMI recognition and reduce treatment times in rural areas, more and more BLS services are obtaining PHECG monitors. BLS providers can be trained in proper PHECG acquisition and transmission of the PHECG to the hospital, where it can be interpreted by the emergency physician. A good example of this rural initiative can be found in South Dakota. In April 2010, the Helmsley Charitable Trust awarded the AHA an $8.4 million grant to build an STEMI system of care in this rural state, which covers nearly 76,000 square miles and has only 6 PCI-capable hospitals (3 in Sioux Falls). Parts of South Dakota are up to 350 miles from a PCI-capable facility. As part of the grant, every EMS system in the state will receive a monitor capable of 12-lead ECG acquisition and transmission. Expansion of this project is under way in North Dakota and is being considered in rural Minnesota.[16]

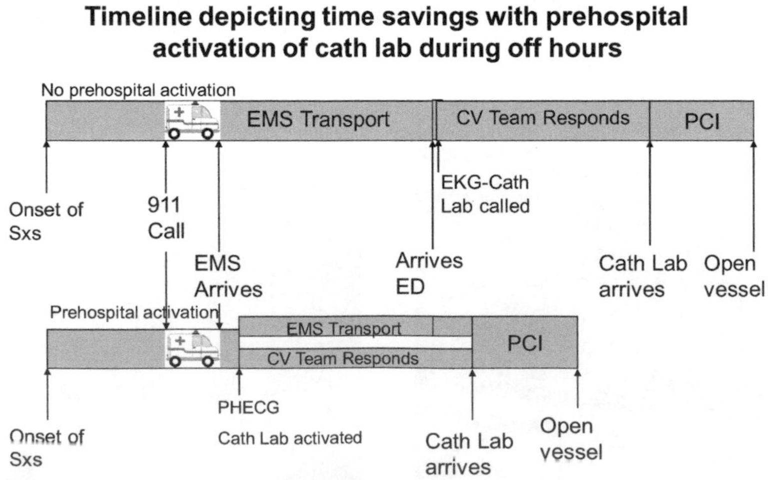

Fig. 4. Time saved during off hours for CCL when cardiac team was activated by EMS system versus waiting to activate until hospital arrival.

Prehospital Destination Protocols in STEMI System

Prehospital diagnosis of STEMI with direct triage to a PCI-capable hospital has been shown to reduce time to treatment (**Fig. 5**). A study from Denmark compared the time from ambulance call to balloon in 3 different groups of patients. Group A patients did not have a prehospital ECG and initially were admitted to a local hospital, followed by transfer to a PCI-capable hospital. Group B patients had a prehospital diagnosis of STEMI and were initially admitted to a local hospital, with subsequent transfer to a PCI-capable hospital. Group C had a prehospital diagnosis of STEMI with triage to a PCI-capable hospital. The time from initial ambulance call to balloon was 168 minutes (179–347) for group A, 127 minutes (115–156) for group B, and 87 minutes (82–102) for group C (*P*<.001), demonstrating the benefit of both prehospital diagnosis and bypass of non–PCI-capable hospitals to PCI-capable hospitals.[17] One of the first cities to organize a prehospital STEMI system was Boston, where paramedics perform prehospital ECGs and reliably transport "definite" patients with STEMI directly to the CCL at PCI-capable hospitals.[18] Their system also performs rigorous quality assessment with feedback to the EMS and hospital providers.

A standardized protocol for primary PCI was implemented for the entire metropolitan area of Ottawa, Ontario, Canada, in 2005. Paramedics were trained to perform and interpret PHECG and patients with STEMI who were diagnosed in the field were transported directly to a PCI-capable hospital. In addition, all patients with STEMI who presented by private vehicle to a non–PCI-capable hospital were transferred according to protocol to

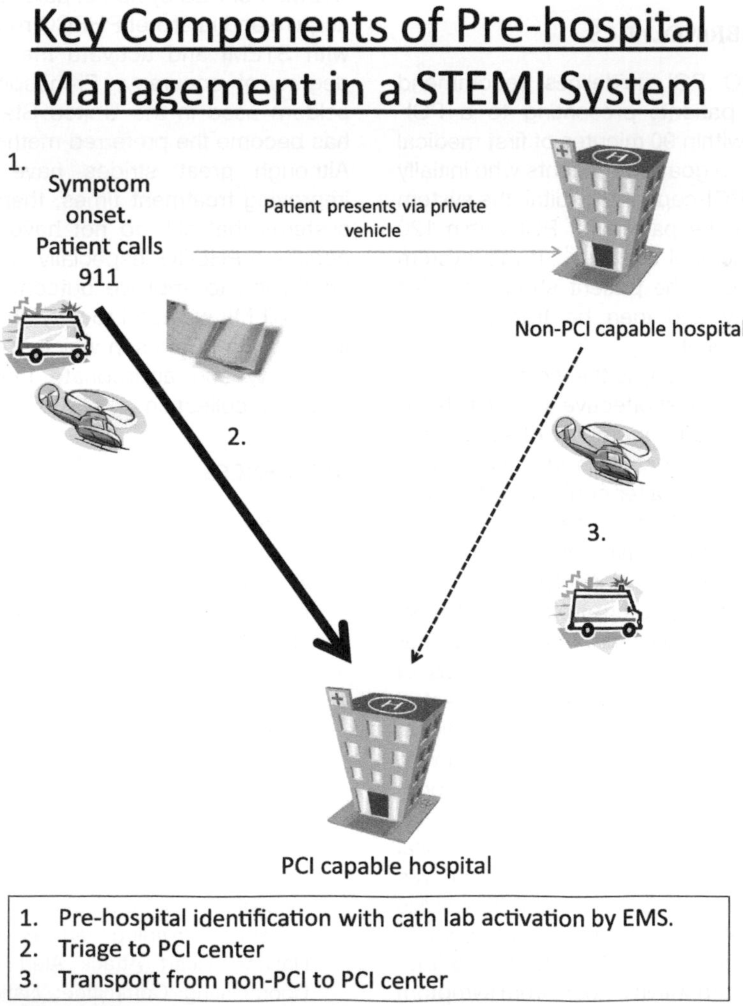

Fig. 5. Patient flow diagram from symptom (Sx) onset to PCI illustrating key components of prehospital care.

a PCI-capable hospital. The median D2B times were significantly shorter for patients triaged directly to the PCI center (69 minutes; interquartile range, 43–87) than for patients undergoing transfer (123 minutes; interquartile range, 101 to 153; $P<.001$). The percentage of patients with a D2B time of less than 90 minutes triaged directly from the field was 79.7% compared with 11.9% for those transferred from a non–PCI-capable hospital ED ($P<.001$).[19]

More recently, the success of a prehospital STEMI system has been demonstrated in several metropolitan areas in the United States. In a pooled analysis of 10 independent regional STEMI receiving center networks, paramedics transported 2712 patients with a PHECG diagnosis of STEMI directly to an STEMI receiving center network (PCI-capable hospital). A PCI was performed in 2053 (76%) of patients with a D2B time of less than 90 minutes in 86% of the cases. Even more remarkable, the PHECG to balloon time was less than 90 minutes in 68% of patients.[20]

PREHOSPITAL FIBRINOLYTICS

Current AHA/ACC PCI guidelines recommend primary PCI for patients presenting to a PCI-capable hospital within 90 minutes of first medical contact as a system goal. For patients who initially present to a non–PCI-capable hospital, the system goal is to transfer the patient for PCI within 120 minutes of first medical contact.[21] If this system goal is not possible, the patient should receive fibrinolytic therapy and then be transferred to a PCI-capable hospital.

When fibrinolytic therapy is the indicated reperfusion strategy, it is most effective if administered as early as possible after the onset of symptoms. Therefore, it seemed reasonable to administer a fibrinolytic in the ambulance after confirming the diagnosis of an STEMI with the use of a PHECG. Several randomized trials have compared prehospital to ED administration of a fibrinolytic.[22–24] These trials indicated shorter symptom-to-treatment intervals with prehospital fibrinolysis but without a clear benefit in mortality. However, a meta-analysis of data from 6 randomized trials ($n = 6434$) suggested a decrease in all-cause mortality among patients treated with prehospital fibrinolysis compared with in-hospital fibrinolysis (odds ratio, 0.83; 95% confidence interval, 0.70–0.98).[25]

The Comparison of Angioplasty and Pre-hospital Thrombolysis in acute Myocardial Infarction was a French study comparing prehospital fibrinolysis (in ambulances staffed by physicians) with primary PCI in patients with STEMI. Patients with STEMI who were randomized within 2 hours from symptom onset had a strong trend toward lower 30-day mortality with prehospital fibrinolysis compared with primary PCI (2.2% vs 5.7%, $P = .058$).[26]

Prehospital fibrinolysis is seldom used in the United States because primary PCI is available in most cities and even in rural areas, where it would be most appropriate, the availability of PHECG and appropriately trained EMS personnel are scarce.[27] Therefore, fibrinolysis is usually administered in the local community hospital rather than in the prehospital setting. In contrast, in Canada and some European countries where ambulances are staffed by physicians, prehospital fibrinolysis is used when primary PCI may not be available in a timely manner.[28]

SUMMARY

Depending on where one lives, a wide variety of combinations of EMS levels of care exist in the United States. The PHECG has been a key factor in reducing time to treatment in the patient with STEMI. For ALS systems, paramedics can reliably acquire and interpret PHECG results in the patient with STEMI and activate the CCL with a high degree of accuracy. Prehospital fibrinolysis is seldom used in the United States because PCI has become the preferred method of reperfusion. Although great strides have been made in improving treatment times, there are many EMS systems that still do not have the capability to acquire a PHECG, especially in the rural areas. In continuing to improve outcomes for the patient with STEMI, we need to strive for an EMS system in the United States in which 100% have PHECG capability and appropriate funding for training and data collection.

REFERENCES

1. Antman EM, Anbe DT, Armstrong PW, et al. ACC/AHA guidelines for the management of patients with ST-elevation myocardial infarction–executive summary: a report of the American College of Cardiology/American Heart Association Task Force on Practice Guidelines (Writing Committee to Revise the 1999 Guidelines for the Management of Patients With Acute Myocardial Infarction). Circulation 2004;110:588–636.
2. Garvey JL, MacLeod BA, Sopko G, on behalf of the National Heart Attack Alert Program (NHAAP) Coordinating Committee. Pre-hospital 12-lead electrocardiography programs: a call for implementation by emergency medical services systems providing advanced life support—National Heart Attack Alert Program (NHAAP) Coordinating Committee; National Heart, Lung, and Blood Institute (NHLBI); National Institutes of

Health. J Am Coll Cardiol 2006;47:485–91. http://dx.doi.org/10.1016/j.jacc.2005.08.072.
3. Moyer P, Ornato JP, Brady WJ, et al. Development of systems of care for ST-elevation myocardial infarction patients. Circulation 2007;116:e43–8.
4. Ting HH, Krumholz HM, Bradley EH, et al. Implementation and integration of prehospital ECGs into systems of care for acute coronary syndromes: a scientific statement from the American Heart Association Interdisciplinary Council on Quality of Care and Outcomes Research, Emergency Cardiovascular Care Committee, Council on Cardiovascular Nursing, and Council on Clinical Cardiology. Circulation 2008;118:1066–79.
5. Mathews R, Peterson ED, Li S, et al. Use of emergency medical service transport among patients with ST-segment-elevation myocardial infarction: findings from the National Cardiovascular Data Registry Acute Coronary Treatment Intervention Outcomes Network Registry—Get With the Guidelines. Circulation 2011;124:154–63.
6. Luepker RV, Raczynski JM, Osganian S, et al. Effect of a community intervention on patient delay and emergency medical service use in acute coronary heart disease: the Rapid Early Action for Coronary Treatment (REACT) Trial. JAMA 2000;284:60–7.
7. McMullan JT, Hinckley WH, Bentley J, et al. Ground emergency medical services requests for helicopter transfer of ST-segment elevation myocardial infarction patients decrease medical contact to balloon times in rural and suburban settings. Acad Emerg Med 2012;19:153–9.
8. Jollis JG, Al-Khalidi HR, Monk L, et al. Expansion of a regional ST-segment elevation myocardial infarction system to an entire state. Circulation 2012; 126(2):189–95.
9. Henry TD, Sharkey SE, Burke MN, et al. A regional system to provide timely access to percutaneous coronary intervention for ST-elevation myocardial infarction. Circulation 2007;116:721–8.
10. Graham KJ, Strauss CE, Boland LL, et al. Has the time come for a national cardiovascular emergency care system? Circulation 2012;125:2035–44.
11. O'Connor RE, Bossaert L, Arntz H- R, on behalf of the Acute Coronary Syndrome Chapter Collaborators. Part 9: acute coronary syndromes: 2010 International Consensus on Cardiopulmonary Resuscitation and Emergency Cardiovascular Care Science With Treatment Recommendations. Circulation 2010;122:S422–65.
12. Williams DM. 2006 JEMS 200-city survey: EMS from all angles. JEMS 2007;32:38–46.
13. Williams DM, Ragone M. 2009 JEMS 200-city survey: zeroing in on what matters. JEMS 2010;35:38–42.
14. Garvey JL, Monk L, Granger CB, et al. Rates of cardiac catheterization for ST-segment elevation myocardial infarction after activation by emergency medical services or emergency physicians: results from the North Carolina Catheterization Laboratory Activation Registry. Circulation 2012;125:308–13.
15. Trivedi K, Schuur JD, Cone DC. Can paramedics read ST-segment elevation myocardial infarction on prehospital 12-lead electrocardiograms? Prehosp Emerg Care 2009;13:207–14.
16. Helmsley Grant to Improve Heart Attack Care in South Dakota. 2010. Retrieved from American Heart Association Mission Life Line. Available at: www.heart.org/HEARTORG/Affiliate/Helmsley-Grant-to-Improve-Heart-Attack-Care-in-South-Dakota_UCM_308139_Article.jsp. Accessed April 16, 2012.
17. Studnek JR, Garvey L, Blackwell T, et al. Association between prehospital time intervals and ST-elevation myocardial infarction system performance. Circulation 2010;122:1464–9.
18. Moyer P, Feldman J, Levine J, et al. Implications of the mechanical (PCI) vs thrombolytic controversy for ST segment elevation myocardial infarction on the organization of emergency medical services: the Boston EMS experience. Crit Pathw Cardiol 2004;3:53–61.
19. Le May MR, So DY, Dionne R, et al. A citywide protocol for primary PCI in ST-segment elevation myocardial infarction. N Engl J Med 2008;358:231–40.
20. Rokos IC, French WJ, Koenig WJ, et al. Integration of pre-hospital electrocardiograms and ST-elevation myocardial infarction receiving center (SRC) networks: impact on door-to-balloon times across 10 independent regions. JACC Cardiovasc Interv 2009;2:339–46.
21. Levine GN, Bates ER, Blankenship JC, et al. 2011 ACCF/AHA/SCAI guideline for percutaneous coronary intervention: a report of the American College of Cardiology Foundation/American Heart Association Task Force on Practice Guidelines and the Society for Cardiovascular Angiography and Interventions. Circulation 2011;124:2574–609.
22. The European Myocardial Infarction Project Group. Prehospital thrombolytic therapy in patients with suspected acute myocardial infarction. N Engl J Med 1993;329:383–9.
23. Weaver WD, Cerqueira M. Prehospital-initiated vs hospital-initiated thrombolytic therapy. The Myocardial Infarction Triage and Intervention Trial. JAMA 1993;270:1211–6.
24. Morrow D, Antman E, Sayah A, et al. Evaluation of the time saved by prehospital initiation of retaplase for ST-elevation myocardial infarction. Results of the Early Retavase-Thrombolysis in Myocardial Infarction (ER-TIMI) 19 Trial. J Am Coll Cardiol 2002;40:71–7.
25. Morrison LJ, Verbeek PR, McDonald AC, et al. Mortality and prehospital thrombolysis for acute myocardial infarction. JAMA 2000;283:2686–92.
26. Steg G, Bonnefoy E. Impact of time to treatment on mortality after prehospital fibrinolysis or primary

angioplasty. Data from the CAPTIM randomized clinical trial. Circulation 2003;108:2851–6.
27. Henry TD, Gersh BJ. Is there a role for prehospital fibrinolysis in North America? JACC Cardiovasc Interv 2011;4:884–6.
28. Huynh T, Birkhead J, Huber K, et al. The prehospital fibrinolysis experience in Europe and North America and implications for wider dissemination. JACC Cardiovasc Interv 2011;4:877–83.

Percutaneous Left Ventricular Assist Devices

Amit B. Sharma, MD, Jason C. Kovacic, MD, PhD,
Annapoorna S. Kini, MD*

KEYWORDS

• P-LVAD • IABP • Hemodynamics • Catheter

KEY POINTS

- Percutaneous left ventricular assist devices (P-LVADs) can be life saving and may permit the stabilization of a patient in cardiovascular collapse who would otherwise face imminent demise.
- For specific patients and clinical indications, or where a greater degree of hemodynamic support is required, numerous studies have demonstrated the feasibility and safety of the newer generation P-LVADs, particularly Impella 2.5 (Abiomed Inc., Aachen, Germany) and TandemHeart (CardiacAssist, Pittsburgh, PA, USA).
- Inotropic and vasopressor agents enabling rapid improvement and stabilization of hemodynamic parameters in patients suffering from cardiovascular compromise are often used in combination with P-LVADs, adding even greater hemodynamic support.
- The potential applications for P-LVADs have continued to expand, now including diverse uses such as support for cardiogenic shock, bridge to and following cardiac surgery, and more novel applications such as complex electrophysiologic mapping and ablation studies of unstable ventricular rhythms.

Percutaneous left ventricular assist devices (P-LVAD) have been in existence for more than 4 decades,[1,2] significantly predating percutaneous coronary intervention (PCI). Used for the correct indication and in a timely fashion, these devices can be life saving and may permit the stabilization of a patient in cardiovascular collapse who would otherwise face imminent demise.

While intra-aortic balloon counterpulsation remains the gold-standard P-LVAD, there has been considerable recent evolution in other supportive technologies, with devices such as the Impella and TandemHeart now being increasingly used in the catheterization laboratory and other settings.[3] This evolution in P-LVAD technology has been paralleled by advances in other adjunctive supportive measures, particularly pharmacological cardiac support. There are now a broad range of inotropic and vasopressor agents enabling rapid improvement and stabilization of hemodynamic parameters in patients suffering from cardiovascular compromise, and these are often used in combination with P-LVADs, adding even greater hemodynamic support. Concurrently, the potential applications for P-LVADs has continued to expand, now including diverse uses, such as support for cardiogenic shock, bridge to and following cardiac surgery, and more novel applications such as complex electrophysiologic mapping and ablation studies of unstable ventricular rhythms.[4]

Device evolution has been constant since the inception of the P-LVAD. However, the constancy and overall track record of the intra-aortic balloon pump (IABP), discussed later in this article, is impressive. Beyond the IABP, numerous other devices have been developed and entered into

No specific funding or grant was used to fund this study. Jason C. Kovacic is supported by National Institutes of Health Grant 1K08HL111330-01.
Cardiac Catheterization Laboratory of the Cardiovascular Institute, Mount Sinai Hospital, One Gustave L. Levy Place, Box 1030, New York, NY 10029, USA
* Corresponding author.
E-mail address: annapoorna.kini@mountsinai.org

Intervent Cardiol Clin 1 (2012) 609–622
http://dx.doi.org/10.1016/j.iccl.2012.07.003
2211-7458/12/$ – see front matter

clinical use. The femoro-femoral cardiopulmonary support system (CPS) was another early device used to provide circulatory support. Although CPS provided adequate hemodynamic assistance, it required a perfusionist to operate, a high level of anticoagulation, and was associated with significant problems, including bleeding and access site complications.[5,6] As a result of these limitations, the CPS device is no longer commercially available. Another P-LVAD, the Hemopump cardiac assist system (Johnson & Johnson Interventional Systems; Rancho Cordova, California, USA) also fell out of favor because of increased morbidity and mortality associated with the use of large-size arterial cannulae, thromboembolic complications, and the need for an anesthesiologist or a perfusionist.[7,8] Currently available P-LVADs that are reviewed in this article include the IABP, TandemHeart, Impella 2.5, and Reitan catheter pump (RCP) (CardioBridge GmbH, Hechingen, Germany) (**Table 1**).

OPTIMAL P-LVAD FEATURES

The constant evolution of P-LVAD technologies has occurred in parallel with the evolution of the role of the catheterization laboratory in the care of stable and unstable patients with cardiovascular disease, and has recently also expanded into the cardiothoracic surgical setting, where the possibility of performing minimally invasive coronary artery bypass graft surgery via small incisions and without cardiopulmonary bypass has opened the door for P-LVADs to be used in the surgical arena. Considering all salient factors, desirable features of contemporary P-LVADs include all of the following:

- Accessibility: the device should be readily accessible and be amenable to rapid placement and operation.
- Simplicity of use: both for insertion and operation, the device should be simple to use and should require a minimum of training and expertise.
- Hemodynamic efficacy: the device should provide adequate hemodynamic support, reduce left ventricular filling pressures, decrease myocardial oxygen consumption, and improve the supply-demand ratio.
- Safety: the device insertion procedure should be simple, ideally without an external blood circuit. Access catheters should be small bore, and devices should be atraumatic to the patient. The likelihood of hemolysis, platelet consumption, disseminated intravascular coagulation, or other blood disorder should be negligible.
- Dwelling time: it should be possible to leave the device in place for a period of several hours to 2 to 3 days without the risk of thrombosis, hemolysis, or infection.
- Weaning and Removal: device removal should be benign without significant pain, bleeding or vascular complications.

INDICATIONS AND COMMON CLINICAL USE

The indications for P-LVAD use are varied and continue to expand. Although their use in situations such as cardiogenic shock in ST-segment myocardial infarction (STEMI) is strongly supported by guideline recommendations, in many contemporary scenarios, guidelines are yet to be formulated. In the catheterization laboratory, other common indications/uses are cardiovascular collapse of any cause or prophylaxis during high-risk PCI.[3] It is currently estimated that the IABP is used in greater than 30% of patients undergoing complex procedures in the United States.[9] Beyond this, P-LVADs have long been a cornerstone of heart failure management, but their role in this field is increasing as patients may now be bridged to a surgically implanted LVAD (or right ventricular assist device) or cardiac transplantation. P-LVADs have also recently been used in the electrophysiology suite and as an adjunct to cardiothoracic surgical procedures. Essentially, a P-LVAD may be considered for any condition in which there is marked hemodynamic compromise.

In the catheterization laboratory, a STEMI patient with cardiogenic shock remains the "classic" indication for the insertion of a P-LVAD. Cardiogenic shock occurs in approximately 7% to 10% of STEMI patients and is the leading cause of in-hospital death. In-hospital mortality rates of STEMI complicated by cardiogenic shock are around 50%, despite reperfusion by PCI.[10] It is strongly reflected in the current American Heart Association/American College of Cardiology guidelines (**Table 2**) that the insertion of an IABP should be performed for STEMI patients presenting with cardiogenic shock or preshock to support the endangered circulation and failing myocardium.[11] For various reasons including ability to be rapidly deployed with minimal personnel present and that it is familiar to any critical cardiac care unit, the IABP remains the device of choice in this setting. Indeed, other devices are not mentioned in the most recent iterations of these guidelines. However, it is thought that there is a niche indication for the Impella P-LVAD in STEMI patients with extremely high left ventricular end-diastolic pressures (>30–35 mm Hg). In these patients, who usually have very sluggish coronary flow and poor myocardial capillary perfusion, the Impella may be

Table 1
Currently available P-LVADs

Percutaneous Ventricular Assist Devices						
Device	**Pump**	**Speed (rpm)**	**Duration**	**Cardiac Support (L/min)**	**Anticoagulation**	**Motor**
IABP	Balloon counterpulsation	n/a	Typically <7 d but may be longer	Variable - difficult to quantitate	Typically not required with current devices	Gas expanded balloon system
TandemHeart	Centrifugal	300–7500	Up to 14 d	Up to 4	Required ACT 250–300 s	Rotor powered by electromagnetic coupling
Impella 2.5	Axial	Up to 50,000	Up to 5 d	Up to 2.5	Required ACT 250–300 s. ACT >300 s if using bivalirudin	Integrated electric motor
RCP	Axial	Up to 13,000	Up to 5.5 h	Up to 20 (in vitro)	Required ACT 250–300 s	Drive unit connected to propeller by wire

Table 2
American Heart Association/American College of Cardiology recommendations for IABP use in STEMI patients

Class I	
Intra-aortic balloon counterpulsation should be used in STEMI patients with hypotension (systolic blood pressure <90 mm Hg or 30 mm Hg below baseline mean arterial pressure) who do not respond to other interventions, unless further support is futile because of the patient's wishes or contraindications/unsuitability for further invasive care.	Level of evidence: B
Intra-aortic balloon counterpulsation is recommended for STEMI patients with low-output state.	Level of evidence: B
Intra-aortic balloon counterpulsation is recommended for STEMI patients when cardiogenic shock is not quickly reversed with pharmacologic therapy. IABP is a stabilizing measure for angiography and prompt revascularization.	Level of evidence: B
Intra-aortic balloon counterpulsation should be used in addition to medical therapy for STEMI patients with recurrent ischemic-type chest discomfort and signs of hemodynamic instability, poor LV function, or a large area of myocardium at risk. Such patients should be referred urgently for cardiac catheterization and should undergo revascularization as needed.	Level of evidence: C
Class IIa	
It is reasonable to manage STEMI patients with refractory polymorphic ventricular tachycardia with intra-aortic balloon counterpulsation to reduce myocardial ischemia.	Level of evidence: B
Class IIb	
It may be reasonable to use intra-aortic balloon counterpulsation in the management of STEMI patients with refractory pulmonary congestion.	Level of evidence: C

From Antman EM, Anbe DT, Armstrong PW, et al. ACC/AHA guidelines for the management of patients with ST-elevation myocardial infarction–executive summary. A report of the American College of Cardiology/American Heart Association Task Force on Practice Guidelines (Writing Committee to revise the 1999 guidelines for the management of patients with acute myocardial infarction). J Am Coll Cardiol 2004;44:671–719.

able to effectively decant the left ventricle and thereby improve coronary flow dynamics.

INTRA-AORTIC BALLOON PUMP

The IABP was the first P-LVAD to gain widespread popularity. The earliest reports of the use of an IABP are traceable to 1968, when Kantrowitz and colleagues[2] reported on its use in a series of patients with cardiogenic shock in the setting of acute myocardial infarction. Since then, its use has progressively increased in providing circulatory support to patients with a broad spectrum of conditions. Progressive technological improvements in balloon design, the bedside counterpulsation pump, triggering mechanisms for balloon inflation/deflation, insertion sheaths, and access requirements have made IABP a simple-to-use device that can be rapidly inserted in any catheterization laboratory or even at the bedside without the use of fluoroscopic equipment. Current generation devices are sold as an over-the-wire system that can be inserted via a 7.5F introducer sheath (**Fig. 1**), which allows for a smaller arteriotomy and occupies decreased cross-sectional area in the iliofemoral vessels, permitting satisfactory distal flow in cases of significant peripheral arterial disease. The catheter is equipped with a fiberoptic sensor that allows timing accuracy and beat-to-beat adjustment depending on the patient hemodynamics. Owing to the ease of percutaneous implantation, the low cost, and the beneficial hemodynamics at a low complication rate, IABP continues to be the most popular P-LVAD in the catheterization laboratory. Major contraindications to its use include severe peripheral vascular disease, severe aortic disease and/or tortuosity, and worse than moderate aortic incompetence.

IAPB Hemodynamic Effects

The hemodynamic effects of the IABP include decreases in heart rate, left ventricular end-diastolic pressure, mean left atrial pressure, afterload, and myocardial oxygen consumption, the latter by up to 30%. The IABP also modestly increases coronary perfusion pressure and decreases the right atrial

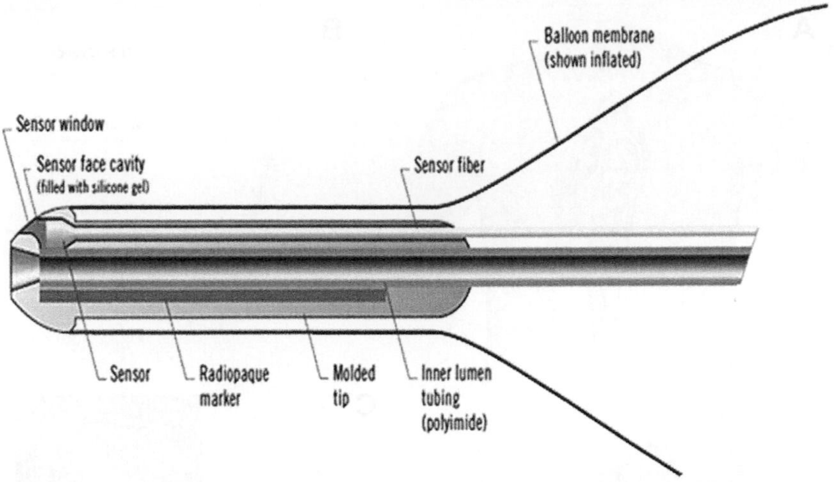

Fig. 1. Schematic diagram of a modern IABP catheter. The fiberoptic sensor facilitates faster calibration and reduces signal delay compared with older fluid-filled systems.

pressure, pulmonary artery pressure, and pulmonary vascular resistance.[12] It has little effect on micro vascular flow in the setting of acute myocardial infarction and provides only modest enhancement in cardiac output. Importantly, and distinguishing it from other P-LVADS, the IABP requires a certain residual level of left ventricular function to be effective.

Recent Pivotal IABP Studies

As discussed earlier, the IABP has a Class I indication for use in various patients with STEMI and cardiogenic shock. Surprisingly, a recent meta-analysis of randomized trials of IABP use in STEMI with cardiogenic shock showed neither a 30-day survival benefit nor improved left ventricular ejection fraction, although being associated with significantly higher stroke and bleeding rates.[13] The use of IABP was apparently beneficial when used as an adjunct to thrombolysis, but the data were limited by potential confounding and bias.[13] Nevertheless, this meta-analysis data have not led to any appreciable chance in practice or practice guidelines at the current time.

In another recent study titled Counterpulsation to Reduce Infarct Size Pre-PCI Acute Myocardial Infarction (CRISP-AMI), the investigators studied initiation of IABP therapy before primary PCI and continuation for more than or equal to 12 hours versus primary PCI alone in anterior wall STEMI patients without cardiogenic shock.[14] The primary outcome, mean infarct size, showed a borderline trend toward being worse in the IABP plus PCI versus the PCI alone group (42.1% [95% confidence interval (CI), 38.7%–45.6%] vs 37.5% [95% CI, 34.3%–40.8%], $P = .06$, respectively). Furthermore, clinical outcomes at 6 months were not significantly different between the 2 groups. However, 8.5% of patients in the PCI alone group crossed over to rescue IABP use. The investigators concluded that the CRISP-AMI study supports standby rather than routine use of IABP therapy during primary PCI in anterior STEMI patients without cardiogenic shock.[14]

TANDEMHEART

The TandemHeart P-LVAD (**Fig. 2**A) is a left atrial-to-femoral artery bypass system that can provide short-term circulatory support.[15] In an animal model of acute myocardial infarction with cardiogenic shock, the TandemHeart device restored endocardial (microvascular) and epicardial blood flow to baseline and resulted in a substantial reduction in infarct size.[16] Unlike the IABP, the TandemHeart device can provide temporary support in the absence of effective left ventricular function. It has been used in a variety of situations, including high-risk PCI, acute myocardial infarction with cardiogenic shock, and decompensated heart failure.[3,17]

There are 3 subsystems that make up the TandemHeart device. The first subsystem is a 21F polyurethane venous transseptal inflow cannula (see **Fig. 2**B). This cannula has a curved design at its end to facilitate tip placement, a large end hole at its distal tip, and 14 side holes to aspirate oxygenated blood from the left atrium. The obturator has a tapered tip to allow for easy insertion into the left atrium. The cannula is attached to a continuous-flow centrifugal pump, which in turn, is driven by a servomotor capable of delivering up to 5.0 L/min of blood flow. The design features a hydrodynamic fluid bearing that supports the

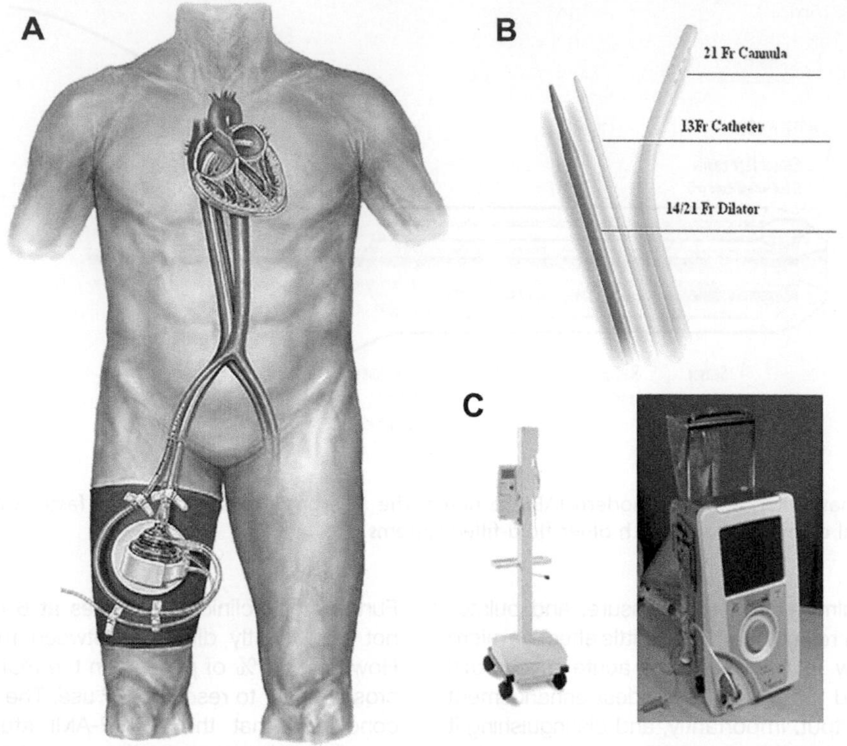

Fig. 2. The TandemHeart P-LVAD. (*A*) The TandemHeart P-LVAD provides circulatory support by continuously withdrawing oxygenated blood from the left atrium by way of a transseptal cannula placed via the femoral vein. The pump then returns blood to the femoral artery. The hemodynamic effects of the TandemHeart include an increase in cardiac output and blood pressure and a decrease in afterload and preload, thus decreasing myocardial oxygen demand. (*B*) Polyurethane 21F venous transseptal inflow cannula with large end hole and 14 side holes to allow aspiration of oxygenated blood from the left atrium. A 2-stage (14/21F) dilator is used to dilate the transseptal puncture after a 0.035 in pigtail guidewire is inserted into the left atrium. The obturator is tapered at its tip to allow easy insertion into the left atrium. (*C*) The TandemHeart controller is a custom designed system for driving the pump and supplying lubrication fluid. (*Courtesy of* CardiacAssist, Pittsburgh, PA; with permission.)

spinning rotor. The fluid bearing is supplied by a lubrication system, which feeds a nominal 10 mL/h of saline to which an anticoagulant (typically heparin) is added. The fluid acts as a coolant and lubricant for the seal that separates the rotor chamber from the blood chamber, and the anticoagulant is delivered to the blood chamber precisely at the seal interface to minimize the risk of thrombus formation. Power is supplied by an electromagnetic motor that operates at 3000 to 7500 rpm. Blood is delivered from the pump to the femoral artery with an arterial perfusion catheter. This catheter ranges from 15F to 17F and pumps blood from the left atrium to the femoral artery. Alternatively, two 12F arterial perfusion catheters may simultaneously pump blood into the right and left femoral arteries. The pump is operated via the dedicated external microprocessor-based controller. A pressure transducer monitors the infusion pressure and identifies any disruption in the infusion line. An in-line air bubble detector monitors for the presence of air in the infusion line.

Patient Selection and Contraindications

Because of the need for venous and arterial access, large cannulae, and more complicated insertion requiring transseptal puncture, the TandemHeart device cannot be inserted as swiftly as an IABP. The presence of left atrial thrombus is an absolute contraindication. Patients who have a ventricular septal defect are not good candidates for the TandemHeart because of the risk of hypoxemia due to right-to-left shunting. Because of the retrograde flow of blood from the femoral return catheters back up the aorta, the left ventricle can become distended in the setting of severe left ventricular dysfunction, and aortic insufficiency is another contraindication to the TandemHeart. Further, because of the retrograde passage of blood into the femoral artery, and the large femoral access catheter, the TandemHeart can induce critical limb ischemia in patients with severe peripheral vascular disease.

In addition to providing hemodynamic support in patients who have cardiogenic shock and in high-risk PCI patients, potential applications for the TandemHeart include to provide cardiovascular support during high-risk aortic valvuloplasty and percutaneous aortic valve replacement. This potential niche application arises because the TandemHeart device (unlike the Impella) does not lie across the aortic valve and permits unrestricted aortic valve access. Also, the TandemHeart device can serve as a percutaneous right ventricular assist device for right heart failure.[18]

Implantation

The TandemHeart is implanted in the cardiac catheterization laboratory or surgical operating suite. With a few minor variations, the typical implantation procedure involves the following steps:

I: Femoral artery preclosure with the Perclose device[3,17]

- An ipsilateral oblique projection femoral artery angiogram using a microaccess catheter is obtained. This angiogram should delineate the anatomy of the iliofemoral system and rule out significant peripheral vascular disease.
- If the vessel anatomy is conducive (stick in the common femoral artery, artery size >5 mm), the microsheath is exchanged for a 6F sheath. If the stick is found to be in the superficial femoral or profunda femoris artery, the microcatheter is removed, manual compression applied, and hemostasis achieved. Using the angiographic anatomy obtained previously, a higher stick is then performed under fluoroscopy, and a 6F sheath is introduced into the common femoral artery.
- A regular "J-tip" wire is inserted through the 6F sheath and the sheath removed, leaving the J-tip wire in the artery. The 2 Perclose devices (Abbott Vascular, Redwood City, CA, USA) are then sequentially deployed at a 60° to 90° angle to each other (2 o'clock and 11 o'clock positions), yielding 2 sets of suture limbs angled 60° to 90° apart. The sutures are harvested and secured using artery forceps, with care taken to avoid advancing the suture knots down to the arterial wall. A 6F sheath (or larger) is then reinserted over the J-wire.[3,17]

II: Transseptal puncture and cannula placement

- The femoral vein is accessed and transseptal puncture performed under fluoroscopic guidance using a Brockenbrough needle and Mullins sheath as is done during balloon mitral valvuloplasty.
- After confirming the position of the Mullins sheath in the left atrium, unfractionated heparin is given to achieve a target-activated clotting time (ACT) greater than 300 seconds.
- The Mullins sheath is exchanged for the 14/21F 2-stage dilator over a 0.038 in J-tip 260 cm Amplatz Super Stiff Guidewire (Boston Scientific Corp., Natick, MA, USA).
- The 21F transseptal cannula is advanced with the 14F obturator over the Amplatz Super Stiff Guidewire and placed in the left atrium.
- The position of the cannula in the left atrium is confirmed by pressure tracing, injecting dye and/or drawing blood and assessing oxygen saturation.
- The obturator and wire are removed and clamps applied for temporary homeostasis. Care should be taken to place all the side holes of the cannula into the left atrium to avoid possible right-to-left shunting during device operation.
- The peripheral end of the cannula is sutured to the skin of the patient's thigh and clamped. The left femoral artery 6F sheath is exchanged for the 15F arterial perfusion cannula with the distal end of the cannula positioned above the aortic bifurcation.
- The peripheral end of the cannula is similarly sutured to the patient's thigh and clamped.

III: Connecting cannulae with the pump, de-airing, and initiation of mechanical support

- After the air is purged from the extracorporeal system, the transseptal cannula is attached to the inflow port of the centrifugal blood pump in the standard wet-to-wet fashion with 3/8 in Tygon tubing.
- The femoral arterial cannula is similarly connected to the outflow conduit of the pump after de-airing.
- A heparinized saline infusate is started according to the product specification, which provides hydrodynamic bearing, anticoagulation, and local cooling for the motor of the pump.
- The pump is connected to the device controller and its speed adjusted to provide support of 2.5 to 3.0 L/min.

- The power supply for the TandemHeart is subsequently connected to the microprocessor-based controller.

In experienced centers, TandemHeart device insertion, assembly, and mechanical circulatory support are accomplished in 30 minutes or less. At the authors' institution, the average time for the entire insertion procedure ranges between 14 and 25 minutes.[17]

Because of the risk of thromboembolic complications, systemic anticoagulation with unfractionated heparin to maintain an ACT of 400 seconds during insertion and 250 to 300 seconds during support is mandatory. The TandemHeart has been used for up to 14 days. A small iatrogenic atrial septal defect is left after the explantation of the transseptal cannula, which typically resolves after 4 to 6 weeks or has no clinically significant left-to-right shunt. Explantation of the device is easily achieved by percutaneous cannula removal after discontinuing the heparin infusion and switching off the pump motor.

Hemodynamic Effects

The TandemHeart provides circulatory support by diverting oxygenated blood from the left atrium into the systemic circulation, which increases cardiac output and blood pressure and decreases afterload and preload, thus decreasing myocardial oxygen demand. The increase in mean arterial pressure may improve the supply and demand of oxygen in the myocardium and increase tissue perfusion.[15]

Potential Complications

The transseptal puncture required for the TandemHeart is a potential source of complications. Inadvertent puncture of the aortic root, coronary sinus, or posterior free wall of the right atrium can lead to catastrophic complications, including death. Thromboembolism is another potential complication. Cerebral thromboembolism has been reported secondary to thrombus formation at the edge of a large ventricular septal defect and at the site of the left atrial puncture, despite anticoagulation. Because unfractionated heparin is needed to achieve a high ACT, bleeding (especially from the groin) may occur. The blood circuit is extracorporeal, and systemic hypothermia can occur if exposure of the circuit to ambient room temperatures leads to the cooling of the extracorporeal blood flowing through the pump. Accidental dislodgement of the arterial cannula has led to acute decompensation and death from cardiogenic shock.[15] Local infections, bacteremia, and sepsis are potential complications with any implantable P-LVAD.

IMPELLA 2.5

The Impella 2.5 is a catheter-based, impeller-driven, axial flow pump, which pumps blood directly from the left ventricle into the ascending aorta. This P-LVAD directly decants the left ventricle and may provide circulatory assistance for up to 5 days in the setting of acute myocardial infarction,[19] cardiogenic shock, low-output states, or for high-risk PCI (**Fig. 3**A).[3] As discussed, the Impella may also have a niche indication for situations with extremely high left ventricular end-diastolic pressures, where this device may effectively decant the left ventricle.

The Impella design involves an intracardiac axial flow pump containing an Archimedes screw-like rotor that is driven by an external electrical motor. The left ventricular pump can provide up to 2.5 L/min of cardiac output, depending on the speed of the rotor (which can operate at up to 50,000 rpm) and the pressure difference across the aortic valve (which is constantly monitored by differential pressure sensors) (see **Fig. 3**B). The appropriate position of the flow pump is confirmed by the pressure difference between the aorta and left ventricle. The catheter is connected to a mobile console that controls the rotational speed of the pump and displays the pressure differential between the left ventricle and aorta (see **Fig. 3**C). The pump is continuously purged with a glucose solution (10%) that is drawn into a 50-mL syringe with heparin (2500 IU). The purge flow rates normally range from 2 to 6 mL/h to continuously rinse the pump and prevent thrombus formation.

Abiomed also produce an Impella 5.0 that is able to provide up to 5 L/min of hemodynamic support. Although the Impella 2.5 requires 13F arterial access, the Impella 5.0 requires 21F arterial access, which effectively limits the 5.0 device to cardiothoracic surgical applications.

Implantation

Similar to the TandemHeart, the Impella 2.5 system is typically placed in the catheterization laboratory. The initial implantation procedure involves iliofemoral angiography to rule out severe peripheral vascular disease and tortuosity. Once suitability of the femoral artery for 13F access has been determined, 2 Perclose sutures are deployed with the preclose technique as described earlier. The following sequence of steps ensures correct device placement and functioning:

- Insert a 7F introducer and administer heparin (ACT between 250 and 300 seconds) or

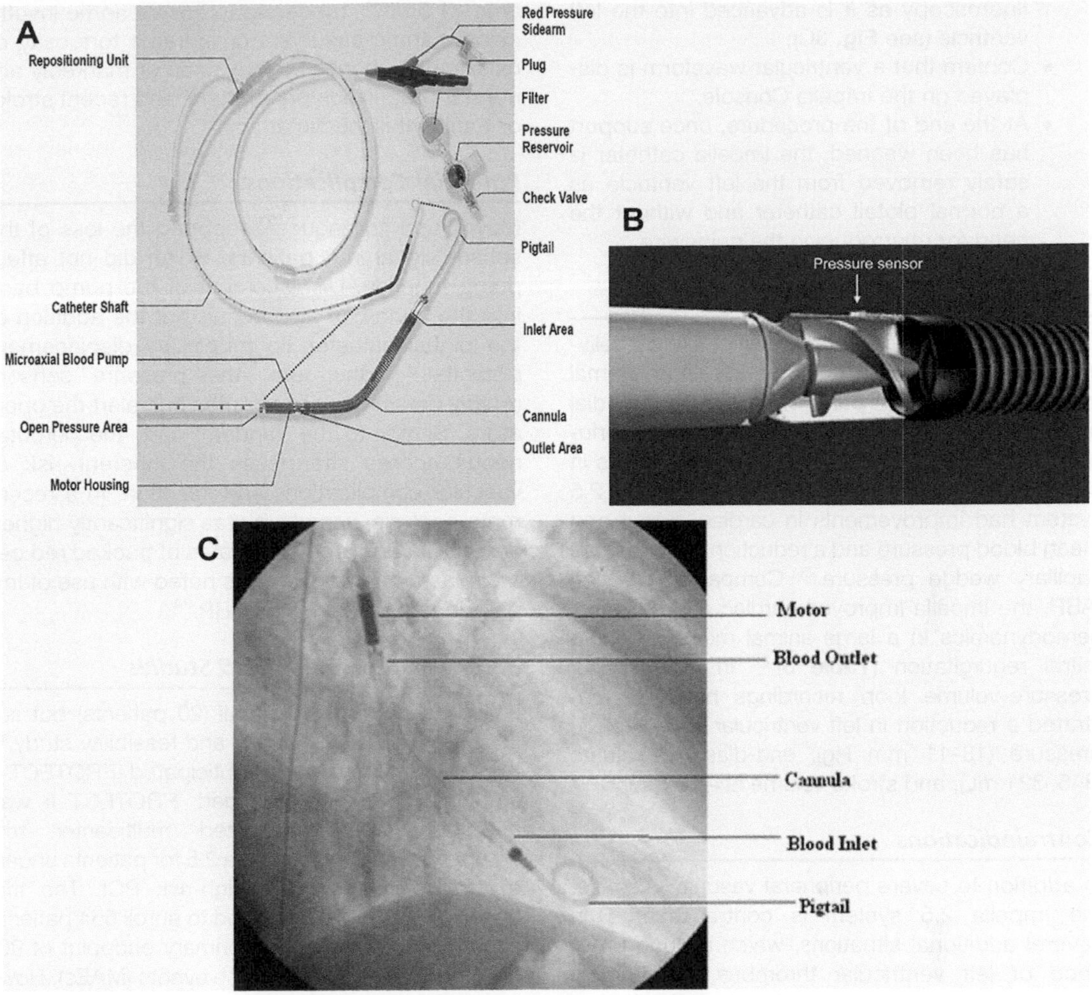

Fig. 3. The Impella 2.5 P-LVAD. (*A*) The Impella 2.5 system is a P-LVAD that provides hemodynamic support by aspirating blood through a pigtail tip positioned in the left ventricle and expelling the blood into the ascending aorta. (*B*) The intracardiac axial flow pump contains a rotor with inflow cannula that is driven by an electrical motor. Blood is drawn in at the tip of the cannula and expelled into the aorta at the sides of the device and upstream from the rotor. A differential pressure sensor measures the difference in pressure between the inflow and outflow of the pump. (*C*) Angiographic appearance of the Impella 2.5 device in correct position. (*Courtesy of* Abiomed Inc., Aachen, Germany; with permission.)

bivalirudin to achieve an ACT of more than 300 seconds.

- After a therapeutic ACT is obtained, remove the 7F introducer over a 0.035 in guidewire and insert the 13F peel-away introducer with dilator.
- Remove the 13F dilator and advance a 6F diagnostic catheter (Judkins right or multipurpose) over a diagnostic 0.035 in guidewire into the left ventricle.
- Remove the 0.035 in guidewire and insert the supplied 0.018 in placement guidewire into the left ventricle, until 3 to 4 cm of the stiffer part of the guidewire is in the left ventricle.
- Remove the 6F diagnostic catheter, leaving the 0.018 in wire in the left ventricle.
- Wet the cannula and backload the pigtail section of the Impella onto the 0.018 in guidewire. Straighten the cannula to ensure the guidewire exits on the inner radius of the cannula.
- Advance the Impella catheter through the hemostatic valve into the femoral artery and along the 0.018 in guidewire into the left ventricle. Follow the catheter under

fluoroscopy as it is advanced into the left ventricle (see **Fig. 3**C).
- Confirm that a ventricular waveform is displayed on the Impella Console.
- At the end of the procedure, once support has been weaned, the Impella catheter is safely removed from the left ventricle as a normal pigtail catheter and without the need for reintroducing the guidewire.

Hemodynamic Effects

The Impella 2.5 unloads the left ventricle by delivering blood into the ascending aorta. In an animal model, the Impella pump reduced myocardial oxygen consumption during ischemia and reperfusion, leading to reduced infarct size.[20] Patients in cardiogenic shock treated with the Impella 2.5 system had improvements in cardiac output and mean blood pressure and a reduction in pulmonary capillary wedge pressure.[21] Compared with the IABP, the Impella improved cardiac and systemic hemodynamics in a large animal model of acute mitral regurgitation (**Table 3**).[22] In clinical use, pressure-volume loop recordings have demonstrated a reduction in left ventricular end-diastolic pressure (18–11 mm Hg), end-diastolic volume (345–321 mL), and stroke volume (94–76 mL).[23]

Contraindications

In addition to severe peripheral vascular disease, the Impella 2.5 system is contraindicated in several additional situations, which include presence of left ventricular thrombus, mechanical aortic valve, moderate aortic stenosis (orifice area <1.5 cm^2), moderate to severe aortic insufficiency, aortic aneurysm or extreme tortuosity or calcification, hepatic dysfunction or markedly abnormal coagulation parameters, and recent stroke or transient ischemic attack.

Table 3
Effect of IABP and Impella 2.5 P-LVADs on hemodynamic parameters in an animal model of acute mitral regurgitation. Values quoted are percentage change from untreated regurgitant state

Hemodynamic Parameter	IABP (1:1)	Impella 2.5 (At Full Support)
Cardiac output	+4	+25
Aortic pressure	+11	+17
Carotid flow	+8	+48
Diastolic coronary pressure	+96	+69
LV work	−4	−46

Data from Reesink KD, Dekker AL, Van Ommen V, et al. Miniature intracardiac assist device provides more effective cardiac unloading and circulatory support during severe left heart failure than intraaortic balloon pumping. Chest 2004;126:896–902.

Potential Complications

Meyns and colleagues[21] reported the loss of the sensor signal in 3 patients, which did not affect pump function. Displacement of the pump back into the aorta can also occur, but the addition of the pigtail catheter tip minimizes displacement potential. Furthermore, the pressure sensors rapidly detect device migration and alert the operators. Similar to the TandemHeart, the percutaneous access site poses the inherent risk of vascular complications and infection. In a recent meta-analysis, hemolysis was significantly higher, and a trend toward higher rates of packed red cell and plasma transfusion was noted with use of Impella in comparison with IABP.[24]

Recent Pivotal Impella 2.5 Studies

Following on from the small (20 patients) but successful PROTECT-I safety and feasibility study,[25] the results of the much anticipated PROTECT-II study have recently emerged. PROTECT II was a prospective, randomized multicenter trial comparing IABP with Impella 2.5 for patients undergoing nonemergent but high-risk PCI. The trial began in late 2007 and aimed to enroll 654 patients across 50 centers, with a primary endpoint of 90-day composite major adverse events (MAEs). However, at an interim analysis of the first 305 patients, the primary endpoint had occurred at a very similar rate in the 2 groups (38% Impella, 45% IABP; P = .40), and a decision was made to terminate the study due to futility.[26] This decision has resulted in much controversy, as there was a marked imbalance between the Impella and IABP groups in rotational atherectomy use, with increased atherectomy use in the Impella group apparently responsible for a higher incidence of periprocedural myocardial infarction. Although the results are yet to be formally published, in a final analysis of 426 patients who met all criteria for the per-protocol analysis, Impella patients had 21% fewer MAEs at 90 days than IABP patients (40.8% vs 51.4%; P = .029).[27] In addition, a post-hoc analysis has identified that although there was no difference in MAEs between Impella and IABP when limited revascularization was performed (59% vs 48%, P = .2), when more extensive revascularization was performed, Impella improved outcomes compared with IABP (90-day MAEs: 33% vs 48%, P = .008, respectively).[28] Finally, although nonrandomized and subject to selection

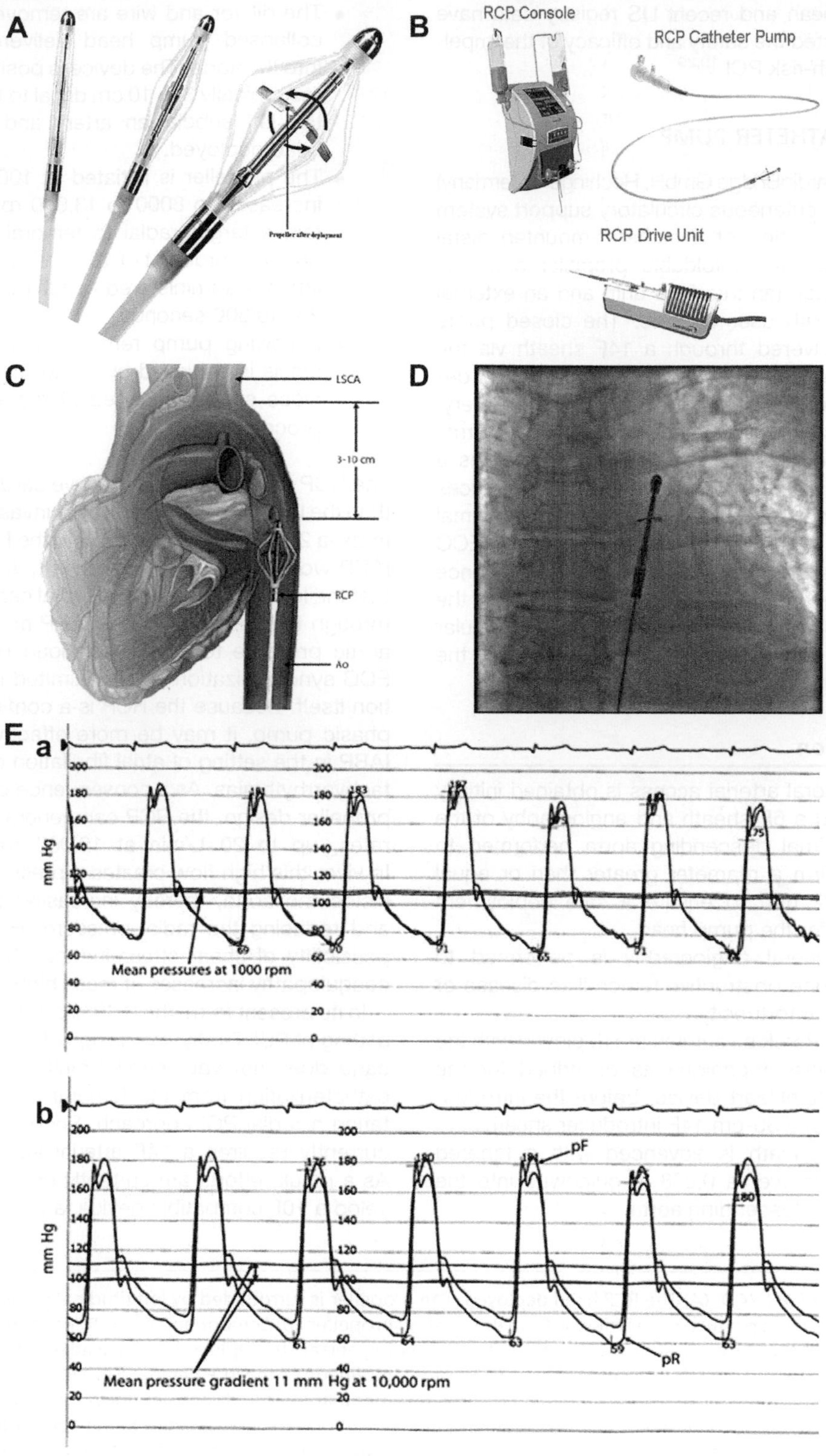
A
Propeller after deployment
B
RCP Console
RCP Catheter Pump
RCP Drive Unit
C
LSCA
3-10 cm
RCP
Ao
D
E
a
mm Hg
Mean pressures at 1000 rpm
b
mm Hg
pF
pR
Mean pressure gradient 11 mm Hg at 10,000 rpm

bias, European and recent US registry data have also supported the safety and efficacy of the Impella 2.5 in high-risk PCI.[19,29]

REITAN CATHETER PUMP

The RCP (CardioBridge GmbH, Hechingen, Germany) is a fully percutaneous circulatory support system (**Fig. 4**) consisting of a catheter-mounted distal pump head with a foldable propeller and surrounding cage (an interface unit) and an external drive unit with user console. The closed pump head is delivered through a 14F sheath via the femoral artery and positioned in the proximal descending aorta, distal to the left subclavian artery. The cage is then deployed, and the propeller arms are extended and rotated. The pump creates a pressure gradient within the aorta that reduces afterload and increases organ perfusion in animal studies.[30,31] The RCP does not require ECG synchronization, and can be used in the presence of aortic regurgitation. In contrast to Impella, the RCP is not deployed within the left ventricular cavity and therefore is not contraindicated in the presence of left ventricular thrombus.

Implantation

- Femoral arterial access is obtained initially using a 6F sheath and angiography of the proximal descending aorta performed to confirm a diameter greater than or equal to 22 mm to ensure a safe deployment site for the pump head.
- Peripheral angiography is performed to exclude obstructive femoroiliac disease or severe tortuosity.
- Two Perclose sutures are deployed with the preclose technique as described for the TandemHeart device, before the introduction of a 30-cm 14F introducer sheath.
- The sheath is advanced with a tapered dilator over a 0.038 in guidewire into the distal descending aorta.
- The dilator and wire are removed, and the collapsed pump head delivered directly into the aorta. The device is positioned fluoroscopically 3 to 10 cm distal to the origin of the left subclavian artery and the pump head deployed.
- The propeller is initiated at 1000 rpm and increased to 8000 to 13,000 rpm to maintain a target radial to femoral transaortic pressure gradient of 10 mm Hg. Anticoagulation is administered to achieve an ACT of 250 to 300 seconds.
- Following pump removal, femoral hemostasis is achieved by deploying the 2 Perclose sutures inserted at the start of the procedure.

The RCP may offer more effective cardiac support than the IABP, although being less invasive than the Impella 2.5 or TandemHeart. Both the RCP and the IABP work in series with the heart, which means that the left ventricle ejects the total cardiac output through the aortic valve. The IABP modifies intra-aortic pressure to reduce afterload but requires ECG synchronization and has limited pump function itself. Because the RCP is a continuous non-phasic pump, it may be more effective than the IABP in the setting of atrial fibrillation or recurrent tachyarrhythmias. As a consequence of its folding propeller design, the RCP can generate high flow rates, up to 20 L/min at 12,000 rpm in vitro. In vivo, this high flow creates a pressure gradient inside the aorta, thereby increasing the femoral and reducing the radial pressure. However, the possibility of shear stress-induced hemolysis or coagulopathy increases at these high flow rates.

In its present form, the RCP has limitations in the setting of PCI. Firstly, the design of the pump head cage does not yet permit simultaneous cardiac catheterization from the femoral route, necessitating a radial PCI approach. Secondly, the RCP currently requires a 14F arterial access sheath. As a result, efforts are currently underway to develop a 10F compatible device, and a mechanism

Fig. 4. The RCP P-LVAD. (*A*) The RCP head deployed. The propeller is surrounded by longitudinal polymer filaments forming a cage that protects the aortic wall from the rotating propeller. (*B*) Components of the RCP system. (*C*) Diagram demonstrating the correct position of the RCP in the descending aorta. The deployed pump head should sit 3 to 10 cm distal to the origin of the left subclavian artery. (*D*) Fluoroscopic image of the RCP deployed in vivo. The pump head is fluoroscopically visualized in the descending aorta. The polymer filaments and cage are not visible. (*E*) Simultaneous radial and femoral pressure traces before and during RCP activation. (*a*) Simultaneous radial and femoral pressure traces are demonstrated before and during pump activation at 1000 rpm. The pump is routinely initiated at 1000 rpm to ensure appropriate function and to reduce thrombotic risk. Radial and femoral pressure traces are superimposed, with no significant pressure gradient. (*b*) The pump is activated when propeller rotation exceeds 8000 rpm. In this case, propeller rotation at 10,000 rpm results in an increase in femoral pressure and a decrease in radial pressure, resulting in a mean pressure gradient of 11 mm Hg. Ao, aorta; LSCA, left subclavian artery; pF, femoral pressure; pR, radial pressure. (*Courtesy of* CardioBridge GmbH, Hechingen, Germany; with permission.)

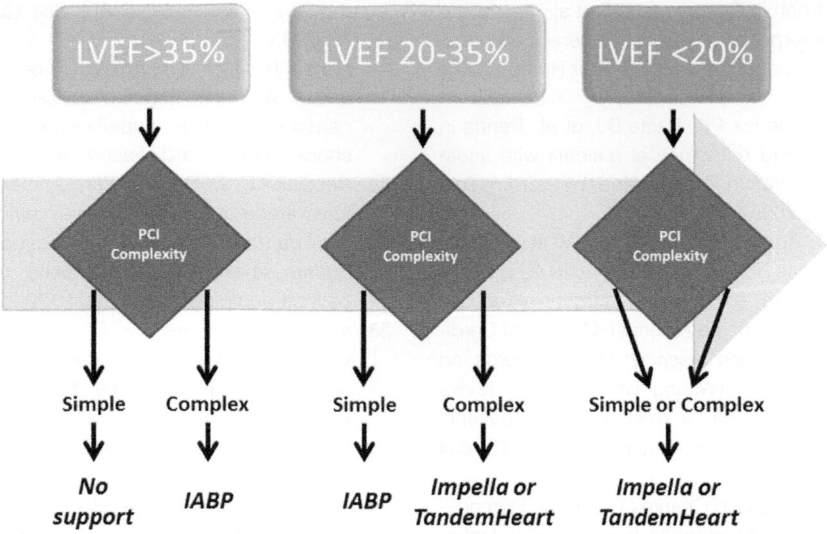

Fig. 5. Suggested P-LVAD selection algorithm.

to provide transverse protection of the propeller to permit femoral catheterization is also being considered. In addition, conversion of the RCP to an over-the-wire technology is being developed, which may further reduce the risk of vascular complications. Although initial clinical experience is promising,[32] further data are awaited, including the ability of the RCP to provide prolonged cardiac support in patients with decompensated chronic left heart failure.

SUMMARY

Several P-LVADs are now available for use in the United States and Europe. These devices continue to evolve and are becoming progressively safer and easier to use. However, the significant track record, familiarity, ease of deployment, and smaller arterial access requirements of the IABP have seen this device continue to enjoy widespread popularity throughout the interventional and wider cardiovascular communities. Nevertheless, for specific patients and clinical indications, or where a greater degree of hemodynamic support is required, numerous studies have demonstrated the feasibility and safety of the newer generation devices, particularly Impella and TandemHeart. Considering all the above data, the authors' suggested algorithm for device selection is shown in **Fig. 5**. Looking ahead, continued technological advances are expected to further enhance P-LVAD design and device profile, and it is widely hoped that this will facilitate enhanced safety and efficacy of complex, unstable, and high-risk PCI cases.

REFERENCES

1. Buckley MJ, Leinbach RC, Kastor JA, et al. Hemodynamic evaluation of intra-aortic balloon pumping in man. Circulation 1970;41:II130–6.
2. Kantrowitz A, Tjonneland S, Freed PS, et al. Initial clinical experience with intraaortic balloon pumping in cardiogenic shock. JAMA 1968;203:113–8.
3. Kovacic JC, Nguyen HT, Karajgikar R, et al. The impella recover 2.5 and TandemHeart ventricular assist devices are safe and associated with equivalent clinical outcomes in patients undergoing high-risk percutaneous coronary intervention. Catheter Cardiovasc Interv August, 2012; [online ahead of print].
4. Miller MA, Dukkipati SR, Mittnacht AJ, et al. Activation and entrainment mapping of hemodynamically unstable ventricular tachycardia using a percutaneous left ventricular assist device. J Am Coll Cardiol 2011;58:1363–71.
5. Vogel RA, Shawl F, Tommaso C, et al. Initial report of the National Registry of Elective Cardiopulmonary Bypass supported coronary angioplasty. J Am Coll Cardiol 1990;15:23–9.
6. Shawl FA, Domanski MJ, Wish MH, et al. Percutaneous cardiopulmonary bypass support in the catheterization laboratory: technique and complications. Am Heart J 1990;120:195–203.
7. Scholz KH, Dubois-Rande JL, Urban P, et al. Clinical experience with the percutaneous hemopump during high-risk coronary angioplasty. Am J Cardiol 1998;82:1107–10 A6.
8. Scholz KH, Tebbe U, Chemnitius M, et al. Transfemoral placement of the left ventricular assist device "Hemopump" during mechanical resuscitation. Thorac Cardiovasc Surg 1990;38:69–72.

9. Cohen M, Urban P, Christenson JT, et al. Intra-aortic balloon counterpulsation in US and non-US centres: results of the Benchmark Registry. Eur Heart J 2003; 24:1763–70.
10. Babaev A, Frederick PD, Pasta DJ, et al. Trends in management and outcomes of patients with acute myocardial infarction complicated by cardiogenic shock. JAMA 2005;294:448–54.
11. Antman EM, Anbe DT, Armstrong PW, et al. ACC/AHA guidelines for the management of patients with ST-elevation myocardial infarction–executive summary. A report of the American College of Cardiology/American Heart Association Task Force on Practice Guidelines (Writing Committee to revise the 1999 guidelines for the management of patients with acute myocardial infarction). J Am Coll Cardiol 2004;44:671–719.
12. Nanas JN, Nanas SN, Charitos CE, et al. Hemodynamic effects of a counterpulsation device implanted on the ascending aorta in severe cardiogenic shock. ASAIO Trans 1988;34:229–34.
13. Sjauw KD, Engstrom AE, Vis MM, et al. A systematic review and meta-analysis of intra-aortic balloon pump therapy in ST-elevation myocardial infarction: should we change the guidelines? Eur Heart J 2009;30:459–68.
14. Patel MR, Smalling RW, Thiele H, et al. Intra-aortic balloon counterpulsation and infarct size in patients with acute anterior myocardial infarction without shock: the CRISP AMI randomized trial. JAMA 2011;306:1329–37.
15. Thiele H, Lauer B, Hambrecht R, et al. Reversal of cardiogenic shock by percutaneous left atrial-to-femoral arterial bypass assistance. Circulation 2001;104:2917–22.
16. Fonger JD, Zhou Y, Matsuura H, et al. Enhanced preservation of acutely ischemic myocardium with transseptal left ventricular assist. Ann Thorac Surg 1994;57:570–5.
17. Rajdev S, Krishnan P, Irani A, et al. Clinical application of prophylactic percutaneous left ventricular assist device (TandemHeart) in high-risk percutaneous coronary intervention using an arterial preclosure technique: single-center experience. J Invasive Cardiol 2008;20:67–72.
18. Rajdev S, Benza R, Misra V. Use of Tandem Heart as a temporary hemodynamic support option for severe pulmonary artery hypertension complicated by cardiogenic shock. J Invasive Cardiol 2007;19:E226–9.
19. Maini B, Naidu SS, Mulukutla S, et al. Real-world use of the Impella 2.5 circulatory support system in complex high-risk percutaneous coronary intervention: The USpella Registry. Catheter Cardiovasc Interv August, 2012; [online ahead of print].
20. Meyns B, Stolinski J, Leunens V, et al. Left ventricular support by catheter-mounted axial flow pump reduces infarct size. J Am Coll Cardiol 2003;41: 1087–95.
21. Meyns B, Dens J, Sergeant P, et al. Initial experiences with the Impella device in patients with cardiogenic shock - Impella support for cardiogenic shock. Thorac Cardiovasc Surg 2003;51:312–7.
22. Reesink KD, Dekker AL, Van Ommen V, et al. Miniature intracardiac assist device provides more effective cardiac unloading and circulatory support during severe left heart failure than intraaortic balloon pumping. Chest 2004;126:896–902.
23. Valgimigli M, Steendijk P, Sianos G, et al. Left ventricular unloading and concomitant total cardiac output increase by the use of percutaneous Impella Recover LP 2.5 assist device during high-risk coronary intervention. Catheter Cardiovasc Interv 2005; 65:263–7.
24. Cheng JM, den Uil CA, Hoeks SE, et al. Percutaneous left ventricular assist devices vs. intra-aortic balloon pump counterpulsation for treatment of cardiogenic shock: a meta-analysis of controlled trials. Eur Heart J 2009;30:2102–8.
25. Dixon SR, Henriques JP, Mauri L, et al. A prospective feasibility trial investigating the use of the Impella 2.5 system in patients undergoing high-risk percutaneous coronary intervention (The PROTECT I Trial): initial U.S. experience. JACC Cardiovasc Interv 2009;2:91–6.
26. PROTECT II study halted for futility: Abiomed explanation meets skepticism. Available at: http://www.theheart.org/article/1161463.do. Accessed July 7, 2012.
27. PROTECT II investigator insists study shows benefits of Impella, despite early termination. Available at: http://www.theheart.org/article/1205543.do. Accessed July 7, 2012.
28. Popma JJ, Moses J, Kleiman N, et al. Impella improves clincial outcomes when extensive revascularization is performed: The Protect II Study. J Am Coll Cardiol 2012;59:E1522.
29. Sjauw KD, Konorza T, Erbel R, et al. Supported high-risk percutaneous coronary intervention with the Impella 2.5 device the Europella registry. J Am Coll Cardiol 2009;54:2430–4.
30. Reitan O, Ohlin H, Peterzen B, et al. Initial tests with a new cardiac assist device. ASAIO J 1999;45: 317–21.
31. Reitan O, Steen S, Ohlin H. Hemodynamic effects of a new percutaneous circulatory support device in a left ventricular failure model. ASAIO J 2003;49: 731–6.
32. Smith EJ, Reitan O, Keeble T, et al. A first-in-man study of the Reitan catheter pump for circulatory support in patients undergoing high-risk percutaneous coronary intervention. Catheter Cardiovasc Interv 2009;73:859–65.

Telemedicine
The Future of Global STEMI Care

Thais Waisman, MD, MBA, PhD[a],
Roberto V. Botelho, MD, PhD[b], Francisco Fernandez, BSc[c],
Sameer Mehta, MD, MBA[d,e,f,*], Estefania Oliveros, MD[f],
Jennifer C. Kostela, MS, MD[g,h], Breno A.A. Falcão, MD[i],
Chabely Cardenas[f]

KEYWORDS

• STEMI • Telemedicine • Thrombolysis • D2B

KEY POINTS

- Telemedicine is the current lead resource to optimize ST elevation myocardial infarction (STEMI) management. It aids the faults in the system of establishing early reperfusion therapy.
- Technology may be a useful tool in decreasing delays in accurate diagnosing of STEMI. Therefore, it provides the basis for an adequate well-timed response when delivering treatment.
- Telecardiology has shown cost beneficial and globally applicable despite economic, geographic, and political differences.
- Prehospital STEMI care plays a pivotal role in patient outcome.

INTRODUCTION

Major advances in the management of STEMI, secondary to widespread use of reperfusion therapies, are critically time-dependent.[1–3] Mechanical reperfusion proves superior to fibrinolysis, although in many countries it is markedly limited by logistic constrains.[1–3] Treatment strategies, including rapid transfer of patients to percutaneous coronary intervention (PCI)-capable centers, results in better outcomes compared with thrombolysis in non-PCI centers.[4,5] In this context, regional and national networks of STEMI treatment, including local hospitals, clinics, ambulances, and PCI-capable facilities, become a public health priority, to provide a global standard of care for acute myocardial infarction (AMI) despite socioeconomic or geographic variables. Applying telemedicine to optimize networks of STEMI treatment can promote rapid integration of the different parts of the system (**Fig. 1**). Networks with a prehospital system equipped with telemedicine (1) provide remote STEMI diagnosis, with

Disclosure: Thais Waisman, Regional IT and Innovation Director, ITMS Telemedicina do Brasil; Roberto V. Botelho, Medical Director, ITMS; Francisco Fernandez, General Manager, MedSolutions; and Sameer Mehta, Chief Medical Officer, Asia-Pacific region, The Medicines Company. The other authors report no conflict of interest regarding the content herein.

[a] Engineering School at University of São Paulo, INTERLAB-EPUSP, Rua Antonio Gonçalves da Cruz, 60/83B, São Paulo 05029060, Brazil; [b] Instituto do Coração do Triângulo, Av Cipriano del Fávero, 659 Ap 1600, Uberlandia, Minas Gerais 38400-106, Brazil; [c] MedSolutions, Rua Desembargador Eliseu Guilherme, 53 cj 121, São Paulo 04004030, Brazil; [d] Miller School of Medicine, University of Miami, 1400 Northwest 12th Avenue, Miami, FL 33136, USA; [e] Mercy Medical Center, 3663 South Miami Avenue, Miami, FL 33133, USA; [f] Lumen Foundation, 55 Pinta Road, Miami, FL 33133, USA; [g] New York Hospital Queens, 56-45 Main Street, Flushing, NY 11355, USA; [h] Ross University School of Medicine, 630 US Highway 1, North Brunswick, NJ 08902, USA; [i] Heart Institute (InCor), University of São Paulo, School of Medicine, Rua Dr. Enéas de Carvalho Aguiar, 44, Pinheiros, São Paulo, CEP 05403-000, Brazil
* Corresponding author. 185 Shore Drive South, Miami, FL 33133.
E-mail address: mehtas@bellsouth.net

Intervent Cardiol Clin 1 (2012) 623–629
http://dx.doi.org/10.1016/j.iccl.2012.07.004
2211-7458/12/$ – see front matter

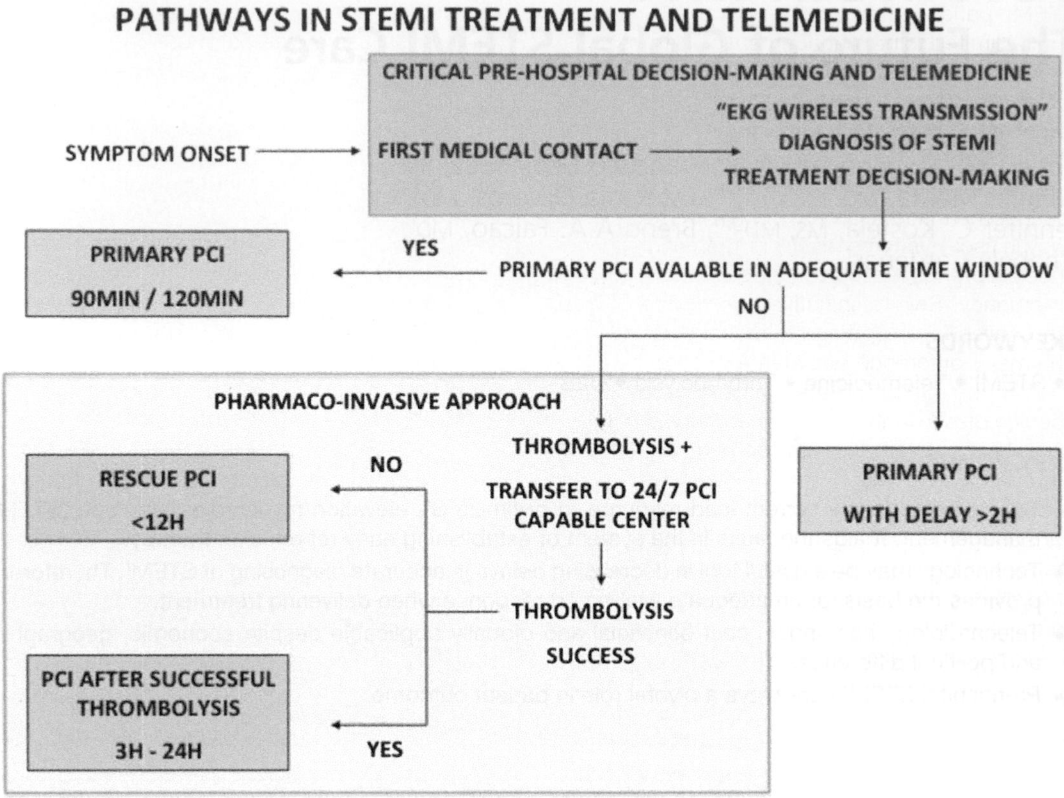

Fig. 1. Telemedicine inserted in the pathway of STEMI treatment.

EKG transmitted and interpreted by a cardiologist; (2) enable prehospital thrombolysis in remote areas; (3) permit rapid activation and immediate transfer of patients to PCI-capable centers, improving time to mechanical reperfusion; and (4) avoid costs and risks of unnecessary transferences.[6–8]

ACCESS TO PREHOSPITAL CARE

An efficient prehospital system is a powerful tool to overcome time pressure for STEMI treatment. Unfortunately, there is a wide variation in prehospital systems quality around the world. Some countries in Europe, such as Denmark and Belgium, have an active and efficient prehospital system capable of providing remote diagnosis, rapid transfer, adequate medical support, and even prehospital thrombolysis in remote areas, whereas in comparison, in other parts of world, such as underdeveloped countries, structured prehospital systems of care are still not available.[6,7]

The prehospital system for STEMI management remains fundamentally dependent on an existing network of ambulance services that provide the initial but critical first step (**Box 1**). Sadly, in most parts of the world, ambulance care for AMI patients merely represents transportation to a hospital. It is pitiful that many patients are transported without a definite diagnosis of AMI. This glaring omission prevents the ambulance from delivering on its aims. In some situations, this is dangerous and the poorly equipped ambulances provide a deceptive sense of security for AMI patients. Suboptimal prehospital AMI care results in (1) a majority of

Box 1
Prehospital STEMI management ambulance roles

1. Prompt recognition and diagnosis
2. Safe transportation to a capable hospital
3. Early pharmacologic management, including use of supplemental oxygen, narcotics, antiplatelets, and intravenous access
4. Management of life-threatening complications, mainly cardioversion of ventricular tachycardia and ventricular fibrillation, intubation to manage cardiopulmonary failure, and external pacing for heart blocks
5. Prehospital alert and triage through wireless or fax modem capability
6. Prehospital thrombolysis

STEMI patients transported to non-PCI centers and (2) limited to no management of in-transit STEMI complications.

Developed and developing countries have different medical assets depending on their economic status. Depending on the resources of the geographic location where the AMI event occurs, management and outcome may vary. The discrepancy in fiscal systems results in international differences in prehospital care in the setting of an STEMI emergency. Several initiatives worldwide address the challenge of optimizing prehospital logistics. The major difference between AMI care in Europe and in the United States emanates from this specific dissimilarity—in Europe, the vast majority of AMI patients are transported to a hospital in an ambulance, whereas in the United States, the larger percentage of patients are still self-transporting (**Table 1**).[9] In various Asian nations, there is a blend of such services, and in some underdeveloped African countries, ambulance services for AMI are unavailable and/or unreliable.

What should patients do if there is no reliable ambulance network to transport them to a hospital? Tragically, this situation occurs in the vast majority of countries in the world.[7,10] In such situations, patients depend on transporting themselves to the hospital and succumb to the large risk that they will not reach urgent care at the hospital to treat their life-threatening AMI. The absence of an ambulance or existence of unreliable and inefficient ambulance systems hugely delays the treatment of AMI. For thrombolytic therapy, a door-to-needle time of less than 30 minutes, and, for primary PCI, a door-to-balloon (D2B) time of less than 90 minutes are the desired goals that are a part of advocated guidelines.[1] With a qualitative and quantitative absence of ambulances, achieving these mandated treatment times is simply not possible, and results with both thrombolytic therapy and primary PCI therefore are suboptimal. Unfortunately, this situation, tragically, is a norm rather than the exception.

TELEMEDICINE

Current knowledge in electronics and technology has transformed the way modern medicine is conducted. Telemedicine effectively facilitates patient assessment and monitoring to provide health care assistance at a distance (**Box 2**). Telecardiology is a tool for populations located in remote geography, because it eliminates the barriers of time and distance. It can even improve the results of thrombolytic therapy and primary PCI by its ability to initiate early management, both within and outside an ambulance. Several reports have demonstrated that prehospital EKG diagnosis in STEMI decreases treatment delays.[10–12] The decrease is due to prompt activation of the catheterization laboratory and bypassing the local non-PCI capable hospitals, in some cases, the emergency department (ED), coronary care unit, and ICU at a primary PCI center. Prehospital diagnosis by telemedicine was implemented in Aarhus County, Denmark. Sorensen and colleagues[7] described their model of prehospital diagnosis of STEMI. They used telemedicine, and the general practitioner, ambulance physician, or emergency medical system paramedics diagnosed with a 12-lead EKG (LIFEPAK-12 defibrillator, Physio-Control, Redmond, Washington). Subsequently, the EKG was transmitted wirelessly to the primary PCI center through the global systems for mobile communications network. The on-call cardiologist at the primary PCI center interpreted the ECG and called the ambulance and did a brief patient interview. If the ECG and the patient interview indicated STEMI, the ambulance was rerouted directly to the prealerted catheterization laboratory at the primary PCI center.

A meta-analysis conducted by de Waure and colleagues[13] reviewed data to demonstrate the efficacy of telemedicine versus standard measures with the aim of reducing mortality in the management of AMI. The relative risk for in-hospital mortality from AMI was 0.65 (95% CI, 0.42–0.99) for the telemedicine group, showing that telemedicine may benefit AMI patients. Early telemetry of the EKGs may improve the health outcomes in patients with coronary artery disease.

ITMS,[14,15] a Brazil-based telemedicine company, showed the cost versus benefit of implementing telecardiology in 698 towns (large cities, countryside, Amazon rainforest, and Indian tribes). The ITMS project also implemented tele-ECG in 338

Table 1
US patients arriving to ED by ambulance

Patients Arriving by Ambulance	Number of Patients	Triaged as Emergent	Resulted in Hospital Admission	Diverted
14.2%	16.2 Million	68%	38%	48%

Box 2
Rationale of using telemedicine in networks of STEMI treatment

Improves network efficiency integrating resources (ambulances, clinics, community hospitals, and PCI-capable centers)

Precise and fast prehospital ECG diagnosis

Allows inputs of a cardiologist in decision making

Enables prehospital thrombolysis in remote areas

Optimizes time to reperfusion through rapid transfer to and early activation of PCI-capable center (bypass community hospitals and bypass unnecessary ED or ICU admissions)

Cost-effectiveness (avoid unnecessary long transportations)

ambulances as well as in rescue helicopters in a joint effort with HCor.[16–18] The communities were equipped with digital and nondigital 12-lead ECG—HeartView (Aerotel Medical Systems, Israel) or Cardioline Cardiette (et Medical Devices, Milan, Italy) electrocardiograph with the capacity of transmitting the ECG tracings through land lines, mobile phones, and computers and forwarding the results to an on-duty cardiologist. The geopolitical design challenge was overcome with the use of telemedicine. The success of the project relied on the capability of transmitting 45,000 ECGs monthly, continuous training for correctly using the technology, medical auditing of the totality of ECGs, and guarantee of a second medical opinion provided in the presence of abnormal ECGs—especially in emergency situations, in an ambulance setting, or when patients came from remote areas. The thorough evaluation by town health teams led to the decrease of unnecessary referrals. The ITMS project reports a successful, feasible experience, with favorable cost-benefit with the implementation of telemedicine in the public health system.

The whole process may be enhanced by using telecardiology applications, sensor technology, wearable monitoring systems, Internet-based peripheral monitoring devices, third-generation mobile phones, cellular videophones, network cameras, a telephone conferencing system, interactive voice response systems, and nanotechnology. One of the concerns of implementing a new system is that inclusion of new equipment may tamper with a previously established diagnostic method. Gonzalez and colleagues[19] showed that cellular videophone–assisted transmission and interpretation in real time of prehospital ECG had high reliability, resembling a printed ECG interpretation.

The ST-Segment Analysis Using Wireless Technology in Acute Myocardial Infarction (STAT-MI) network evaluated a fully automated, field-based wireless network that transmitted 12-lead ECGs from the emergency medical services personnel to the offsite cardiologists for the early evaluation and triage of patients with STEMI. Shorter D2B times were present in STAT-MI patients compared with a control group (63 minutes vs 119 minutes, $P<.00004$) as were significantly decreased peak troponin I levels (39.5 ng/mL vs 290.3 ng/mL, $P = .001$), higher left ventricular ejection fractions (50% vs 35%, $P = .004$), and shorter length of hospital stay (3 days vs 5.5 days, $P<.001$).[20]

The Regime of Explicit Health Guarantees (Regimen de Garantias Explicitas en Salud), also known as Plan AUGE, is a health program conceived and implemented within a social guarantee framework in Chile.[1] It is the first example in Latin America of the legal installment of a rights-based social guarantee that incorporates and defines the principles of access, quality, opportunity, and financial protection. Plan AUGE guarantees a certain set of services for all users. Since 2005, every person with confirmation of AMI has had access to medical treatment coronary bypass or primary PCI and secondary prevention. Patients are evaluated through the chest pain protocol, which includes algorithms of ECG transmitted through telemedicine in hospitals types 3 and 4.[21,22] ECGs are transmitted to an expert or trained physician, while in the meantime, patients are monitored 24 hours by a physician or nurse. Thrombolysis was given in emergency centers in the primary care facilities where patients hads the first initial medical contact. In Chile, the Ministry of Health created collaborative efforts that included elaboration of systematic revisions from the universities of the practice guidelines according to the Appraisal of Guideline Research and Evaluation collaboration. Passage of the explicit health guarantees law was associated with an increment in the percentage of in-hospital deaths in women (relative risk 0.95; 0.92–0.97).[23]

Several models and innovative pathways enable telemedicine in the following ways.

Enabling Prehospital Thrombolysis

In the telemedicine pathway devices are places strategically in an ambulance, remote and inaccessible locations, or in places where patients with an AMI traditionally present (primary clinics, private nursing homes, and offices of general practitioners). This strategy eliminates the huge barriers of inefficient or nonexistent ambulance systems while preserving an ability to administer early, prehospital thrombolytic therapy. In such a model, a general physician performs a 12-lead ECG from a remote location that is wirelessly transmitted to a Web-based platform, where it is immediately transmitted electronically and interpreted by a trained cardiologist. Subsequently, the information is sent back electronically with a diagnosis and additional verbal or written communication in case of emergencies or when a second medical opinion is required. Various such regional networks can also be created between small clinics with dedicated and 24/7-available cardiology networks. Through such reliable, immediate, and efficient diagnosis, prehospital thrombolysis is initiated and arrangements are made to transfer patients using a host of transfer mechanisms (local ambulance services). ITMS has initiated 2 pilot studies to test the model of prehospital thrombolytic therapy in India, a country that is seized with an epidemic of diabetes and AMI presenting in young adults. Two models using telemedicine to advance prehospital thrombolytic therapy are being tested. In the first model, the telemedicine device is placed in ambulances. In the second model, the telemedicine device is strategically placed in small, private nursing homes. With both models, an integrated telemedicine platform is used to initiate thrombolytic therapy.

Improving D2B Outcomes

There are 2 standard methods of prehospital triage and transfer currently used for ambulance management of STEMI, with mandated D2B times of less than 90 minutes. Both these methods are flawed. In the first model, there is placement of a wireless device in the ambulance. This pathway, considered innovative and transformational, is hampered by several drawbacks that are successfully overcome by telemedicine. The wireless transmission model is a pure software diagnosis of an STEMI that is hampered by both false-positive and true negative results. The telemedicine model, in comparison, provides both the performance of a 12-lead ECG and its interpretation by a cardiologist, in real time, without instituting any delays. It is the existence of dedicated and integrated platforms with a network of cardiologists at the end of the transmission that makes telemedicine an attractive option in this situation. The second model of prehospital triage uses either advanced paramedics (Ottawa, Canada) or physicians (France) who travel in an ambulance. This is an inefficient and expensive method that has not gained greater acceptance globally. Finally, the cost of telemedicine devices (ITMS) is considerably less than the cost of standard wireless transmission devices (**Fig. 2**).

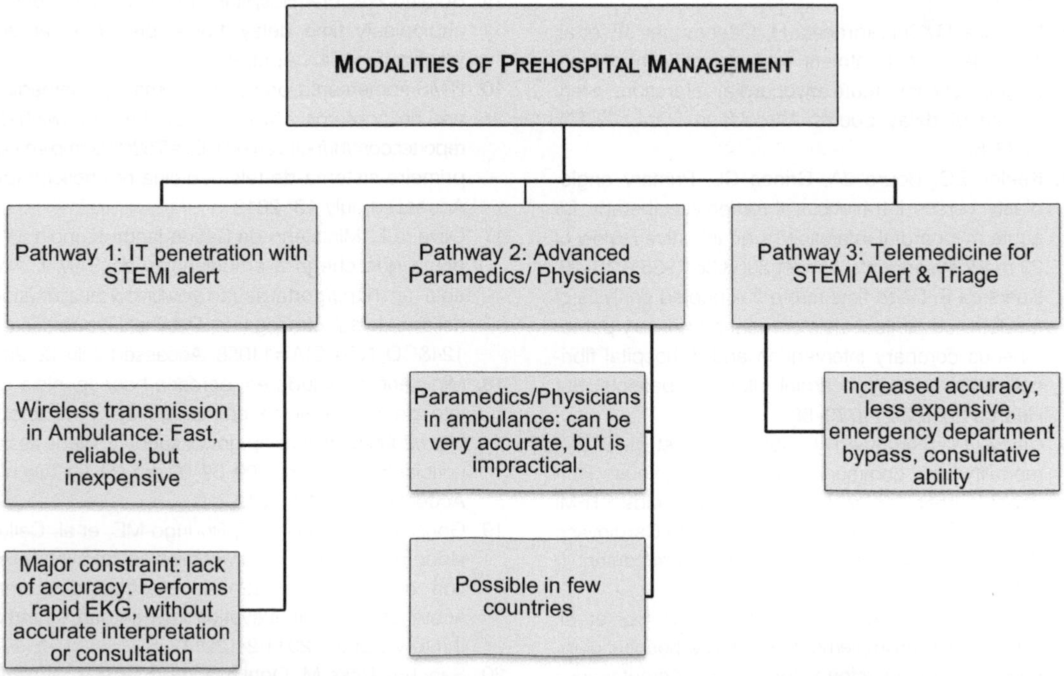

Fig. 2. Modalities of prehospital management.

THE FUTURE OF STEMI CARE

Through the telemedicine network, a global standard of AMI care can be provided to all patients regardless of socioeconomics status. To provide unlimited access to basic STEMI care, such diagnostic and pharmacologic interventions should be the goal of all global STEMI initiatives.

REFERENCES

1. Antman EM, Hand M, Armstrong PW, et al. 2007 focused update of the ACC/AHA 2004 guidelines for the management of patients with ST-elevation myocardial infarction: a report of the American College of Cardiology/American Heart Association Task Force on practice guidelines: developed in collaboration with the Canadian Cardiovascular Society endorsed by the American Academy of Family Physicians: 2007 Writing Group to review new evidence and update the ACC/AHA 2004 guidelines for the management of patients With ST-Elevation myocardial infarction, writing on behalf of the 2004 Writing Committee. Circulation 2008; 117(2):296–329.
2. Van de Werf F, Bax J, Betriu A, et al. Management of acute myocardial infarction in patients presenting with persistent ST-segment elevation: the task force on the Management of ST-segment elevation acute myocardial infarction of the European Society of Cardiology. Eur Heart J 2008;29(23): 2909–45.
3. De Luca G, Suryapranata H, Ottervanger JP, et al. Time delay to treatment and mortality in primary angioplasty for acute myocardial infarction: every minute of delay counts. Circulation 2004;109(10): 1223–5.
4. Keeley EC, Boura JA, Grines CL. Primary angioplasty versus intravenous thrombolytic therapy for acute myocardial infarction: a quantitative review of 23 randomised trials. Lancet 2003;361(9351):13–20.
5. Boersma E. Does time matter? A pooled analysis of randomized clinical trials comparing primary percutaneous coronary intervention and in-hospital fibrinolysis in acute myocardial infarction patients. Eur Heart J 2006;27(7):779–88.
6. Claeys M, Sinnaeve PR, Convens C, et al. STEMI mortality in community hospitals versus PCI-capable hospitals: results from a nationwide STEMI network programme. Eur Heart J: Acute Cardiovasc Care. 2012;1:40. http://acc.sagepub.com/content/1/1/40.full.
7. Sorensen JT, Terkelsen CJ, Norgaard BL, et al. Urban and rural implementation of pre-hospital diagnosis and direct referral for primary percutaneous coronary intervention in patients with acute ST-elevation myocardial infarction. Eur Heart J 2011; 32(4):430–6.
8. Andrade MV, Maia AC, Cardoso CS, et al. Cost-benefit of the telecardiology service in the state of Minas Gerais: Minas Telecardio Project. Arq Bras Cardiol 2011;97(4):307–16.
9. Burt CW, McCaig LF, Valverde RH. Analysis of ambulance transports and diversions among US emergency departments. Ann Emerg Med 2006; 47(4):317–26.
10. Pedersen SH, Galatius S, Hansen PR, et al. Field triage reduces treatment delay and improves long-term clinical outcome in patients with acute ST-segment elevation myocardial infarction treated with primary percutaneous coronary intervention. J Am Coll Cardiol 2009;54(24):2296–302.
11. Le May MR, So DY, Dionne R, et al. A citywide protocol for primary PCI in ST-segment elevation myocardial infarction. N Engl J Med 2008;358(3):231–40.
12. Escobar E. Real-time EKG telemonitoring shows massive rise in lesions during Chile 2010 earthquake. Paper presented at: European Society Of Cardiology (ESC). Paris, August 30, 2011.
13. de Waure C, Cadeddu C, Gualano MR, et al. Telemedicine for the reduction of myocardial infarction mortality: a systematic review and a meta-analysis of published studies. Telemed J E Health 2012; 18(5):323–8.
14. Botelho RV. The impact of Tele-electrocardiogram for Emergency Chest Pain approach in the third world. Paper presented at: ATA. Washington, DC, April 8, 2008.
15. Botelho RV. Pre Hospital EKG impact on primary angioplasty time delay. Paper presented at: ATA. Washington, DC, April, 2008.
16. ITMS implementa primeiro sistema de telemedicina em helicopteros. Available at: http://www.ehealthreporter.com/br/noticia/verNoticia/752/itms-implementa-primeiro-sistema-de-telemedicina-em-helicopteros. Accessed July 13, 2012.
17. Oliveira L. Ministério da Saúde lança tecnologia de ponta que chega a ambulâncias do SAMU. Available at: http://portal.saude.gov.br/portal/aplicacoes/noticias/default.cfm?pg=dspDetalheNoticia&id_area=124&CO_NOTICIA=11058. Accessed July 12, 2012.
18. Ministério da sáude em parceria hcor-sp inicia projeto de telemedicina em campinas. Available at: http://2009.campinas.sp.gov.br/saude/unidades/samu/noticias/not_2009/not_09_09_09/not_09_09_09a.html. Accessed July 12, 2012.
19. Gonzalez MA, Satler LF, Rodrigo ME, et al. Cellular video-phone assisted transmission and interpretation of prehospital 12-lead electrocardiogram in acute st-segment elevation myocardial infarction. J Interv Cardiol 2011;24(2):112–8.
20. Sanchez-Ross M, Oghlakian G, Maher J, et al. The STAT-MI (ST-Segment Analysis Using Wireless

Technology in Acute Myocardial Infarction) trial improves outcomes. JACC Cardiovasc Interv 2011; 4(2):222–7.

21. Ministerio de Salud. Guía Clínica Infarto Agudo del Miocardio y Manejo del Dolor Torácico en Unidades de Emergencia. 1st edition. Santiago (Chile): Misal; 2005.
22. Escobar E. Telemedicine and Teleelectrocardiography in Chile. Available at: http://www.slideshare.net/antroponet/presentacin-itms. Accessed July 13, 2012.
23. Alonso FT, Nazzal C, Alvarado ME. Mortalidad por cardiopatía isquémica en Chile: quiénes, cuántos y dónde. Rev Panam Salud Publica 2010;28(5):319–25 [in Spanish].

Index

Note: Page numbers of article titles are in **boldface** type.

Intervent Cardiol Clin 1 (2012) 631–637
http://dx.doi.org/10.1016/S2211-7458(12)00124-1
2211-7458/12/$ – see front matter

Printed and bound by CPI Group (UK) Ltd, Croydon, CR0 4YY
03/10/2024
01040351-0003